Tropical Neurology

Tropical Neurology

Edited by

Raad A Shakir
*Department of Neurology, Middlesbrough General Hospital,
Middlesbrough, Cleveland, UK*

Peter K Newman
*Department of Neurology, Middlesbrough General Hospital,
Middlesbrough, Cleveland, UK*

and

Charles M Poser
*Neurological Unit, Harvard Medical School and Beth Israel Hospital,
Boston, Massachusetts, USA*

WB SAUNDERS COMPANY LTD
London Philadelphia Toronto
Sydney Tokyo

W.B. Saunders Company Ltd   24–28 Oval Road
London NW1 7DX, UK

The Curtis Center
Independence Square West
Philadelphia, PA 19106-3399, USA

Harcourt Brace & Company
55 Horner Avenue
Toronto, Ontario M8Z 4X6, Canada

Harcourt Brace & Company, Australia
30–52 Smidmore Street
Marrickville, NSW 2204, Australia

Harcourt Brace & Company, Japan
Ichibancho Central Building, 22-1 Ichibancho
Chiyoda-ku, Tokyo 102, Japan

British Library Cataloguing in Publication Data is available

ISBN 0–7020–1922–4

This book is printed on acid-free paper

Typeset by J&L Composition Ltd, Filey, North Yorkshire
Printed and bound in Great Britain by the University Press, Cambridge

Foreword

Lord Walton of Detchant, Kt, MD, MA, DSc, FRCP

When I first became involved with the World Federation of Neurology as Chairman of its Research Group on Neuromuscular Diseases, Charles Poser, one of the distinguished editors of this volume, was appointed by the first WFN President, Ludo van Bogaert, as the editor of the Federation's first journal, *World Neurology*. The papers which he was able to publish in that journal demonstrated to the full what many of us had already realized, namely that the special problems of disorders of the nervous system in tropical countries were receiving relatively little attention at a time when interest in neurology was burgeoning throughout the developed world. As the authors say in their Preface, Spillane in his book on tropical neurology published in 1973 said that 'it will be many years before a comprehensive account of tropical neurology can be undertaken'. Through its Research Group on Tropical Neurology, the WFN and its Research Committee have made strenuous efforts over the succeeding years to further research in this challenging field, and the three divisions of the Research Group based respectively on Asia and the Far East, the Middle East and Africa, and South America, have each made significant contributions to our understanding of the subject. But still the topic continues to be something of a 'Cinderella' and hence I am confident that this book, written by acknowledged experts in the field, will be widely welcomed.

It opens with a scholarly article on the history of the subject and then in five sections the individual chapters examine first viral conditions, then those resulting from bacterial and fungal infections, then parasitic disorders, fourthly environmental conditions, and finally a concluding section deals with some of the commoner neurological disorders which raise special problems in tropical and developing countries. I warmly congratulate the editors in bringing together such a distinguished group of contributors. Raad Shakir, former Professor of Neurology and Academic Vice-Dean of the Medical School in Kuwait until the time of the Gulf War, but now well established in his new neurological career in the United Kingdom, has been one of the leaders, along with a number of other authors of chapters in this volume, in revitalizing the activities of the Tropical Neurology Research Group of the WFN; Charles Poser's international reputation in neurology stands so high that it needs no elaboration from myself; and Peter Newman, a former colleague of mine in Newcastle upon Tyne, has taken an increasing interest in this field over the last few years. Their skilful editing of the varied and disparate contributions written by authors of acknowledged ability and distinction, many of them household names in the field, has assured that this book will in my opinion prove to be a great success. One can but hope that it will reach those many neurologists, physicians and paediatricians in the tropical countries and in the developing world who are faced with the problem of diagnosing and managing the many conditions described in this comprehensive volume. Without doubt, tropical neurology has come of age, as this splendid volume testifies, and I am confident that it will be widely welcomed.

John Walton
Oxford

Preface

Writing in 1973 in the introduction to his book on tropical neurology, Spillane said 'there was a time when tropical medicine and neurology were poles apart' and furthermore, that 'it will be many years before a comprehensive account of tropical neurology can be undertaken'. These statements were then followed by more than 400 fascinating pages describing almost every imaginable tropical neurological disorder, as well as erudite accounts of their geographical variations. A quarter of a century has passed since these essays were gathered together and there have been many changes in tropical and geographical neurology.

The developing countries have a burden of illness that differs drastically from the rest of the world. The major health problems are generally related to warm climates, overcrowding, conditions in rural areas, severe poverty, illiteracy and high infant mortality. Social and economic deprivation in many areas has led to further spread of parasitic and infectious diseases which could have been eradicated, whereas sustained growth in other countries has introduced the very best of medical technology and care to the fortunate populace.

Some diseases that had been found in the West but have virtually disappeared, such as poliomyelitis and subacute sclerosing panencephalitis, are still taking their toll in the developing world. Conversely, some of the protozoan and helminthic infections that are so characteristic of the tropics are now being seen in the West with increasing frequency. Rapid and efficient means of transportation which have additionally the undesirable potential of introducing disease vectors, along with large-scale military ventures and expanding overseas business enterprises, have all contributed to the spread or the reintroduction of some of these diseases in the Western world. The scourge of AIDS has affected developed and developing countries in equal measure, often with local clinical peculiarities, and is particularly devastating in Africa.

This book aims to distil current knowledge in a form which will be valuable to the neurologist practising in tropical zones and in temperate regions where imported cases are seen. Modern investigations and treatments that may not be available in developing countries are described, but the various chapters also emphasize low technology approaches which may be more relevant for many practitioners. Most of the subject matter concerns disorders indigenous to the tropics or developing nations, but inevitably there is some straying into the field of general infectious disease. In the final section of the book are several essays dealing with non-tropical topics such as epilepsy or rehabilitation, placing these in the context of the developing world.

We will not attempt to enter into the debate of the definition of tropical neurology but we feel that the special circumstances that prevail in the developing world, which is mainly situated in the warmer parts of the globe, warrant specific attention from the point of view of the neurologist. In recognition of the varying patterns of disease in the tropics, the different approaches to the diseases in developed and developing countries, and the distribution of expertise in tropical neurology, the editors have incorporated contributions from all over the world, making this a genuinely international and comprehensive book.

R.A. Shakir
P.K. Newman
C.M. Poser

Contributors

Mathew Alexander Department of Neurological Sciences, Christian Medical College and Hospital, Vellore 632 004, India

Mohammed-Zuheir Al-Kawi Department of Medicine, King Faisal Specialist Hospital and Research Centre, PO Box 3354, Riyadh 11211, Saudi Arabia

Milne Anderson Midland Centre for Neurosurgery and Neurology, Holly Lane, Smethwick, Warley, W. Midlands, B67 7XJ, UK

Samir Atweh Professor of Neurology, Faculty of Medicine, American University of Beirut, PO Box 113-6044, Beirut, Lebanon

Nadir E Bharucha Chief, Department of Neuroepidemiology, 15th Floor Medical Research Centre, Bombay Hospital, 12 Marine Lines, Bombay 400 020, India

Suranjan Bhattacharji Associate Professor and Head, Rehabilitation Department, Christian Medical College and Hospital, Vellore, India

Pierre Louis Alfred Bill Professor and Head of Neurology, Neurology Unit, Wentworth Hospital, Private Bag Jacobs 4026, Durban, Natal 4026, South Africa

Paulo RM de Bittencourt Hosp Nossa Senhora das Gracas & Unidade de Neurologia Clinica, Padre Anchieta 155, 80410-030 Curitiba, Brazil

Robert Colebunders Institute of Tropical Medicine, Nationalestraat 155, B-2000 Antwerp, Belgium

Gordon C Cook Department of Clinical and Tropical Medicine, Hospital for Tropical Diseases, 4 St Pancras Way, London NW1 0PE, UK

Michel Dumas Director, Institute of Neurological Epidemiology and Tropical Neurology, Faculty of Medicine, Limoges University, 2 rue du Docteur Marcland, 87025 Limoges Cedex, France

M Gourie-Devi   Department of Neurology, National Institute of Mental Health and Neurosciences, Post Bag 2779, Bangalore 560 029, India

John B Harris   Professor of Experimental Neurology, Head School of Neurosciences, Newcastle General Hospital, Newgate Road, Newcastle, NE4 6BE, UK

Patricia L Hibberd   Infectious Diseases and Transplantation Units, Massachusetts General Hospital, Fruit Street, Boston, MA 02114, USA

Mustafa Khogali   Department of Community Medicine, Faculty of Medicine, American University of Beirut, PO Box 113-6044, Beirut, Lebanon

KS Mani   Retired Professor of Neurology, Neurological Clinic, 1 Old Veterinary Hospital Road, Basavanagudi, Bangalore 560 004, India

Ammar Mubaidin   PO Box 926442, Amman, Jordan

Peter K Newman   Consultant Neurologist, Department of Neurology, Middlesbrough General Hospital, Middlesbrough, Cleveland, UK

Charles M Poser   Department of Neurology, Harvard Medical School and Beth Israel Hospital, 330 Brookline Avenue, Boston, MA 02215, USA

Subhashini Prabhakar   Department of Neurological Sciences, Christian Medical College and Hospital, Vellore 632 004, India

Geeta Rangan   Associate Professor of Neurology, Neurological Clinic, 1 Old Veterinary Hospital Road, Basavanagudi, Bangalore 560 004, India

Roberta H Raven   'The Beacon', Flat 5, 140 Backbay Reclamation, Opposite Mantralaya, Bombay 400 021, India

Gustavo C Román   Clinical Neurophysiology Department, International Spinal Neurosurgical Clinic, Suite 204, Rosa Verde Towers, 343 West Houston Street, San Antonio, TX 78205, USA

Hans Rosling   Unit for International Child Health, University Hospital, S-751 85 Uppsala, Sweden

Thomas D Sabin   Department of Neurology, Medical College of Georgia, 1459 Laney Walker Blvd, Augusta, GA 30912, USA

Marcos C Sandmann   Hosp Nossa Senhora das Gracas & Unidade de Neurologia Clinica, Padre Anchieta 155, 80410-030 Curitiba, Brazil

Michael Saunders Consultant in Neurological Rehabilitation, Medical Director and Consultant Neurologist, Friarage Hospital, Northallerton, North Yorks, UK

Nimal Senanayake Senior Professor of Medicine, Faculty of Medicine, University of Peradeniya, Peradeniya, Sri Lanka

Raad A Shakir Consultant Neurologist, Department of Neurology, Middlesbrough General Hospital, Middlesbrough, Cleveland, UK

Antonio Spina-França Neurology Investigation Centre, Faculty of Medicine, The University of Sao Paulo, PO Box 5199, 01051-970 Sao Paulo, Brazil

Thomas R Swift Chairman, Department of Neurology, Medical College of Georgia, 1459 Laney Walker Blvd, Augusta, GA 30912, USA

Redda Tekle-Haimanot Department of Internal Medicine, Faculty of Medicine, Addis Ababa University, PO Box 4147, Addis Ababa, Ethiopia

Michele Trucksis Division of Geographic Medicine, Center for Vaccine Development, Department of Medicine, University of Maryland School of Medicine, 10 South Pine Street, Baltimore, MD 21201, USA

Thorkild Tylleskär Unit for International Child Health, University Hospital, S-751 85 Uppsala, Sweden

Jean-Claude Vernant Neurology Service, CHU de Fort de France, Hopital Zobda Quitman, 97240 Fort de France, Martinique

Noshir H Wadia A/1 Ben Nevis, 100 Bhulabhai Desai Road, Bombay 400 036, India

David A Warrell The Centre for Tropical Medicine, University of Oxford, John Radcliffe Hospital, Headington, Oxford, OX3 9DU, UK

Margaret J Warrell The Centre for Tropical Medicine, University of Oxford, John Radcliffe Hospital, Headington, Oxford, OX3 9DU, UK

Contents

Section 5   Selected Aspects of Neurological Conditions

1

The History of Tropical Neurology

Charles Poser[1], Michel Dumas[2] and Antonio Spina-França[3]

[1] Harvard Neurological Unit, Beth Israel Hospital, Boston, MA, USA; [2] Institut d'Epidémiologie Neurologique et de Neurologie Tropicale Limoges, France; [3] Department of Neurology, University of São Paulo, São Paulo, Brazil

INTRODUCTION

Many of what we now call tropical diseases at one time were spread throughout the world: leprosy, malaria, cholera and the plague were well known in Western countries and temperate climates. Until recently most research on these diseases and the resulting discoveries were carried out in the West. It is no accident that Hansen described *Mycobacterium leprae* in Bergen, Norway, in 1871.

The best description of the origins of the discipline of tropical medicine was provided by Garrison in his *History of Medicine (1929)*: 'Tropical medicine, vaguely rooted in antiquity, came into being largely through the exploration of the globe by navigators and the settlements made in tropical and torrid regions by Spain, England, Holland, France and Germany. It had its authentic start with the organization of the Indian Medical Service of the British Army in 1764.' It is not surprising that many major contributions were made by military medical officers working in the far-flung colonies of Western powers.

One of the prime movers was Patrick Manson (1844–1922), who made many significant contributions to the field and founded a school of tropical medicine in Hong Kong in 1886, and in 1898, the London School of Tropical Medicine. Others followed in short order: the schools of tropical medicine in Liverpool and Edinburgh (1899); in Hamburg (1900); in Lisbon (1902); in Brussels (1906), which was later moved to Antwerp and became the Institute of Tropical Medicine; in Manila (1914); and in San Juan, Puerto Rico (1917). Other specialized institutions included the Instituto Oswaldo Cruz in Rio de Janeiro (1901); the Wellcome Tropical Research Laboratory in Khartoum, the Sudan; the Gorgas Memorial Institute of Tropical Medicine in Chicago (1921); and the Ross Institute and Hospital for Tropical Diseases in London (1923). The first governmental agency concerned with tropical diseases was the Tropical Disease Bureau established in the British Colonial Office in London in 1908. Scientific societies devoted to this new specialty began to form: first was the American Society of Tropical Medicine (1903), followed by the French Société de Pathologie Exotique (1905) and the Royal Society of Tropical Medicine and Hygiene (1907). The first meeting of the latter devoted to tropical neurology was organized by Raad Shakir in London in 1993.

Neurological complications of tropical diseases were being observed and recorded all along, but it was not until some time after World War II, as neurology was establishing itself as an independent specialty, that the study of tropical neurology started to come into its own.

THE ORIGINS OF TROPICAL NEUROLOGY

Tropical neurology can be traced back many centuries; only a few examples will serve to introduce the subject. Rumler found cysticerci in the human brain in 1558. Bontius, a Dutch physician, was the first to describe beriberi in 1642. Other tropical conditions affecting primarily the nervous system had also been known for a long time. African sleeping sickness (trypanosomiasis) was described by Winterbottom in 1803 in Sierra Leone. It was redescribed by Clarke in 1840 but it was not until 1901 that Dutton and Ford discovered the trypanosome. On the other hand, the American form of the disease was described by Chagas in Brazil in 1909. Lathyrism was reported by Sleeman in 1844. The peripheral nerve disturbances of leprosy had been observed by Danilssen and Boeck in 1848 but the classical study by Monrad-Krohn of Oslo did not appear until 1925. Strachan's seminal report on 510 cases of 'a strange peripheral neuropathy' in Jamaica was published in 1888.

Although many textbooks of medicine mentioned neurological aspects of tropical diseases, the first, most extensive descriptions appeared in August Hirsch's encyclopaedic *Geographical and Historical Pathology*, published in London in 1886.

TROPICAL NEUROLOGY AS A SEPARATE DISCIPLINE

The birth of the study of tropical neurology is often dated from the appearance of John Spillane's famous *Tropical Neurology* in 1973. Indeed it was the first textbook on the subject and included contributions from many of the most prominent clinicians and investigators of tropical neurology of that time.

It is probably impossible to credit a single individual with the establishment of the discipline of tropical neurology, but the one who comes closest to qualifying is Henri Collomb, who in 1958 founded a department of tropical neuropsychiatry at the Fann Hospital of Dakar, Senegal. After he left neurology to devote himself to ethnopsychiatry, he was succeeded as professor of neurology by Michel Dumas in 1969. In 1962 Collomb and Dumas, along with Girard and Giordano, also of Dakar; Ruberti of Kenya; Oduku and Dada of Nigeria; and

Sorour of Egypt founded the Pan-African Association of the Neurological Sciences, a bilingual group of neuroscientists, neurologists and neurosurgeons which is still active today.

Simultaneously, a powerful and highly productive group of tropical neurologists was developing in Latin America. Their activity culminated in 1961 in the First Congress of Tropical Neurology in Buenos Aires. This meeting was sponsored by the World Federation of Neurology (WFN) and organized by Ludo van Bogaert of Belgium (the President of the WFN), Jose Pereyra-Käfer and Gustavo Poch of Argentina. The proceedings of this Congress were published in 1963 and constitute the first collection of papers dealing exclusively with tropical neurology. Contributors included van Bogaert, who for many years was associated with Antwerp's Institute of Tropical Medicine; A.B. Baker of Minneapolis, the founder of the American Academy of Neurology; Antonio Spina-França, Walter Maffei and Deolindo Couto of Brazil; Julio Trelles of Peru; Roman Arana-Iniguez of Uruguay; Henri Collomb of Senegal; Neville Proctor of South Africa; John Spillane of England; G. Monekosso of Nigeria; Hatai Chitanondh of Thailand and Noshir Wadia of India. During the Congress, van Bogaert, Trelles and Pereyra-Kafer formed the Research Group on Tropical Neurology of the WFN. Its official journal, the *Journal of Tropical and Geographical Neurology*, started publication in 1991 but did not survive the economic rigours of the early 1990s.

Many others throughout the world, in addition to those already named, had made contributions to tropical neurology. In Africa there were Hall in Ethiopia; Lambo, Howard and Osuntokun in Nigeria; Haddock in Tanzania; Muwezi, Trowell, Billinghurst and Hutton in Uganda; Sharp in Ghana; Goldstein, Harries and Foster in Kenya; Levy, Rachman and Gelfand in Rhodesia; Ben Hamida in Tunisia; and Cosnett, Cochrane and Berman in South Africa. Two important books from Africa must be mentioned because they contain relevant material, although they were not specifically concerned with neurology: Gelfand's *The Sick African* (1943) and Trowell's *Non-Infective Disease in Africa: The Peculiarities of Medical Non-Infective Diseases in the Indigenous Inhabitants of Africa South of the Sahara* (1969). Prominent in India were Bharucha, Mani, Dastur, Ramamurthi and Wadia who ably chaired the WFN Research Group in Tropical Neurology for many years; in Malaysia, Gwee, Selby, Pettit and Ransome; in Thailand, Vejjajiva; in Indonesia, Verhaart, Palthe and De Vries; in the Dutch Indies, Moffie; in Martinique, Vernant; and in Jamaica, Cruickshank and Montgomery. Many important developments of tropical neurology are a result of the excellent work of general physicians working in tropical medicine. This is best exemplified by the work of Warrell on malaria and rabies, both in the Oxford Tropical Medicine Research programme in Thailand and the Centre for Tropical Medicine and Infectious Diseases in Oxford.

An important event in the evolution of tropical neurology studies was the publication in 1983 of the Spanish-language *Neurologia Tropical* by Gabriel Toro, Gustavo Roman-Campos and Lydia Navarro de Roman of Bogota, Colombia.

One of the landmarks in the history of tropical neurology was the foundation in 1982 by Michel Dumas of the Institut d'Epidémiologie Neurologique et de Neurologie Tropicale in Limoges, France. This unique research and training centre is dedicated to the neurological education of African physicians who will return to their native countries and carry on teaching, treatment and research in tropical neurology. The Institute organized an international congress of tropical neurology in Limoges in 1991. Its proceedings were published in French in 1994, at the time of the second such meeting, which was attended by almost 300 participants from all over the world, an impressive testimonial to the breadth and growth of the specialty.

Interest in tropical neurology is not restricted to the classic areas of Africa, Asia, the Western Pacific and Central and South America. New diseases have been discovered in the tropics such as konzo, kuru, the motor neurone disease and Parkinson–dementia complex of the Guamanian Chamorros and the eosinophilic meningitis of Tahiti. These and other diseases that have so far appeared only in the tropics may in time provide important clues regarding the aetiology of diseases seen in temperate areas. AIDS, which started as an African disease, has become a world-wide scourge. Slowly but surely, tropical neurology is being incorporated into general neurology.

Section 1
VIRAL CONDITIONS

2

Viral Encephalitides

Gustavo C. Román

University of Texas at San Antonio, USA

INTRODUCTION

There is a dearth of aetiological information regarding viral encephalitides in the tropics due to lack of proper diagnostic facilities. The most common sporadic forms include herpes simplex virus (HSV), mumps, rabies and enteroviral infections, as well as acute post-measles encephalopathy and subacute sclerosing panencephalitis. Arboviruses, such as Japanese encephalitis and dengue, usually present as epidemic outbreaks.

In the last decade, the discovery of the human retroviruses clarified the aetiology of tropical spastic paraparesis (TSP), produced by the human T-lymphotropic virus type I (HTLV-I), and of the current pandemic of acquired immunodeficiency syndrome (AIDS), due to infection with another retrovirus, the human immunodeficiency virus type 1 and 2 (HIV-1, HIV-2). AIDS has also increased the frequency of opportunistic viral infections of the nervous system, in particular due to cytomegalovirus (CMV), varicella–zoster virus, and the human papovavirus JC, the agent of progressive multifocal leukoencephalopathy (PML).

The unconventional viruses (prions) are the agents of the transmissible spongiform encephalopathies, which include in the human, kuru, Creutzfeldt–Jakob disease and the Gerstmann–Sträussler syndrome. Some progress has been achieved in the treatment of viral encephalitides, in particular herpes encephalitis and other herpesvirus infections (Toro *et al.*, 1983).

HUMAN HERPESVIRUSES

The human herpesviruses are DNA viruses which include HSV types 1 and 2, varicella–zoster virus, cytomegalovirus and Epstein–Barr virus. All the herpesviruses are characterized by producing persistent latent infection for the duration of the lifetime of the host.

Herpes Simplex Virus Encephalitis (HSVE)

HSVE is considered the most common form of non-epidemic viral encephalitis in the world with an annual incidence of 1–3 cases per million population. All age groups may be affected, including newborns infected at birth (usually with herpes genitalis, HSV-2).

Pathogenesis and Pathology

All human herpesvirus infections are characterized by primary infection of the susceptible host through a mucous membrane portal of entry. In childhood most primary infections are asymptomatic, but in the young adult gingivostomatitis, keratitis or genital herpes are usually severe, painful and with systemic manifestations.

The virus replicates at the portal of entry and then travels to the sensory ganglia by intra-axonal spread. Circulating antibodies and cell-mediated immunity develop and last for life. The virus remains in latency in sensory neurones, mainly in the trigeminal ganglia, superior cervical sympathetic and jugular vagus ganglia, as well as in sacral ganglia. Latency in brain neurones has also been demonstrated in the olfactory system and mesencephalic trigeminal nucleus. Viraemia with systemic dissemination of the virus may occur in the newborn and in the immunocompromised host. Latent HSV-DNA persists in the cells in a non-encapsidated circular form. Transcription is probably repressed since low HSV mRNA is found in extracts from infected ganglia.

Reactivation occurs in response to a number of non-specific stimuli such as fever (fever blisters, cold sores, herpes labialis), ultraviolet radiation and stress, as well as immunosuppression with cyclophosphamide, X-irradiation or steroids. Trigeminal neuralgia has been strongly associated with HSV infection, and therapeutic neurectomy or rhizotomy produced postoperative recurrence of herpes labialis. Pregnancy in young women has been a risk factor for HSVE.

Herpes encephalitis is typically focal, localized preferentially to the temporal lobe, medial frontal lobe, or rarely to the brainstem. There is significant oedema, necrosis, microscopic haemorrhages, and perivascular cuffing and parenchymal infiltrates composed of T lymphocytes (T4$^+$, T8$^+$), macrophages and granulocytes. Meningeal inflammation is usually prominent. The most typical feature is the presence of intranuclear, eosinophilic Cowdry type A inclusions, predominating in oligodendroglia.

Clinical Features, Diagnosis and Treatment

In adults, HSVE presents as an acute febrile illness, with headache, changes in behaviour – sometimes with visual hallucinations, progressive decrease in the level of alertness, and focal neurological signs such as speech difficulties, hemiparesis, seizures, facial weakness, cranial nerve deficits and papilloedema.

The differential diagnosis is with focal neurological lesions such as brain abscess, tumour, stroke or toxic encephalopathies (Whitley, 1990).

Brain imaging (CT, MRI, isotopic brain scan) usually demonstrates an area of decreased tissue intensity in the typical temporal lobe location, with alteration of the blood–brain barrier (BBB), focal brain oedema and often petechial haemorrhages.

The electroencephalogram (EEG) is helpful, showing unilateral bursts of slow activity of high amplitude overlying the affected area, and presence of periodic epileptiform lateralized discharges (PLEDs), with spikes and slow waves. A periodic pattern of epileptiform discharges and burst suppression is highly suggestive of HSVE (Lai and Gragasin, 1988).

Examination of the cerebrospinal fluid (CSF) is usually abnormal, with increased pressure, presence of pleocytosis (10–100 WBC mm^{-3}), and increased proteins. Low CSF glucose occurs in only 5% of patients. However, early in the disease, up to 11% of patients may have no pleocytosis, and up to 18% have normal protein levels in the CSF.

Intrathecal production of antibodies against HSV results in increased levels of IgG in the CSF, usually in an oligoclonal pattern. IgG and IgM immunoglobulins are also increased in the CSF. The diagnosis of HSVE can be confirmed by comparing serum and CSF antibody titres against HSV in order to confirm the intrathecal antibody production in response to the CNS infection. A ratio serum: CSF anti-HSV of $\leq$ 20:1 is consistent with HSVE. The antibody index, defined as:

$$CSF\ HSV\ antibody/serum\ HSV\ antibody \div CSF\ albumin/serum\ albumin$$

takes into account the alteration of BBB resulting from inflammation. Rarely, no antibody response may be present in HSVE (McKendall, 1989).

Brain biopsy of the affected temporal lobe may demonstrate the presence of meningoencephalitis and inclusions by histopathologic examination, and of HSV particles by fluorescent antibody techniques or electronmicroscopy. Biopsy also allows cultivation of HSV to confirm the diagnosis, or defines the true nature of the process. However, because of the low toxicity of acyclovir, the drug of choice for HSVE, brain biopsy is currently seldom used.

HSVE mortality used to reach close to 90% with devastating sequelae in the days prior to specific antiviral therapy. Adenine arabinoside decreased mortality to about 50%, and acylovir to less than 20% (Whitley *et al.*, 1986). Acyclovir (acycloguanosine) is phosphorylated by viral thymidine kinase resulting in acyclovir triphosphate which then inhibits herpes-specific DNA polymerase. Acyclovir is not taken up by uninfected cells and this explains its remarkably low toxicity. The drug is also useful in infections by the varicella–zoster virus.

Acyclovir is given in doses of 10 mg kg^{-1} infused intravenously over 1 hour, repeated every 8 hours (30 mg kg^{-1} day^{-1}), at least for 10 days. In patients with acute or chronic renal failure the frequency of the doses should be decreased. Early treatment is associated with better results; lethargic patients have less morbidity than those who are comatose at the onset of acyclovir therapy.

Treatment of increased intracranial pressure with mannitol or corticosteroids, control of seizures with parenteral lorazepam and phenytoin, appropriate ventilation and oxygenation of the patient, and adequate fluid and electrolyte balance and nutrition, should be maintained in the usually critically ill patients.

Other Neurological Infections by Herpesgroup Viruses

Herpes Simplex Virus (HSV)

Primary infection with HSV-2 (herpes genitalis) may be accompanied by lymphocytic meningitis in up to 25% of patients. Rarely HSV-1 is the cause of the genital lesions. Meningitis may also occur in recurrent genital herpes.

Varicella–Zoster Virus (VZV)

Varicella infection may be complicated by meningoencephalitis, sometimes with a prominent cerebellar syndrome, optic neuritis and ophthalmoplegia. Acute haemorrhagic leukoencephalitis and acute transverse myelitis may also occur following varicella infection. Devic's syndrome (neuromyelitis optica) has been reported.

A congenital varicella syndrome occurs in about 12% of infants born to mothers who suffer varicella (chickenpox) during the first trimester of pregnancy. Limb hypoplasia and mental retardation are observed. Maternal zoster during pregnancy is not associated with fetal lesions.

Neurological complications of herpes zoster include segmental motor weakness, encephalomyelitis, cranial nerve lesions and a syndrome of herpes zoster ophthalmicus with contralateral hemiplegia due to vasculitis of internal carotid artery and other intracerebral arteries (Hilt *et al.*, 1983). This last complication is observed with some frequency in patients with AIDS.

Epstein–Barr Virus (EBV)

Infectious mononucleosis can be rarely complicated with lymphocytic meningitis, encephalitis and meningoencephalitis (Gautier-Smith, 1965). Cerebral and cerebellar manifestations, ataxia and seizures are common. Focal EEG manifestations similar to those of HSVE may also occur. Isolated cerebellar ataxia, transverse myelitis, acute deafness, Bell's palsy, and Guillain–Barré syndrome have been described following infectious mononucleosis.

EBV is the cause of African Burkitt's lymphoma and has been associated with nasopharyngeal carcinoma in South-East Asia and North Africa, as well as with lymphoma in the immunosuppressed, including patients with AIDS. Neoplastic invasion of cranial nerves and spinal cord compression may occur in Burkitt's lymphoma and nasopharyngeal carcinoma.

Primary CNS lymphoma, formerly a very rare lesion, is becoming one of the most common intracranial lesions of AIDS patients. Primary CNS lymphoma usually develops late in HIV infection, in patients with CD4 counts below 100 cells mm^{-3}, presenting with confusion, decreased level of alertness, headache, signs of increased intracranial pressure and focal neurological findings. Brain imaging studies show contrast-enhancing lesions, single or multiple, surrounded by oedema. Differential diagnosis with toxoplasmosis may be difficult. Lesions respond to radiotherapy but prognosis is poor.

Cytomegalovirus (CMV)

Congenital infection due to viraemia during maternal infection with CMV produces a severe syndrome called cytomegalic inclusion body disease, manifested by hepatitis, splenomegaly, pneumonitis, anaemia and petechial rash. Lesions in the CNS in congenital CMV infection cause diffuse encephalitis manifested by seizures, mental retardation, spasticity and chorioretinitis followed by microcephaly, periventricular calcifications, optic atrophy and encephalomalacia.

Around 90% of AIDS patients have evidence of CMV infection at autopsy, and up to 40% of those with AIDS dementia have CMV focal encephalitis with microglial nodules and cytomegalic inclusions. CMV may also cause choroidoretinitis, vasculitis, ventriculoencephalitis, meningoencephalitis and radiculomyelitis in AIDS patients. CMV encephalitis is indistinguishable clinically from AIDS dementia, although abrupt onset and the association with adrenal insufficiency and retinal lesions are suggestive of CMV infection. CMV encephalitis usually occurs late in the disease in patients with CD4 counts below 50 mm^{-3}. Retinitis responds to treatment with ganciclovir. However, recurrences are common and life-long treatment is required; resistant strains often develop (Laskin *et al.*, 1987). Treatment with foscarnet (trisodium phosphonoformic acid) may be used.

Simian Herpesviruses

Herpesviruses from infected monkeys, in particular *Herpesvirus simiae* of rhesus monkeys (*Macaca mulatta*), Asian macaques and African green monkeys, may produce encephalitis and transverse myelitis following bites and other forms of infection in humans. Acyclovir is active against *H. simiae*.

RABIES

Rabies (from the Latin *rabere*, to rage) is one of the most important viral encephalitides in the tropics (Warrell and Shope, 1990; Phelps *et al.*, 1994) and is covered in Chapter 5.

MUMPS AND MEASLES

Mumps and measles are RNA paramyxoviruses. Mumps is a frequent cause of aseptic meningitis and mild encephalitis predominating in males. Measles, the cause of rubeola, produces postinfectious encephalomyelitis and subacute sclerosing panencephalitis. Rare complications of measles include transverse myelitis, polyneuritis, toxic encephalopathy and acute hemiplegia of childhood.

Measles Encephalomyelitis

Typically, onset of the neurological symptoms occurs 2–7 days after the onset of the rash in an afebrile child. Fever, involuntary movements, hemiparesis, cerebellar signs and depression of consciousness are seen. Paraparesis occurs in a third of patients. Boys and girls are affected with the same frequency. Mortality reaches 25% and neurological sequelae occur in 60% of survivors (Johnson *et al.*, 1984).

Neuropathological examination shows brain oedema and typical perivenous demyelination accompanied by perivascular infiltrates. In acute haemorrhagic leukoencephalitis diffuse haemorrhages are seen in the white matter. There is fibrinoid necrosis of blood vessels and extravasation of red blood cells.

Treatment includes corticosteroids (despite unproved efficacy) and supportive measures including anticonvulsants. The use of childhood vaccination has decreased significantly the frequency of this condition.

Subacute Sclerosing Panencephalitis (SSPE)

SSPE is due to infection of the CNS by a defective measles virus. Multiple mutations cause defective virus expression; in particular, the matrix (M) protein of measles virus is not synthesized. The topic is covered in Chapter 6.

PROGRESSIVE MULTIFOCAL LEUKOENCEPHALOPATHY (PML)

PML is caused by the JC virus, a human papovavirus belonging to the DNA papovavirus family. PML is currently observed in 4% of AIDS patients. It is manifested by mental alterations, visual fields disturbances, speech difficulties, focal motor deficits and abnormal gait. MRI images in T2 sequences typically show large confluent areas of increased signal intensity involving the white matter. Histological examination shows perivascular cuffing of inflammatory cells and bizarre oligodendroglial cells containing nuclear inclusions. Electron-microscopy or in situ hybridization show the presence of JC virions. Intravenous and intrathecal cytarabine (Ara-A) therapy has been recommended.

ARBOVIRUSES

The arthropod-borne viruses comprise a large group of RNA viruses transmitted by mosquitoes and ticks, belonging to the togavirus, flavivirus, bunyavirus and reovirus families. World-wide, the most important cause of encephalitis transmitted by mosquitoes in the tropics is Japanese encephalitis virus. In the Americas, the arboviruses capable of causing human encephalitis include Western and Eastern equine encephalitis, Venezuelan equine encephalitis, St Louis encephalitis viruses and dengue virus. West Nile virus, a flavivirus, is a cause of mosquito-borne encephalitis in Africa and the Middle East. Tickborne encephalitides occur in the Far East, Central Europe, India (Kyasanur Forest) and the Rocky Mountains (Colorado tick fever) (Johnson, 1989).

Japanese Encephalitis (JE)

JE is the most common cause of epidemic encephalitis world-wide. It occurs in epidemic outbreaks and approximately 50 000 cases are reported annually from China, Japan, Korea, Bangladesh, Burma, India, Nepal, southern Thailand, the Philippines and Vietnam. It causes significant mortality and neurologic morbidity among children below 15 years of age and the elderly in many countries in Asia (Umenai *et al.*, 1985). In endemic areas the annual incidence is 1–10/10 000. JE may also affect tourists and travellers to the Far East producing either encephalitis or fever of unknown origin.

Pathogenesis

The disease is caused by the Japanese encephalitis virus (JEV), an RNA flavivirus whose main reservoirs are migratory water birds such as herons and egrets. Pigs are an important amplifying host because of their capacity to develop asymptomatic high viraemias which allow mosquitoes to become infected. The role of cattle, in particular water buffalo is less clear. Man is an incidental dead-end host, infected by *Culex* mosquitoes, in particular *Culex tritaeniorhyncus* which breeds in flooded rice fields. Isolation of JEV in mosquito larvae suggests the possibility of vertical transovarial transmission of the virus (Dhanda *et al.*, 1989).

JEV affects mainly children and non-immune adults. Most infections are inapparent or subclinical (Monath, 1988). The inapparent:apparent infection ratio ranges from 25:1 to 1000:1 being greater in children (> 500:1) than in adults, with a 210:1 ratio among troops in Vietnam.

Clinical Features

The incubation period ranges from 4 to 14 days. Prodromal signs include fever, headache and malaise, respiratory and gastrointestinal symptoms. This is followed in 2 or 3 days by the development of meningeal signs, confusion, rapid decrease in the level of consciousness and coma. Focal or generalized seizures are common in children. Focal motor weakness in the upper limbs and facial muscles may be present. Ataxia, tremor, dystonia, parkinsonian features and other abnormal movements are common.

Diagnosis

In endemic areas the seasonal occurrence of meningoencephalitis among susceptible children is characteristic. CSF examination shows lymphocytic pleocytosis but the virus is rarely isolated from the CSF in non-fatal cases. CT and MRI of the brain reveal abnormalities of thalami and basal ganglia which are quite characteristic (Misra *et al.*, 1994). The lesions appear to be haemorrhagic in the majority. Factors associated with poor outcome include absence or low levels of JE virus-specific IgG and IgM in CSF and serum, as well as deep stupor and coma (Burke *et al.*, 1985a, b). JE is a severe disease with mortality ranging from 15 to 40%. Neurological sequelae, in particular paralyses with muscle atrophy, extrapyramidal signs, mental retardation and behavioural changes are frequent. Seizures may occur in up to 20% of survivors.

Pathology

In fatal cases, JEV can be demonstrated in the brain by immunofluorescent antibody techniques, localized mainly in neurones of the thalamus and brainstem (Johnson *et al.*, 1985). Histologic examination of the brain shows prominent perivascular infiltrates and focal necrosis in brainstem, basal ganglia and cervical spinal cord. The distribution of lesions explains the frequent occurrence of coma, respiratory distress, abnormal movements and lower-motor neurone paralysis.

Treatment and Prevention

Treatment is supportive controlling brain oedema, hyperthermia and seizures. The use of leukocyte α-interferon appears promissory. Preventive measures include the use of vaccines in non-immune children, vaccination of young pigs and control of the vector mosquitoes.

DENGUE AND DENGUE HAEMORRHAGIC FEVER

The spread of this mosquito-borne viral disease is increasing. The haemorrhagic variety is deadly and in many tropical countries it is one of the leading causes of death among the young. In South-East Asia, for example, the attack rate was as high as 5400 per 100 000 in Vietnam in 1987. The disease is seen throughout the tropics and subtropics with an estimate of 150–200 mild or clinically asymptomatic dengue cases for each case of dengue haemorrhagic fever (DHF) or dengue shock syndrome. The vectors *Aedes aegypti* and *A. albopictus* are spreading in spite of control measures. The criteria for diagnosis for DHF include high fever for 2–7 days, haemorrhagic diathesis, hepatomegaly, thrombocytopenia (up to 100 000 mm^{-3}), haemoconcentrations (increase haematocrit by 20%) and shock. Signs of encephalitis can be seen in the evolution of the syndrome. The management is symptomatic and depends on early diagnosis, volume replacement to prevent plasma leak, haemoconcentration and shock.

LASSA FEVER

This is an acute and severe viral haemorrhagic febrile illness due to an Arenavirus which is spread by a West African rodent (*Mastomys natalensis*). The illness may be fatal in about a fifth of the patients. Neurological involvement is seen in the acute phase with confusion, convulsions and coma. In the convalescent stage, deafness probably due to cochlear damage is reported in about 20%. Ataxia is another convalescent complication which does not seem to occur together with deafness in the same patient. The diagnosis is made by CSF pleocytosis and rising serum Lassa IgG and IgM antibodies. Ribavirin has been found effective in treatment (McCormick *et al.*, 1986).

HUMAN RETROVIRUSES

The retroviruses (family Retroviridae) are comprised of three subfamilies: (1) *Oncoviruses*, formerly called RNA tumour viruses, induce malignant transformation of cells in culture and cause leukaemias, lymphomas and other tumours in animals. The first human retrovirus, HLTV-1, produces adult T-cell leukaemia–lymphoma. HTLV-2 was isolated in a patient with hairy cell leukaemia. These two human oncoviruses have been associated also with tropical spastic paraparesis and spinocerebellar syndromes (Román *et al.*, 1990). (2) *Lentiviruses* are lytic to cells in culture and produce 'slow viral infections': chronic diseases of the nervous system and other organs after unusually long incubations. The prototype lentivirus, visnamaedi, causes two diseases in sheep: maedi, a pulmonary disease, and visna, an encephalomyelopathy with extensive demyelination, oligodrendroglial damage and inflammation. HIV types 1 and 2 have been classified as lentiviruses. (3) *Spumaviruses*, or foamy viruses, are similar to oncoviruses and produce foamy cytopathology in cell cultures. Spumaviruses are not pathogenic but have been isolated from the brains of normal chimpanzees.

AIDS in the Tropics

In the tropics, the human immunodeficiency syndrome (AIDS) presents some peculiar characteristics (Simpson and Tagliati, 1994). WHO estimates that more than half (67%) of the world's three million AIDS cases have occurred in Africa (see Chapter 4) There are high rates of infection in some groups, such as 30% of all pregnant women and 90% of prostitutes in some parts of Africa. Some nine million adults have been infected with HIV in Sub-Saharan Africa, mainly from heterosexual transmission. AIDS is the leading cause of adult death in Ivory Coast, Zaire and Uganda. Isolation of HIV from the brain and CSF of patients with AIDS, and the presence of a subacute encephalitis in this condition led to the description of AIDS dementia (Pajeau and Román, 1992). Nearly 25% of all AIDS patients eventually develop HIV encephalopathy.

CONCLUSION

Viral diseases are a main cause of neurological morbidity and mortality, the best example is the scourge of HIV and its tremendous toll throughout the world. The diagnosis of various viral infections is primarily clinical but may require techniques which are expensive and labour intensive which may not be available in many developing countries.

REFERENCES

Burke DS, Lorosomrudee W, Leake CJ, Hoke CH, Nisalak A, Chongswasdi V and Laorakpongse T (1985a) Fatal outcome in Japanese encephalitis. *American Journal of Tropical Medicine and Hygiene* **34**: 1203–1210.

Burke DS, Nisalak A, Ussery MA, Laorakpongse T and Chantavibul S (1985b) Kinetics of IgM and IgG responses to Japanese encephalitis virus in human serum and cerebrospinal fluid. *Journal of Infectious Diseases* **151**: 1093–1099.

Dhanda V, Monrya DT, Mishra AC, Ilkal MA, Part U, George Jacob P and Bhat HR (1989) Japanese encephalitis infection in mosquitoes reared from field collected immatures and wild caught males. *American Journal of Tropical Medicine and Hygiene* 732–734.

Gautier-Smith PC (1965) Neurological complications of glandular fever (infectious mononucleosis). *Brain* **88**: 323–334.

Hilt DC, Buchholz D, Krumholz A and Weiss H (1983) Herpes zoster opthalmicus and delayed contralateral hemiplegia caused by cerebral angiitis: diagnosis and management approaches. *Annals of Neurology* **14**: 543–553.

Johnson RT (1989) Arboviral encephalitis. In: *Tropical and Geographical Medicine*, 2nd edn (eds KS Warren and AAF Mahmoud), pp 691–700. New York: McGraw-Hill.

Johnson RT, Griffin DE, Hirsch RL *et al.* (1984) Measles encephalomyelitis – clinical and immunologic studies. *New England Journal of Medicine* **310**: 137–141.

Johnson RT, Burke DS, Elwell M, Leake CJ, Nisalak A, Hoke CH and Lorosomrudee W (1985) Japanese encephalitis: immunocytochemical studies of viral antigen and inflammatory cells in fatal cases. *Annals of Neurology* **18**: 567–573.

Lai CW and Gragasin ME (1988) Electroencephalography in Herpes simplex encephalitis. *Journal of Clinical Neurophysiology* **5**: 87–103.

Laskin OL, Cederberg DM, Mills J, Eron LJ, Mildvan D and Spector SA (1987)

Ganciclovir for the treatment and suppression of serious infections caused by cytomegalovirus. *American Journal of Medicine* **83**: 201–207.

McCormick J, King IJ, Webb PA *et al.* (1986) Lassa fever. Effective therapy with ribavirin. *New England Journal of Medicine* **314**: 20.

McKendall RR (1989) Herpes simplex. In: *Handbook of Clinical Neurology*, vol. 12(56). *Viral Disease* (eds PJ Vinken, GW Bruyn and HL Klawans), pp 207–227. Amsterdam: Elsevier.

Misra UK, Kalita J, Jain SK and Mathur A (1994) Radiological and neurophysiological changes in Japanese encephalitis. *Journal of Neurology Neurosurgery and Psychiatry* **57**: 1484–1487.

Monath TP (1988) Japanese encephalitis – a plague of the Orient. *New England Journal of Medicine* **319**: 641–643.

Pajeau AK and Román GC (1992) HIV encephalopathy and dementia. *Psychiatric Clinics of North America* **15**: 455–466.

Phelps R, Collins DE, Kram JA *et al.* (1994) Human rabies – California, 1994. *Morbidity and Mortality Weekly Report* **43**: 455–457.

Román GC, Román LN and Osame M (1990) Human T lymphotropic virus type I neutropism. *Progress in Medical Virology* **37**: 190–210.

Simpson DM and Tagliati M (1994) Neurologic manifestations of HIV infection. *Annals of Internal Medicine* **121**: 769–785.

Toro G, Román GC and Navarro de Román L (1983) *Neurologia Tropical: Aspectos Neuropatológicos de la Medicina Tropical*. Printer: Bogota.

Umenai T, Krzysko R, Bektimirov TA and Assaad FA (1985) Japanese encephalitis: current worldwide status. *Bulletin of the World Health Organization* **63**: 625–631.

Warrell DA and Shope RE (1990) Rabies. In: *Tropical and Geographical Medicine* (eds KS Warren and AAF Mahmoud), pp 635–644. New York: McGraw-Hill.

Whitley RJ (1990) Viral encephalitis. *New England Journal of Medicine* **323**: 242–250.

Whitley RJ, Alford CA, Hirsch MS *et al.* (1986) Vidarabine versus acyclovir therapy in herpes simplex encephalitis. *New England Journal of Medicine* **314**: 144–149.

3

HTLV-I

Jean-Claude Vernant

Neurology Service, CHU de Fort de France, Hopital Zobda Quitman, Fort de France, Martinique

INTRODUCTION

The human T lymphotropic virus type I (HTLV-I) was isolated in 1980 from cutaneous lesions of American patients suffering from T leukaemias (Poiesz *et al.*, 1980). It was quickly established that this human retrovirus was responsible for adult T-cell leukaemia (ATL) which had been described in 1977 among natives of Southern Japan (Takatsuki *et al.*, 1977). In 1982, the Caribbean endemia was identified (Catovsky *et al.*, 1982; Vyth-Dreese *et al.*, 1982) and in Martinique in 1984 it was found that this virus was also responsible for paraplegias which had been considered to be of unknown origin (Gessain *et al.*, 1985). These paraplegias had previously been mentioned by neurologists in other tropical areas (Cruickshank, 1956; Montgomery *et al.*, 1964; Vernant *et al.*, 1990a) and had been designated under the term 'tropical spastic paraparesis' (TSP) (Roman *et al.*, 1985). Since then, the same retroviral infection has been reported outside tropical areas such as in Japan (Osame *et al.*, 1986a), Chile (Inostroza *et al.*, 1991) and Canada (Oger *et al.*, 1993), demonstrating that HTLV-I endemic regions exist, regardless of climate.

HTLV-I

HTLV-I is a type C retrovirus. Its genome is characterized by regulatory sequences named long terminal repeats (LTR 5′ and LTR 3′), between which are located a *gag* gene which encodes the viral core, a *pol* gene which encodes reverse transcriptase and an *env* gene which encodes glycoproteins in the envelope. HTLV-I belongs to the oncovirus subfamily but shares some distinctive features with the bovine leukaemia virus (BLV) and the simian T-cell leukaemia virus (STLV). These oncogenic retroviruses do not possess a specific oncogene sequence in the genome, and their oncogenicity is not related to the site of their integration in the genome of the host cell. They also have two regulatory genes: the *tax* gene which encodes a protein acting on LTR 5' and is responsible for the activation of viral replication, and the *rex* gene which encodes a protein which, conversely, inhibits replication. It is believed that the status of viral replication is dependent upon the dominant activity of one of these two genes. In addition, it has been shown that *tax* products enhance other promotors and particularly those of IL-2 and R-IL2 which may be implicated in the interdevelopment of ATL. Another striking feature of HTLV-I is its weak genomic variation in the different endemic areas. This very low degree of genetic drift could be an index of ancient human migration patterns (Gessain *et al.*, 1994).

HTLV-II is also present in numerous HTLV-I endemic areas and the two viruses have similar epidemiologic characteristics. However, the pathogenicity of the former has not been clearly established and will not be discussed here.

EPIDEMIOLOGY

Transmission and Seropositivity Studies

Although the overall seropositivity rates vary from one endemic area to another, the seroprevalence increases with age in both sexes but more so in women than

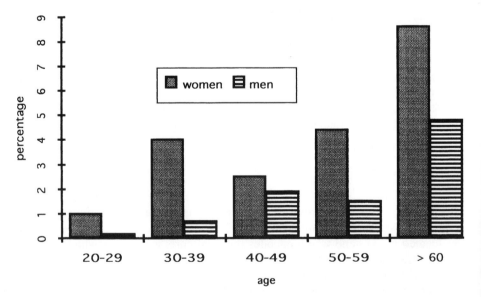

Figure 3.1 Percentage of HTLV-I seropositive blood donors in Martinique, showing increasing seropositivity with age more marked in women (N. Monplaisir, CTS Fort de France, 1987).

men (Figure 3.1), except in Africa (Verdier *et al.*, 1994) and in Papua New
Guinea (Imai *et al.*, 1990).

Epidemiological studies have shown three main modes of transmission:
transfusion of contaminated blood products, sexual intercourse and breast
feeding. Transfusion of HTLV-I infected blood products was first reported in
Japan (Osame *et al.*, 1986b) and was quickly confirmed elsewhere. Kajiyama *et
al.* (1983, 1986) then demonstrated, again in Japan, that sexual transmission is
mostly from male to female while the reverse is rare, indeed questionable, and
probably insignificant from an epidemiological point of view. Breast feeding is
the third well-established mode of transmission. Hino and Doi (1989) showed
that 22% of children between the ages of 3 and 10 breast-fed by a contaminated
mother were seropositive for HTLV-I. But some seronegative children born to
seropositive mothers were also found to be carriers of HTLV-I when polymerase
chain reaction (PCR) technology is used (Monplaisir *et al.*, 1993). This suggests
that other mechanisms for mother to child transmission may exist.

Geographic Distribution

It is not necessary to carry out an extensive survey of the various epidemiologic
studies carried out in regard to HTLV-I to note certain characteristics of its
endemia (Figure 3.2). Japan and Africa were the first two important foci to have
been reported. In the latter continent, HTLV-I is found in central, western and
southern areas where cases of unexplained paraparesis had been described long

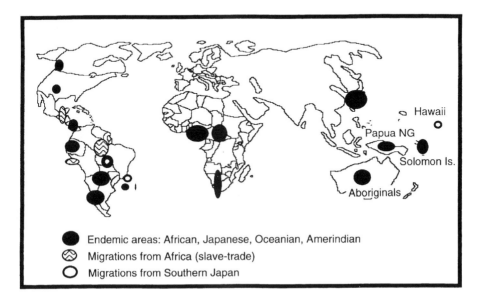

Figure 3.2 Main HTLV-I endemic areas identified.

before HTLV-I was known (Cosnett, 1965; Kayembe, 1990). In Japan, HTLV-I is found mainly in Kiushu and the southern islands, but also in a small, very ancient Aïnhu community in Hokkaïdo. Human migrations originating from these two major endemias are responsible for the establishment of secondary foci on the American continent. The slave trade explains the endemia found in black and mixed-blood people of the Caribbean basin and North America. Small foci in Brazil (Kitagawa *et al.*, 1986), Bolivia (Ohtsu *et al.*, 1987) and Hawaii (Blattner *et al.*, 1986) can be traced to Japanese immigrants. In addition the HTLV-I endemia is present amidst isolated Amerindian populations spread over the American continent (Reeves *et al.*, 1990; Zamora *et al.*, 1990; Oger *et al.*, 1993; Zaninovic *et al.*, 1981, 1994). It can also be found in the Seychelles (Roman *et al.*, 1987), among Papous in New Guinea, Australian aborigines and other insular groups in Melanesia and Micronesia (Garruto *et al.*, 1990). In all these instances, the HTLV-I infection is characterized by the fact that it is scattered in different, isolated foci, even microfoci, within the endemic area, with great variability in the frequency of seropositivity between villages. One example of this occurs on the island of Tsushima (Tajima *et al.*, 1987). Finally, the recent study of Iran-born Mashhadi Jews (Achiron *et al.*, 1993) illustrates the importance of geographic and/or cultural isolation which seems to be required for the propagation of this mildly contagious virus.

CLINICAL ASPECTS

Neurological Involvement

HTLV-I Associated Paraplegia (HAP)

HAP, also called 'tropical spastic paraparesis' (TSP), or 'HTLV-I associated myelopathy' (HAM), or 'HAM/TSP' is the most commonly encountered neuro-logical syndrome (Vernant *et al.*, 1986, 1987). It consists of a progressive paraparesis which is usually spastic but careful examination may reveal involve-ment of the peripheral nerves and muscles as well as other organs suggesting widespread systemic involvement.

The neurological symptoms usually begin during adulthood, most frequently after the age of 30. Although onset above the age of 70 is not unusual, it is extremely rare in childhood or adolescence (Figure 3.3). There is a female predominance, e.g. 237 of 345 Martinican cases.

In most cases the onset is slowly progressive and usually consists of pain involving the low back, the thighs, the sciatic or crural nerves distribution, mimicking rheumatic disease. In other instances, urinary disturbances may be the only symptoms for the first few months until motor disturbances or distal paraesthesias call attention to the neurological system. The diagnosis of HTLV-I related infection is rarely made at this stage except in endemic areas where,

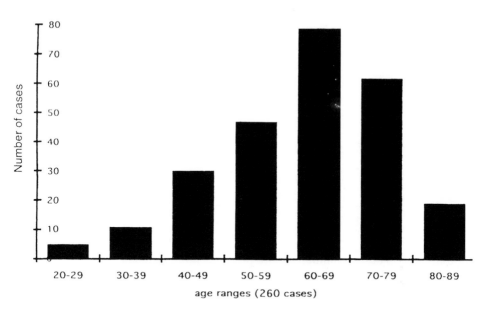

Figure 3.3 Age of onset of neurological disease (260 cases of HTLV-I associated paraplegia).

during the last decade, physicians have become very much aware of this disease. After this initial progressive course, the pace of the illness becomes slower and may even become arrested. In some instances the patients may erroneously be considered as asymptomatic, or indeed, never correctly diagnosed. In most cases, however, a slow deterioration ensues.

The degree of handicap in this chronic stage is highly variable, some patients continue to work, but others are confined to a wheelchair or bedridden. In the mildest cases, the only complaint is that of leg stiffness which may interfere with walking and climbing stairs, but in the more severe ones, there is a spastic gait associated with a certain degree of waddling due to a proximal weakness of the legs. Examination in those patients reveals signs of pyramidal tract involvement with hyperreflexia in all four limbs. Ankle jerks, however, may be normal, depressed or absent suggesting involvement of peripheral nerves. In most cases, bilateral Babinski sign is present. Strength is usually normal in the arms and decreased in the legs with weakness more marked proximally, possibly due to involvement of the muscles themselves. Sensory disturbances consist mainly of paraesthesias of the feet, sometimes of the hands. Objective hyperaesthesia to pin prick is inconstant involving the legs and sometimes the trunk, but disturbances of position sense and gait ataxia are never seen. The striking difference between the mild sensory disturbances and the more obvious motor signs and symptoms is characteristic of the disease. Some authors have noted tremor or nystagmus, which are usually quite mild. Vertigo, diplopia and pronounced cerebellar disturbances are so unusual that their presence suggests that another diagnosis should be considered.

In some rare instances, the onset may be rapidly progressive, in particular in cases resulting from transfusional contamination, especially after open heart surgery (Desgranges *et al.*, 1990; Gout *et al.*, 1990), complete paraplegia being present within a few weeks after seroconversion. Sudden onset, due to involvement of the anterior spinal artery by an inflammatory HTLV-I-induced vasculitis is exceptional and associated with marked elevation of erythrocyte sedimentation rate (Vernant *et al.*, 1994).

Peripheral Neuropathies and Myositis

The coexistence of peripheral nerve involvement had already been noted by some authors prior to the definition of HAP (Montgomery *et al.*, 1964). The involvement of the peripheral system was again noted by Saïd *et al.* in 1988, and dermatomyositis (DM) or polymyositis (PM) by Mora *et al.* in 1988. Both of these conditions were found in cases of HAP by Vernant *et al.* (1990b) (Figures 3.4 and 3.5). These combinations are probably more frequent than suspected as indicated by a retrospective survey carried out in Martinique of 276 cases of HAP which revealed symptoms of peripheral neuropathy in 42 patients, of myositis in 8 others and a combination of these in 20 or more. When the peripheral involvement is particularly marked, it will alter the usual clinical picture since it may result in atrophy of the hand muscles giving the appearance of pseudoamyotrophic lateral sclerosis (pseudo-ALS) (Vernant *et al.*, 1989; Roman *et al.*, 1991). In the same way, when muscle involvement is promi-

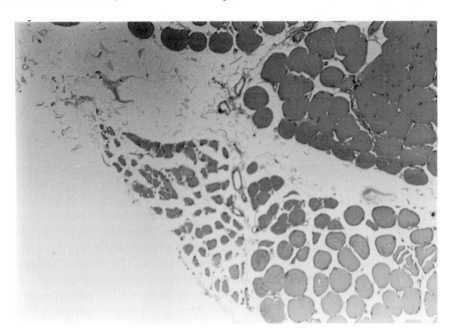

Figure 3.4 Muscle biopsy with neurogenic atrophy (haematoxylin–eosin stain).

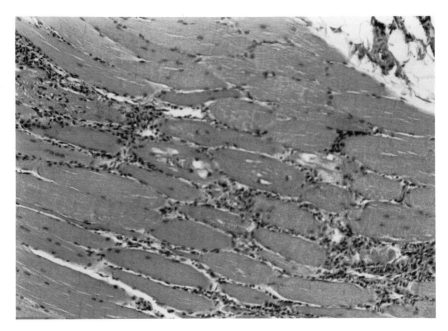

Figure 3.5 Muscle biopsy showing mononuclear cell infiltrates in a case of HTLV-I associated polymyositis.

nent, the clinical picture is that of DM or PM. In those instances, other abnormalities can be found which, in endemic areas, render the differentiation from ALS and DM/PM possible: the common bladder disturbances, the rarity of bulbar involvement, and the presence of minor sensory changes militate against the diagnosis of ALS. In addition, abnormalities of the CSF or the presence of inflammatory changes demonstrated by muscle biopsy, also may be used to rule out ALS. Similarly, HTLV-I myositis has features that distinguish it from primary DM such as the existence of slight peripheral nerve or pyramidal tract signs, the absence of dysphagia and the tendency to chronicity (Figures 3.4 and 3.5).

Associated Systemic Symptoms

The existence of systemic symptoms in addition to the neurological syndrome is one of the striking features of this HTLV-I associated pathology. Most of these, for example, uveitis, lymphocytic alveolitis, sicca syndrome, were noted in the original description of the disease in Martinique (Vernant *et al.*, 1986) and have now been found in most other cases in other endemic areas.

Lymphocytic alveolitis coexists with neurological disturbances in 80% of cases (Sugimoto *et al.*, 1987; Vernant *et al.*, 1988). It is usually clinically silent and abnormalities are rarely seen on X-ray. The diagnosis is made by a bronchoalveolar lavage which shows alveolar lymphocytosis. HTLV-I can be demonstrated in these lymphocytes by PCR technology (Desgranges *et al.*, 1989). Sicca syndromes are found in two-thirds of Martinicans with neurological symptoms (Vernant *et al.*, 1988).

Patients may complain of a sensation of ocular and/or oral dryness, with a feeling of sand or foreign body in the eye. The diagnosis can always be confirmed using the Schirmer test or a biopsy of an accessory salivary gland showing lymphocytic infiltration. In addition to ocular symptoms related to the sicca syndrome, uveitis is probably more common than suspected. Nakao and Ohba (1993) found that 40% of Japanese subjects affected by uveitis of unknown origin were HTLV-I seropositive but traces of the virus were found in only 15.8% of cases of uveitis of known aetiology. The latter percentage is the same as that of the general population of the region. In a systematic survey of our own patients with HAP, we found uveitis in 15% of cases which in one individual was associated with papillitis (Merle *et al.*, 1993, 1994).

Rheumatological features are of two types, atypical lumbosacral back and root pain (Jean-Baptiste *et al.*, 1990), or arthritis and polyarthritis (Nishioka *et al.*, 1989) which may be difficult to differentiate from other inflammatory poly-arthritides, in particular rheumatoid arthritis. The demonstration of HTLV-I antibody synthesis in the affected joint fluid is diagnostic.

Two types of cutaneous manifestation which are different from those of ATL, have been reported in HTLV-I infection. The first (Hashiguchi *et al.*, 1989) consists of xerosis and hypohidrosis observed in patients with HAP, which is probably secondary to the involvement of the autonomic nervous system. The second one was reported by Jamaican authors (La Grenade *et al.*, 1990) who demonstrated a prevalence of 100% HTLV-I seropositivity in children with an infective dermatitis which is described as 'a chronic eczema associated with refractory non-virulent staphylococcus aureus or β haemolytic streptococcus infection of the skin and nasal vestibule'.

The systemic symptoms of this illness can dominate the clinical picture and mask mild or absent neurological symptoms. This is probably why Japanese authors describe cases of lymphocytic alveolitis or Sjögren syndromes possibly associated with uveitis (Eguchi *et al.*, 1992) without recognizing the neurological features of HTLV-I infection. Moreover, outside HTLV-I endemic areas, the aetiologic role of this retrovirus has been strongly suspected in primary Sjögren's syndromes (Green *et al.*, 1989; Iwakura *et al.*, 1991; Mariette *et al.*, 1993).

PATHOPHYSIOLOGY

In all endemic regions, the vast majority of HTLV-I seropositive individuals remain asymptomatic throughout their lives and only a small number develop ATL or HAP. Interestingly, the percentage of the latter varies in different areas. For example, the prevalence of HAP in Japan is estimated to be one case per

1000 seropositive subjects, whereas in Martinique we observe five cases per 100 seropositive subjects. Studies carried out in Japan as well as in Martinique revealed that the risk of developing clinical features may be related to HLA haplotypes, but these results need confirmation from other endemic areas. The coexistence in the same patient of ATL and HAP is sufficiently rare to be fortuitous and probably due to different mechanisms. Contrary to what is observed in ATL, in most cases of HAP, anti-HTLV-I antibodies are produced in great quantity, making serological diagnosis easy and unquestionable. In post-transfusional infection where the infecting viral load is significant, the incubation period is short, followed in a few weeks by seroconversion and, quickly thereafter, by the appearance of neurological signs and symptoms. On the other hand, symptoms appear quite late in patients contaminated by breast feeding.

It is of interest that the age of onset of HAP is identical with that of the proportion of asymptomatic HTLV-I seropositive individuals when grouped by age. In two of our cases, the clinical onset of HAP occurred within a few weeks of seroconversion. This suggests that the appearance of neurological and systemic symptoms is in some way related to the immunological phenomena which occur at the time of seroconversion. However, some difficult cases of HAP, seronegative but PCR positive, have been reported, a situation which is inconsistent with this hypothesis (d'Auriol et al., 1990; Nishimura et al., 1993). A recent study (Monplaisir et al., 1993) of mother to child transmission shows that approximately one-third of seronegative children born to seropositive mothers were PCR positive. We can, therefore, expect that a number of HTLV-I carriers will remain seronegative for several decades and will seroconvert later in life, some of them developing neurological and systemic symptoms at that time. The application of PCR technology in epidemiological studies should reveal a proportion of seronegative carriers in the various age groups in endemic areas.

NEUROPATHOLOGY

Necropsy Findings

Autopsy of the central nervous system shows that the brain is macroscopically normal whereas some atrophy of the spinal cord is generally present. It is more marked in the thoracic portion but may be present either above or below and rarely in the brainstem. The leptomeninges adjacent to the atrophic areas may be thickened. Microscopic lesions are more prominent in the lower thoracic region and consist of loss of myelin sheaths and axons, associated with a proliferation of capillaries and perivascular infiltration with lymphocytes and macrophages. Vacuolar changes have been described in rapidly progressive cases (Yoshioka et al., 1993), whereas in advanced and chronic cases, gliosis is present. Demyelination and remyelination have been observed by electron microscopy by Ohama et al. (1993). Some authors have indicated that demyelination and axonal loss are more marked in the lateral columns at the lumbar level and in the posterior columns in the cervical cord. Perivascular cuffing with lymphocytes without loss of myelin or axons, has been observed in the hemispheric white matter, cerebellum and pons by Izumo *et al.* (1989). The type of lymphocytes in the cuffs varies, consisting of CD8 cells in some cases, CD4 in others or both, as well as CD8 cytotoxic in a case autopsy at an early stage (Yoshioka *et al.*, 1993). Viral antigens have rarely been identified in autopsy material (Moore *et al.*, 1989), but Bhigjee *et al.* (1991) showed the presence of proviral DNA in the spinal cord using PCR technology.

Neuromuscular Biopsy

Saïd *et al.* (1988) described abnormalities of peripheral nerve consisting of perivascular lymphocytic infiltrates associated with demyelination and remyelination as well as axonal degeneration. Mora *et al.* (1988) reported a high prevalence of HTLV-I seropositivity among Jamaican patients suffering from polymyositis and numerous publications have confirmed the frequency of abnormal muscles and peripheral nerves noted in neuromuscular biopsy even when they produce no symptoms (Vernant *et al.*, 1990b). In some of the cases of pseudo-ALS, muscle biopsy shows fascicular atrophy compatible with anterior horn cell disease (Roman *et al.*, 1991).

METHODS FOR THE DETECTION OF HTLV-I INFECTION

Serology

Several diagnostic methods are available for the detection of HTLV-I infection, which include enzyme-linked immunoassay (ELIA), Western blot (WB), immunofluorescence assay (IFA), radioimmunoprecipitation assay (RIPA), and in vitro amplification by PCR. Although antibodies to most HTLV-I gene products have been detected, the serological assays usually measure antibodies to *gag* encoded proteins (p 19, p 24, p 53) and *env* encoded proteins (gp 46 and gp 61/68). Cost-effective, easy to use with high sensitivity, ELIA has been the procedure of choice for screening donated blood. It is an indirect immunoenzymatic method which uses peroxidase-labelled antihuman IgG and IgM antibodies. ELIA is prone to false positive results and these must be confirmed by a supplementary test such as WB or RIPA. WB is the most commonly used confirmatory test because of its easy use and specific reactivity to the individual gene products of HTLV-I. RIPA is labour intensive and requires cell culture facilities as well as radiolabelled nucleotides so that it is primarily a research tool with limited use in routine diagnostic testing. IFA is a simple assay used for the detection of HTLV-I antibodies but does not discriminate between antibodies to particular gene products. Like ELIA, the IFA is subject to false positive results and requires a subjective interpretation of the results. PCR detects infection by the exponential amplification of a nucleic acid sequence of the HTLV-I proviral DNA. This amplified DNA is demonstrated by a hybridization with a specific HTLV-I oligonucleotide marked probe. Since PCR reacts directly with viral DNA, it can detect the retrovirus with great sensitivity regardless of the host's immune response. Discrimination between HTLV-I and HTLV-II is accomplished using probes specific to each virus.

Other Laboratory Data

In the typical cases of HAP, red and white blood cell counts are normal but CD4/CD8 T cell ratio may vary slightly from one patient to another. The erythrocyte sedimentation rate is normal or slightly elevated except in cases with inflammatory vasculitis. In many cases, however, a few abnormal ATL-like lymphocytes with multilobulated nuclei may be found, but they have no prognostic value. Muscle enzymes, particularly creatine kinase (CK), may be elevated, reflecting the degree of inflammatory muscle involvement. Protein electrophoresis may be of the inflammatory type but antinuclear antibodies are absent.

In most instances, the CSF shows moderate lymphocytosis but rarely enough to suggest lymphocytic meningitis. The protein content is moderately elevated and oligoclonal bands and intrathecal synthesis of anti-HTLV-I antibodies may be demonstrated.

Neuroimaging

Neuroradiological examination of individuals who have progressive spastic paraplegia is indicated for the purpose of eliminating a treatable compression of the spinal cord. Myelography is the procedure of choice because more recent techniques such as computer tomography and magnetic resonance imaging (MRI) are most often not available in HTLV-I endemic areas. Atrophy of the spinal cord is seen in longstanding cases. MRI may be normal or show areas of high signal intensity on T2-weighted images in the cervical/thoracic areas in the cord and/or in the periventricular cerebral white matter (Figures 3.6 and 3.7). Such abnormalities may actually exist in asymptomatic seropositive individuals (Mattson *et al.*, 1987).

DIFFERENTIAL DIAGNOSIS

Before 1985, when patients suffering from HAP were seen in Europe or North America, they were most often considered to have multiple sclerosis (MS), while in tropical areas, it was well known under the term of tropical spastic paraplegia

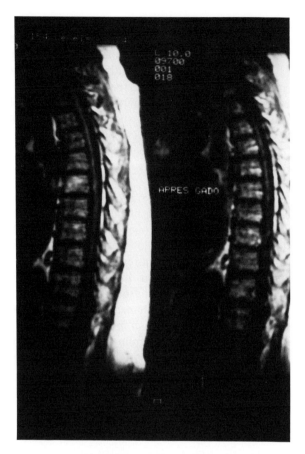

Figure 3.6 MRI showing spinal cord atrophy in cervical and thoracic areas.

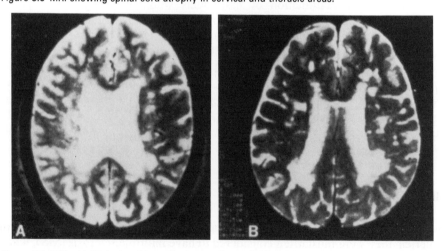

Figure 3.7 MRI with high signal intensity images in cerebral white matter.

(TSP). Most HTLV-I endemic regions have a low prevalence of MS, although it unquestionably exists as shown in Martinique (Poser and Vernant, 1993). It should be noted, however, that HTLV-I positive serology may coexist in a patient with MS in an HTLV-I endemic area (Poser *et al.*, 1990). Commonly found abnormalities in MS such as ataxia, oculomotor disturbances, major sensory disturbances, spontaneous remission, are absent in HAP while involvement of the peripheral nervous system, and myositis do not occur in MS. Similarly, the existence of sicca syndromes and lymphocytic alveolitis is characteristic of HLTV-I and helps in distinguishing between the two ailments (Poser *et al.*, 1990). Diagnostic problems may differ in various endemic regions. In Martinique, there is a high prevalence of cervical spondylosis and spinal stenosis which produces a neurological syndrome closely similar to HAP and the two may coexist (Rivierez *et al.*, 1993).

TREATMENT

All medicinal treatments to date have been disappointing. Corticosteroids may be beneficial when first used, but rapidly lose their efficacy. However, they are clearly indicated in the rare cases of inflammatory vasculitis. Zidovudine is useless. Confirmation is needed of reports of benefit with high doses of vitamin C. The importance of physiotherapy and the treatment of bladder dysfunction must be stressed. In fact, orthopaedic negligence and infections of the urinary tract prove to be the main cause of death in patients who, for one reason or another, escape medical attention. Physiotherapy, therefore, remains the principal means of treatment, whilst the development of more specific therapy is awaited.

CONCLUSION

Rare and often unknown outside endemic areas, HTLV-I associated neurological symptoms have appeared as a public health problem in certain endemic regions. In this way, they represent 90% of inflammatory pathology of the nervous system in Martinique. They most frequently take on the form of a multisystemic inflammatory illness, of which the exact mechanism remains uncertain, but in which HTLV-I induced autoimmune mechanisms certainly play a decisive part.

ACKNOWLEDGEMENTS

Thanks to Didier Smadja, Philippe Cabre, Remi Bellance, Agnes Lezin for their clinical and laboratory help, to Viviane Lenoir and Charles Poser for the translation from French to English.

REFERENCES

Achiron A, Pinhas-Hamiel O, Doll L *et al.* (1993) Spastic paraparesis associated with human T-lymphotropic virus type I: a clinical, serological, and genomic study in Iranian-born Mashhadi Jews. *Annals of Neurology* **34**: 670–675.

Bhigjee AI, Wiley CA, Wachsman W *et al.* (1991) HTLV-I associated myelopathy: clinicopathologic correlation with localization of provirus to spinal cord. *Neurology* **4**: 1990–1992.

Blattner WA, Nomura A, Clark JW *et al.* (1986) Modes of transmission and evidence for viral latency from studies of human T-cell lymphotropic virus type-I in Japanese migrants populations in Hawaï. *Proceedings of the National Academy of Sciences, USA* **83**: 4895–4898.

Catovsky D, Graves MF, Rose M *et al.* (1982) Adult T-cell lymphoma/leukemia in blacks from the West Indies. *Lancet* **i**: 639–643.

Cosnett JE (1965) Unexplained spastic myelopathy. *South Africa Medical Journal* **39**: 592.

Cruickshank EK (1956) A neuropathic syndrome of uncertain origin. Review of 100 cases. *West Indies Medical Journal* **5**: 147–158.

d'Auriol L, Vernant J-C, Ouka M *et al.* (1990) Diagnostic of HTLV-I infected seronegative neurological patients by PCR amplification in Martinique. *Nouvelle Revue Française d'Hématologie* **32**: 113–116.

Desgranges C, Bechet JM, Couderc J, Caubarrere I and Vernant J-C (1989) Detection of HTLV-I DNA by polymerase chain reaction in alveolar lymphocytes of patients with tropical spastic paraparesis. *Journal of Infectious Diseases* **160**: 162–163.

Desgranges C, Winter C and Delzant G (1990) Screening for HTLV-I. *Lancet* **ii**: 1517 (letter).

Eguchi K, Matsuoka N, Ida H *et al.* (1992) Primary Sjögren's syndrome with antibodies to HTLV-I: clinical and laboratory features. *Annals of Rheumatic Diseases* **51**: 769–776.

Garruto RM, Slover M, Yanagihara R *et al.* (1990) High prevalence of human T-lymphotropic virus type 1 infection in isolated population of the Western Pacific region confirmed by Western immunoblot. *American Journal of Human Biology* **2**: 439–447.

Gessain A, Vernant J-C, Barin A, Gout O and De Thé G (1985) Antibodies to human-lymphotropic virus type 1 in patients with tropical spastic paraparesis. *Lancet* **ii**: 407–410.

Gessain A, Koralnik I, Fullen J *et al.* (1994) Phylogenetic study of ten new HTLV-I-strains from the Americas. *AIDS Research and Human Retroviruses* **10**: 103–106.

Gout O, Baulac M, Gessain A *et al.* (1990) Rapid development of myelopathy after HTLV-I infection acquired by transfusion during cardiac transplantation. *New England Journal of Medicine* **322**: 383–388.

Green J, Hinrichs H, Vogel J and Jay G (1989) Exocrinopathy resembling Sjögren's syndrome in HTLV-I tax transgenic mice. *Nature* **341**: 72–74.

Hashiguchi T, Osame M, Arimura K *et al.* (1989) Skin manifestations in HTLV-I associated myelopathy (HAM): xerosis and erythema. In: *HTLV-I and the Nervous System* (eds G Roman, J-C Vernant and M Osame), pp 443–448. New-York: Alan R Liss.

Hino S and Doi H (1989) Mechanisms of HTLV-I transmission. In: *HTLV-I and the*

Nervous System (eds G Roman, J-C Vernant and M Osame), pp 495–501. New-York: Alan R Liss.

Imai J, Terashi S, Talonu T *et al.* (1990) Geographic distribution of subjects seropositive for human T-cell leukemia virus type I in Papua New Guinea. *Japanese Journal of Cancer Research* **81**: 1218–1221.

Inostroza J, Diaz P and Saunier C (1991) Prevalence of antibodies to HTLV-I in South American Indians (Mapuches) from Chile. *Scandinavian Journal of Infectious Diseases* **23**: 507–508.

Iwakura Y, Tosu M, Yoshida E *et al.* (1991) Induction of inflammatory arthropathy resembling rheumatoid arthritis in mice transgenic for HTLV-I. *Science* **253**: 1026–1028.

Izumo S, Usuku K, Osame M *et al.* (1989) The neuropathology of HTLV-I-associated myelopathy in Japan: report of an autopsy case and review of the literature. In: *HTLV-I and the Nervous System* (eds GC Roman, J-C Vernant and M Osame), pp 261–267. New York: Alan R Liss.

Jean-Baptiste G, Arfi S, Horreard A *et al.* (1990) Lomboradiculalgies atypiques associées au HTLV-I. *La Revue du Rhumatisme* **57**: 869–872.

Kajiyama W, Kashiwagi S, Ikematsu H *et al.* (1983) Intrafamilial transmission of adult T-cell leukemia virus. *Journal of Infectious Diseases* **154**: 851–857.

Kajiyama W, Kashiwagi S, Hayashi J *et al.* (1986) Intrafamilial clustering of anti-ATLA-positive persons. *American Journal of Epidemiology* **124**: 800–806.

Kayembe K, Goubeau P, Desmyter J, Vlietinck R and Carton H (1990) A cluster of HTLV-I associated tropical spastic paraparesis in Equateur (Zaïre): ethnic and familial distribution. *Journal of Neurology, Neurosurgery, and Psychiatry* **53**: 4–10.

Kitagawa T, Fujishita M, Tagushi H and Miyoshi I (1986) Antibodies to HTLV-I in Japanese immigrants in Brazil. *Journal of the American Medical Association* **256**: 2342.

La Grenade L, Hanchard B, Flechter V, Cranston B and Blattner W (1990) Infective dermatitis of Jamaican children: a marker for HTLV-I infection. *Lancet* **ii**: 1345–1347.

Mariette X, Agbalika F, Daniel M-T *et al.* (1993) Detection of human T lymphotropic virus type 1 *tax* gene in salivary gland epithelium from two patients with Sjögren's syndrome. *Arthritis and Rheumatism* **36**: 1423–1428.

Mattson DH, Mc Farlin DE, Mora C and Zaninovic V (1987) Central-nervous-system lesions detected by magnetic resonance imaging in an HTLV-I antibody positive symptomless individual. *Lancet* **ii**: 49.

Merle H, Smadja D, Bera O, Grolier-Bois L and Vernant J-C (1993) Uvéopapillite associée à une paraparésie due au HTLV-I. *La Presse Médicale* **22**: 1179–1182.

Merle H, Smadja D, Bera O, Cabre P and Vernant J-C (1994) Manifestations ophtalmologiques au cours de la myelopathie due au HTLV-I. *Journal Français d'Ophtalmologie* **17**: 403–413.

Monplaisir N, Neisson-Vernant C, Bouillot M *et al.* (1993) HTLV-I maternal transmission in Martinique, using serology and polymerase chain reaction. *AIDS Research and Human Retroviruses* **9**: 869–874.

Montgomery RD, Cruickshank K, Robertson WB and McMenemey WH (1964) Clinical and pathological observations on Jamaican neuropathy. *Brain* **87**: 425–462.

Moore W, Traugott U, Scheinberg L and Raine C (1989) Tropical spastic paraparesis: a model of virus-induced, cytotoxic T-cell-mediated demyelinisation? *Annals of Neurology* **26**: 523–530.

Mora CA, Garruto RM, Brown P *et al.* (1988) Seroprevalence of antibodies to HTLV-I in patients with chronic neurological disorders other than tropical spastic paraparesis. *Annals of Neurology* (supplement) **235**: S192–195.

Nakao K and Ohba N (1993) Clinical features of HTLV-I associated uveitis. *British Journal of Ophthalmology* **77**: 274–279.

Nishimura M, Mingioli E, McFarlin DE and Jacobson S (1993) Demonstration of human T-cell lymphotropic virus type 1 (HTLV-I) from HTLV-I seronegative South Indian patient with chronic, progressive spastic paraparesis. *Annals of Neurology* **34**: 867–870.

Nishioka K, Maruyama I, Sato K *et al.* (1989) Chronic inflammatory arthropathy associated with HTLV-I. *Lancet* **i**: 441–442.

Oger J, Werker D, Foti D and Dekaban G (1993) HTLV-I associated myelopathy: an endemic disease of Canadian Aboriginals of the North-West Pacific coast. *Canadian Journal of Neurological Sciences* **20**: 302–306.

Ohama E, Horikawa Y, Shimizu T *et al.* (1993) Demyelinisation and remyelinisation in spinal cord lesions of human lymphotrophic virus type-1-associated myelopathy. *Acta Neuropathologica* **81**: 78–83.

Ohtsu T, Tsugane S, Tobinai K *et al.* (1987) Prevalence of antibodies to human T-cell leukemia/lymphoma virus type 1 and human immunodeficiency virus in Japanese immigrants colonies in Bolivia and Bolivian natives. *Japanese Journal of Cancer Research* **78**: 1347–1353.

Osame M, Usuku K, Izumo S *et al.* (1986a) HTLV-I associated myelopathy: a new clinical entity. *Lancet* **i**: 1031–1032.

Osame M, Isumoi S, Igata A *et al.* (1986b) Blood transfusion and HTLV-I associated myelopathy. *Lancet* **ii**: 104–105.

Poiesz BJ, Ruscetti FW, Gazdar AF *et al.* (1980) Detection and isolation of type C retroviruses particles from fresh and cultured lymphocytes of a patient with cutaneous T-cell lymphoma. *Proceedings of the National Academy of Sciences, USA* **77**: 7415–7419.

Poser CM and Vernant J-C (1993) La sclerose en plaques dans la race noire. IV° Congrès International de Médecine Tropicale de Langue Française. Fort de France (Martinique), 15–18 Novembre 1993. Sous presse in: *Bulletins de la Société de Pathologie Exotique de Langue Française.*

Poser CM, Román GC and Vernant J-C (1990) Multiple sclerosis or HTLV-I myelitis? *Neurology* **40**: 1020–1022.

Reeves WC, Cutler JR, Gracia F *et al.* (1990) Human T-cell lymphotropic virus infection in Guaymi Indians from Panama. *American Journal of Tropical Medicine and Hygiene* **43**: 410–418.

Rivierez M, Vernant J-C, Randrianbolona J, Buisson G, Smadja D *et al.* (1993) Cervicarthrosis and spinal stenosis associated paraplegias: is surgery indicated? *Abstracts of the X° International Congress of Neurological Surgery.* Acapulco (Mexico), October 17–22. F750–Q64, p 281.

Román GC, Spencer PS and Schoenberg BS (1985) Tropical myeloneuropathies: the hidden endemias. *Neurology* **35**: 1158–1170.

Román GC, Schoenberg BS, Madden DL *et al.* (1987) Human T-lymphotropic virus type I antibodies in the serum of patients with tropical spastic paraparesis in the Seychelles. *Archives of Neurology* **44**: 605–607.

Román G, Vernant J-C and Osame M (1991) HTLV-I-associated motor neuron disease. In: *Handbook of Clinical Neurology*, vol. 15 (59) *Diseases of the Motor System* (ed. JMBV de Jong), pp 447–457. Amsterdam: Elsevier Science Publishers B.V.

Saïd G, Goulon-Godeau C, Lacroix C *et al.* (1988) Inflammatory lesions of peripheral nerve in a patient with human T-lymphotropic virus type 1 associated myelopathy. *Annals of Neurology* **24**: 275–277.

Sugimoto M, Nakashima H, Watanabe S *et al.* (1987) T-lymphocyte alveolitis in HTLV-I associated myelopathy. *Lancet* **ii**:1220.

Tajima K, Kamura S, Ito S *et al.* (1987) Epidemiologic features of HTLV-I carriers and incidence of ATL in an ATL-endemic island: a report of the community based cooperative study in Tsushima. Japan. *International Journal of Cancer* **40**: 741–746.

Takatsuki K, Uchiyama T, Sagawa K *et al.* (1977) Adult T-cell leukemia in Japan. In: *Topics in Hematology* (eds S Seno, F Takaku and S Irion), pp 73–77. Amsterdam: Excerpta Medica.

Verdier M, Bonis J and Denis F (1994) The prevalence and incidence of HTLVs in Africa. In: *AIDS in Africa* (eds M Essex, S M'Boup, P Kanki, M Kalengayi), pp 173–193. New York: Raven Press.

Vernant J-C, Gessain A, Gout O *et al.* (1986) Paraparésies tropicales en Martinique: haute prévalence d'anticorps HTLV-I. *La Presse Medicale* **15**: 419–422.

Vernant J-C, Maurs L, Gessain A *et al.* (1987) Endemic tropical spastic paraparesis associated with the human T-lymphotropic virus type 1: a clinical and seroepidemiological study of 25 cases. *Annals of Neurology* **21**: 123.

Vernant J-C, Buisson G, Magdeleine J *et al.* (1988) T-lymphocyte alveolitis, tropical spastic paraparesis and Sjögren syndrome. *Lancet* **i**: 177.

Vernant J-C, Buisson G, Bellance R *et al.* (1989) Pseudo amyotrophic lateral sclerosis, peripheral neuropathy and chronic polyradiculoneuritis in patients with HTLV-I associated paraplegias. In: *HTLV-I and the Nervous System* (eds G Roman, J-C Vernant and M Osame), pp 361–365. New York: Alan R Liss.

Vernant J-C, Buisson GG, Monplaisir N and Hugon J (1990a) From tropical paraparesis to neurological manifestations of HTLV-I infection. In: *Advances in Neurology. Proceedings of the XIVth World Congress of Neurology*, New Delhi, October 22–27, 1989 (eds JS Chopra, K Jagannathan IMS Sawhney), pp 257–264. Amsterdam: Excerpta Medica.

Vernant J-C, Bellance R, Buisson G *et al.* (1990b) Peripheral neuropathies and myositis associated by HTLV-I infection in Martinique. In: *Human Retrovirology: HTLV-I* (ed. WA Blattner), pp 225–235. New York: Raven Press.

Vernant J-C, Smadja D, Deforges-Lasseur C *et al.* (1994) Vascularites et manifestations neurologiques associées au virus HTLV-I. *La Presse Médicale* **23**: 1421–1425.

Vyth-Dreese FA and De Vries JE (1982) Human T-cell leukemia virus in lymphocytes from T-cell leukemia patient originating from Surinam. *Lancet* **ii**: 407–411.

Yoshioka A, Hirose G, Ueda Y, Nishimura Y and Sakai K (1993) Neuropathological studies of the spinal cord in early stage HTLV-I-associated myelopathy (HAM). *Journal of Neurology, Neurosurgery and Psychiatry* **56**: 1004–1007.

Zamora T, Zaninovic V, Kajiwara M *et al.* (1990) Antibody to HTLV-I in indigenous inhabitants of the Andes and Amazon Regions in Colombia. *Japanese Journal Cancer Research (Gann)* **81**: 715–719.

Zaninovic V, Biojo R and Barreto P (1981) Paraparesia Espastica del Pacifico. *Colombia Médica* **12**: 111–117.

Zaninovic V, Sanzon F, Lopez F *et al.* (1994) Geographic independence of HTLV-I and HTLV2 foci in the Andes Highland, the Atlantic Coast, and the Orinoco of Colombia. *AIDS Research and Human Retroviruses* **10**: 97–101.

4

HIV

Robert Colebunders

Institute of Tropical Medicine, Nationalestraat 155-2000 Antwerp, Belgium

INTRODUCTION

The human immunodeficiency (HIV) epidemic is rapidly spreading in tropical countries. In 1994 the World Health Organization (WHO) estimates that there are 9 million persons with HIV infection in Africa, 2 million in Asia and 1.5 million in South America (WHO, 1994). Neurological manifestations occur in at least 40% of HIV-infected patients at some stage of their disease and at autopsy 80–90% of patients have some degree of neuropathological abnormality (Anders *et al.*, 1986). Therefore, physicians working in tropical countries confronted with neurological problems often will have to consider an underlying HIV infection.

Neurological manifestations are seen at all stages in patients with HIV-1 as well as HIV-2 infection (Ramiandrisoa *et al.*, 1991). These include a wide variety of disorders affecting all parts of the nervous system (Table 4.1). In the tropics, because diagnostic facilities are often limited, it is difficult to determine the presence of these neurological complications. Probably for this reason so far relatively few studies have been carried out in this part of the world concerning the neurological manifestations associated with HIV infection (Belec *et al.*, 1989a, b; Conlon, 1989; Howlett *et al.*, 1989, 1994; Pallangyo *et al.*, 1992; Perriens *et al.*, 1992; Ramiandrisoa *et al.*, 1991) (Table 4.2).

NEUROLOGICAL DISORDERS DURING ACUTE HIV INFECTION

Neurological disorders may develop within 10 weeks of HIV infection (Carne *et al.*, 1985). Early central nervous system infection with HIV is usually asymptomatic or responsible for only mild symptoms such as headache and meningism. Severe neurological involvement is relatively rare. Disorders that have been observed during acute HIV infection are: encephalitis, meningitis, myelopathy with subacute or acute onset, cranial neuropathy, brachial plexopathy or peripheral neuropathy (Portegies and Brew, 1992). Most patients recover from these

TABLE 4.1 Neurological complications in HIV-infected patients

Brain
  Predominantly non-focal
    Acute HIV-related encephalitis
    Metabolic encephalopathies
    AIDS–dementia complex
    Cytomegalovirus encephalitis
    Herpes encephalitis

  Predominantly focal
    Progressive multifocal leukoencephalopathy
    Cerebral toxoplasmosis
    Primary central nervous system lymphoma
    Tuberculosis brain abscess/tuberculoma/cryptococcoma
    Varicella–zoster virus encephalitis
    Multiple sclerosis-like illness
    Vascular disorders

Spinal cord
    Vacuolar myelopathy
    Varicella–zoster virus myelitis
    Spinal epidural or intradural lymphoma

Meninges
    Aseptic meningitis
    Cryptococcal meningitis
    Tuberculous meningitis (*Mycobacterium tuberculosis*)
    Lymphomatous meningitis

Peripheral nerve and root
    Inflammatory neuropathies
    Distal predominantly sensory polyneuropathy
    Cranial neuropathies
    Mononeuritis multiplex
    Cytomegalovirus polyradiculopathy
    Varicella–zoster virus infection
    Toxic neuropathies
    Autonomic neuropathy

Muscle
    HIV-related myopathy
    Zidovudine-related myopathy
    Pyomyositis

TABLE 4.2 Postmortem study among 247 persons with HIV infection who died in Abidjan, Côte d'Ivoire: cerebral pathology

Tuberculous meningitis	49 (20)
Cerebral toxoplasmosis	37 (15)
Purulent meningitis	12 (5)
Cryptococcal meningitis	6 (2)
Progressive multifocal leukoencephalopathy	3 (1)
Multinuclear giant-cell encephalitis	8 (3)
Primary cerebral lymphoma	3 (1)
Cytomegalovirus encephalitis	3 (1)

Values in parentheses are percentages

neurological manifestations within several weeks. However, focal deficits and cognitive disorders may persist in some patients with encephalitis.

NON-FOCAL CENTRAL NERVOUS SYSTEM DISEASE

Central Nervous System Disease With Concomitant Decrease of Alertness

This category includes a wide range of conditions, such as metabolic disorders (e.g. hepatic encephalopathy, hypoxia, renal insufficiency, electrolyte imbalances) and side-effects of drugs (sedatives, anticonvulsants, narcotics, foscarnet, etc.).

Central Nervous System Disease Without Concomitant Decrease of Alertness

AIDS–Dementia Complex (ADC)

This is the most common central nervous system complication of HIV infection. ADC affects between a third and two-thirds of AIDS patients in industrialized countries (Price and Brew, 1988).

The American Academy of Neurology and the WHO have developed a definition for ADC (WHO, 1990). A criterion of this definition is that central nervous system opportunistic infections or malignancies have to be excluded by appropriate laboratory and radiological investigations. Because in most tropical countries these diagnostic facilities are not available, it is difficult to define ADC in these countries. Moreover in the tropics certain parasitic diseases, such as trypanosomiasis, may present with ADC-like symptoms. Therefore, the incidence of ADC in developing countries is difficult to ascertain. In a study performed in Tanzania, an incidence of ADC similar to that observed in the West was reported (Howlett et al., 1989). In Zaïre, however, a lower incidence was observed (Perriens et al., 1992).

Clinical manifestations of HIV dementia include cognitive, motor and behavioural disorders. The earliest symptoms of ADC are cognitive and patients complain of difficulties in concentration, forgetfulness and cognitive slowing. Occasionally agitation and mania may be the initial manifestations (Price and Brew, 1988). These early symptoms are difficult to recognize and are confused with psychiatric complaints. Usually judgement is reserved until late. Complex tasks become more difficult and take longer to complete. Cognitive dysfunction is often missed in the early stages, but becomes more apparent with disease progression. Motor abnormalities which are frequently noted early, include ataxia, hyperreflexia and the appearance of frontal lobe release reflexes such as a snout response. Grasp and Babinski reflexes are also commonly present. In late stages paraparesis with faecal and urinary incontinence may develop.

Behavioural dysfunction includes personality change and apathy. Disorientation develops in advanced stages of the disease and in the end stages there may be complete mutism. A staging system for ADC is shown in Table 4.3.

ADC is often associated with a vacuolar myelopathy (see later). In these

TABLE 4.3 Staging scheme for the AIDS–dementia complex (ADC)

ADC stage	Characteristics
Stage 0 (normal)	Normal mental and motor function
Stage 0.5 (equivocal, subclinical)	Either minimal or equivocal symptoms of cognitive or motor dysfunction characteristic of ADC, or mild signs (snout response, slowed extremity movements), but without impairment of work or capacity to perform activities of daily living (ADL). Gait and strength are normal
Stage 1 (mild)	Unequivocal evidence (symptoms, signs, neuropsychological test performance) of functional intellectual or motor impairment characteristic of ADC, but able to perform all but the more demanding aspects of work or ADL. Can walk without assistance
Stage 2 (moderate)	Cannot work or maintain the more demanding aspects of daily life, but able to perform basic activities of self care. Ambulatory, but may require a single prop
Stage 3 (severe)	Major intellectual incapacity (cannot follow news or personal events, cannot sustain complex conversation, considerable slowing of all output), or motor disability (cannot walk unassisted, requiring walker or personal support usually with slowing and clumsiness of arms as well)
Stage 4 (end stage)	Nearly vegetative; intellectual and social comprehension and response are at a rudimentary level. Nearly or absolutely mute. Paraparetic or paraplegic with double incontinence.

patients motor abnormalities may predominate over cognitive impairment. Some patients also develop tremor, myoclonus and chorea.

Children with AIDS may also develop HIV encephalopathy which is characterized by loss of previously acquired motor and cognitive milestones, spastic paraparesis or quadriparesis with pseudobulbar palsy and rigidity.

ADC generally only develops in the presence of severe immune deficiency (CD4 lymphocyte count below 200 cells mm^{-3}). The majority of patients with ADC will have cerebrospinal fluid abnormalities. An elevated protein level is found in about 65% of the cases, and often there is a mild lymphocytic pleocytosis. These cerebrospinal fluid abnormalities are, however, non-specific as they are also frequently observed in neurologically normal HIV carriers. CT and MRI reveals widened cortical sulci and enlargement of the ventricles with subcortical white matter abnormalities. In children, calcification of the basal ganglia can be seen.

The pathology of ADC is heterogeneous; in some patients there develops a multinucleated-cell encephalitis whereas in others multinuclear cells are absent and only a diffuse myelin pallor is observed. The associated vacuolar myelopathy resembles subacute combined degeneration caused by vitamin B_{12} deficiency. Possibly these different pathological manifestations are caused by different mechanisms. A direct infection of neurones and glial cells by neurotropic HIV strains is proposed, or HIV infection of monocytes–macrophages may occur resulting in release of inflammatory products causing tissue destruction.

The use of zidovudine seems to decrease the incidence of ADC (Portegies *et al.*, 1989). Moreover, some clinical improvement in ADC as well as in HIV encephalopathy in children has been observed during zidovudine treatment. As in most tropical countries zidovudine is not available, treatment of ADC in those countries should mainly be supportive.

Vacuolar Myelopathy

Spinal cord lesions are less common than those affecting the brain. Pathologically the myelopathy is characterized by vacuolar changes in the lateral and posterior columns (Budka, 1991). Clinical findings include hyperreflexia, spastic paraparesis, ataxia, incontinence and occasionally sensory deficits. The differential diagnosis in tropical countries should include other non-traumatic spastic paraparesis such as paraparesis caused by HTLV-I infection (Ramiandrisoa *et al.*, 1991) and cassava-cyanide poisoning. (See Chapters 3 and 21.)

FOCAL CENTRAL NERVOUS SYSTEM DISORDERS

Focal central nervous system disorders caused by opportunistic infections or malignancies develop generally only in the presence of severe immune deficiency (CD4 lymphocyte count < 200 cells mm^{-3}). Certain opportunistic infections are more prevalent in particular geographic areas.

Cerebral Toxoplasmosis

Toxoplasma gondii is the most frequent opportunistic infection causing a focal central nervous system disorder, occurring in 5–20% of AIDS patients (Luft and Remington, 1988). In a postmortem study in Abidjan (Ivory Coast), 23% of people with AIDS were shown to have cerebral toxoplasmosis (Lucas *et al.*, 1993). Cerebral toxoplasmosis usually presents as a subacute illness with focal neurological deficits, which may vary according to the localization of the abscess (e.g. hemiparesis, ataxia, aphasia, hemisensory loss, central loss of vision). Patients often have low-grade fever and complain of headache (Luft and Remington, 1988). Unusually a patient may present with a diffuse (encephalitic) form of toxoplasmosis with multiple microabscesses. The diagnosis is made on the basis of clinical symptoms and radiological findings. Both CT and MRI usually show contrast-enhancing spherical lesions in the basal ganglia or cortex (Figure 4.1), which are surrounded by oedema and show signs of some mass effect.

Serological tests are not very helpful in the diagnosis of cerebral toxoplasmosis in AIDS patients. IgM antibodies are usually absent and IgG antibodies are only indicative of a previous toxoplasma infection. The absence of IgG antibodies is, however, an argument against the diagnosis of cerebral toxoplasmosis. The diagnosis of cerebral toxoplasmosis in tropical countries should be made on clinical grounds, including the response to treatment, as usually patients respond within a few days of starting therapy. The treatment of choice (Leport *et al.*, 1988) is with pyrimethamine 200 mg orally the first day, followed by 50 mg day^{-1} orally thereafter, combined with sulphadiazine given at a dose of 200 mg kg^{-1} day^{-1} orally. Folinic acid 10–50 mg day^{-1} should be added to prevent leukopenia caused by the pyrimethamine. Treatment should be continued at this dose for 3–6 weeks and should be followed by maintenance therapy consisting of pyrimethamine 25–50 mg day^{-1} and sulphadiazine 2 g day^{-1}. Many patients will develop an allergic reaction to the sulphadiazine. For these patients the sulphadiazine should be replaced by clindamycin 600 mg orally four times daily. Long-term anticonvulsant therapy is also necessary, because of the high frequency of epilepsy. Corticosteroids should only be given in the presence of significant cerebral oedema. Recently, the new drug atovaquone has been shown to have some efficacy in patients unable to take the pyrimethamine–sulphadiazine treatment (Kovacs, 1992).

Progressive Multifocal Leukoencephalopathy

Progressive multifocal leukoencephalopathy (PML) is an opportunistic infection caused by a human papova virus (JC virus). In the West, PML occurs in 2–5% of AIDS patients. Its incidence in AIDS patients in the tropics is unknown.

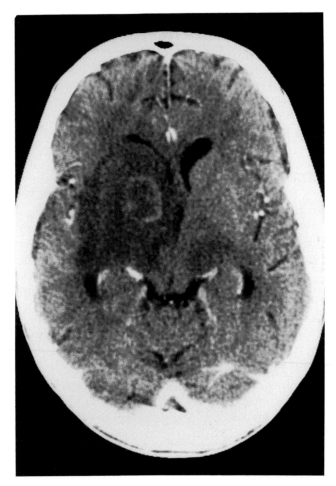

Figure 4.1 Cerebral toxoplasmosis abscess. CT scan showing ring enhancement of the contrast and oedema surrounding the abscess, causing compression of the lateral ventricle.

Symptoms develop over several weeks or a few months. Focal symptoms and signs include hemiparesis, aphasia, visual loss, sensory loss and ataxia. MRI and CT scans generally demonstrate single or multiple lesions of the white matter. On CT usually there is no enhancement on contrast in the lesions and there is no mass effect. There is no therapy for this disorder, but spontaneous remissions may occur (Berger and Mucke, 1988).

PRIMARY CENTRAL NERVOUS SYSTEM LYMPHOMA

In a postmortem study among AIDS patients in Abidjan (Ivory Coast) central nervous system lymphoma was observed in 1% (Lucas *et al.*, 1993). These lymphomas are of B cell type. Symptoms may develop insidiously and focal neurological deficits may be the same as for cerebral toxoplasmosis. The CT and MRI lesions are often single, generally less dense and more diffusely enhancing than toxoplasma abscess, and usually surrounded by oedema. Patients do not respond to antitoxoplasma therapy and brain biopsy is needed for a definitive diagnosis. Steroids and radiotherapy are used in the treatment (Baumgarter *et al.*, 1990). With or without treatment the prognosis of the patient with a cerebral lymphoma is very poor.

OTHER FOCAL CENTRAL NERVOUS SYSTEM DISEASES

Mycobacterium tuberculosis brain abscess is reported (Bishburg *et al.*, 1986), but atypical mycobacterial infection of the brain is rare. Among the viruses, cytomegalovirus (CMV) usually causes a diffuse microscopic infection with or without symptoms and signs. Only occasionally a CMV encephalitis may cause discrete small macroscopic spherical lesions detectable by MRI (Masden *et al.*, 1988). A varicella–zoster virus encephalitis also may cause multifocal lesions suggestive of PML (Morgello *et al.*, 1988). Herpes simplex virus also may cause encephalitis with focal neurological abnormalities (Dix *et al.*, 1985). Occasionally a patient with HIV infection may develop a multiple sclerosis-like illness of unknown origin (Berger *et al.*, 1989).

Cerebrovascular disease has been reported in patients with HIV infection in industrialized countries and in the tropics (Berger *et al.*, 1990). This may present as transient ischaemic attacks and strokes both in adults and in children, and in adults often has a benign outcome. The pathogenesis of these ischaemic events remains unclear.

MENINGITIS

Cryptococcal Meningitis

The most important cause of meningitis in AIDS patients is *Cryptococcus neoformans* and this seems to be more frequent in certain geographic regions. In Central Africa it occurs in 5–15% of AIDS patients (Howlett *et al.*, 1994) who usually present with low-grade fever and headache, without meningismus initially (Powderly, 1993). However, if the diagnosis of cryptococcal meningitis is delayed then neck stiffness, photophobia and vomiting may appear. In the late stages of the disease, confusion and an alteration in the level of consciousness may develop. Other organs such as the lungs or the skin may also be involved.

The diagnosis of cryptococcal meningitis is made at lumbar puncture when the cerebrospinal fluid shows in general a small increase in white cell count, fewer

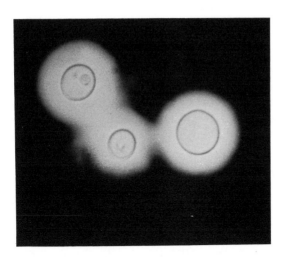

Figure 4.2 Cryptococcal meningitis. Indian ink preparation of the cerebrospinal fluid showing numerous cryptococci.

than 20 cells mm^{-3} (mainly lymphocytes), some elevation of protein levels (less than 2 g l^{-1}) with normal or slightly decreased glucose levels. By examination of the cerebrospinal fluid with indian ink the cryptococci appear as rounded or budding forms with a distinct capsule (Figure 4.2).

Cryptococci can also be cultured from the CSF. A cryptococcus antigen can be demonstrated in both the serum and the CSF in 95% of the patients with cryptococcal meningitis. In a study performed in Zaïre, cryptococcus antigen testing was found to be more sensitive than the detection of cryptococci in the CSF using indian ink (Desmet *et al.*, 1989). Cryptococcal meningitis is treated by amphotericin B alone (0.3–0.6 mg kg^{-1} day^{-1} intravenously) for 6 weeks or amphotericin B together with flucytosine (150 g kg^{-1} day^{-1} in four divided daily doses). Fluconazole, 600 mg day^{-1} orally for 2–3 weeks followed by fluconazole 400 mg day^{-1} for 3 weeks is probably as effective. Lifelong maintenance therapy with fluconazole 100–200 mg day^{-1} is needed. Fluconazole has less side-effects and is much easier to administer than amphotericin but it is very expensive and unavailable in most tropical countries.

Mycobacterium tuberculosis Meningitis

In tropical countries this is a relatively frequent complication of HIV infection (Lucas *et al.*, 1993), and often such infection is undiagnosed. The diagnosis and treatment is covered in Chapter 9.

Neurosyphilis

Several studies have suggested that HIV may cause accelerated progression of early syphilis infection to neurosyphilis (Aronow *et al.*, 1988). While the average time from primary to tertiary syphilis in HIV seronegative individuals is 7 years, in HIV seropositive persons this period may be as short as a few months. However, HIV-infected people with syphilis may have a false negative treponema test (Hicks *et al.*, 1987). The treatment of neurosyphilis in HIV-infected individuals requires 20 million U of penicillin intravenously daily for 10–14 days.

PERIPHERAL NERVE DISORDERS

One quarter to a third of HIV-infected individuals will develop a peripheral nerve disorder (Simpson and Wolfe, 1991). The pathophysiology of this disorder is not fully understood and varies from autoimmunity, as in the Guillain–Barré syndrome, to a possible direct HIV infective distal polyneuropathy. A peripheral nerve disorder may develop during any stage of HIV infection.

Inflammatory Polyneuropathies

These include the Guillain–Barré syndrome and a chronic inflammatory demyelinating polyneuropathy. A Guillain–Barré syndrome may be the first manifestation of HIV infection (Cornblath *et al.*, 1991). Demyelinating polyneuropathies are characterized by development of paresis of legs and arms. In the Guillain–Barré syndrome this paresis may develop in a matter of hours or days. In chronic inflammatory demyelinating polyneuropathy, paresis develops over weeks or months. The presenting clinical features of these demyelinating polyneuropathies are similar to those seen in non-HIV infected cases. The pathogenesis of these polyneuropathies is unclear, but may have an autoimmune basis. Some patients may respond favourably to plasmaphoresis or corticosteroid administration.

Cranial Neuropathies

An isolated paralysis of the 7th cranial nerve is a relatively frequent complication of HIV infection (Belec *et al.*, 1989b) and may develop quickly, within 24 hours. Patients usually make a spontaneous full or partial recovery. Other cranial nerves, particularly the 3rd, 4th, 5th and 6th, may also be involved.

Distal, Predominantly Sensory Polyneuropathy (DSPN)

This is an axonal neuropathy and commonly occurs in the late stage of HIV disease (So *et al.*, 1988). Patients complain of symmetrical paraesthesias, numbness and painful burning in the feet. The clinical course is usually slowly progressive. The treatment of the neuropathy is symptomatic, zidovudine has no effect, amitriptyline is sometimes effective, in some the pain may respond to carbamazepine or phenytoin, but analgesics and narcotics are often needed.

Toxic Neuropathies

Isoniazid is increasingly used in the tropics not only for treatment of tuberculosis but also as prophylaxis for tuberculosis in HIV-infected individuals. The nucleoside analogues dideoxyinosine (DDI) and dideoxycytidine (DDC) may cause axonal neuropathy (Lambert *et al.*, 1990; Fischl *et al.*, 1993). In most cases these neuropathies regress once the drug is discontinued.

Vincristine, a chemotherapeutic agent used for the treatment of Kaposi's sarcoma and non-Hodgkin lymphoma, also may cause polyneuritis.

Cytomegalovirus Infection of the Nerves

CMV is able to infect endothelial cells (leading to angiopathic damage to the nerve) and Schwann cells (leading to Schwann cell death and demyelination), thus causing a demyelinating neuropathy, multiple mononeuropathy and polyradiculopathy (Behar *et al.*, 1987; Fuller *et al.*, 1989). Cytomegalovirus polyradiculopathy occurs in patients who are severely immunocompromised (De Gans *et al.*, 1990). The symptoms include pain in the back and lower extremities with rapidly developing flaccid paraparesis. There may also be bladder and bowel dysfunction and sensory loss in the extremities. Early recognition of this polyradiculopathy is important because ganciclovir or foscarnet treatment can reverse the condition in some patients (De Gans *et al.*, 1990).

Varicella–zoster Infection

Shingles is observed in about 10–15% of patients with HIV infection in the tropics (Howlett *et al.*, 1994). In certain patients with advanced immune deficiency, a generalized form of varicella–zoster infection occurs. Neurological complications are unusual but include encephalitis, myelitis, radiculitis and cranial nerve palsy. Postherpetic neuralgia is, however, frequent, and can be very painful.

Autonomic Neuropathy

Abnormal autonomic functions tests as well as symptoms suggestive of autonomic dysfunction are frequently observed in AIDS patients (Welby *et al.*, 1991).

MYOPATHIES

An idiopathic inflammatory myopathy has been observed during HIV infection (Buskila and Gladman, 1990) causing progressive proximal and distal muscle weakness, myalgia, muscle tenderness and leg cramps. In certain patients there may be an asymptomatic elevation of the serum creatinine kinase. HIV myopathy may lead to severe muscle wasting. The pathogenesis of this myopathy remains unknown, but an autoimmune process has been suggested. Certain patients respond to corticosteroid treatment. Zidovudine may also cause a toxic myopathy which is indistinguishable from the AIDS myopathy, except that after stopping zidovudine the myopathy disappears. In Africa, staphylococcal pyomyositis is also a relatively frequent complication of HIV infection (Pallangyo *et al.*, 1992).

SEIZURES

Seizures occur relatively frequently in HIV-infected individuals, caused by focal or non-focal central nervous system disease, but in many cases the cause is not found (Wong *et al.*, 1990).

PSYCHIATRIC MANIFESTATIONS

Psychiatric disorders are frequent in HIV-infected individuals (Maj, 1990; Miller and Riccio, 1990) but so far few reports concerning the psychiatric manifestations in the tropics have been published (Howlett *et al.*, 1994). They may be related to adjustment or stress reactions and it is often difficult to determine whether or not the psychiatric disorder is related to an underlying organic disease (Maj, 1990). Indeed, AIDS–dementia complex may cause behavioural abnormalities and episodes of mania or depression. Certain medication such as zidovudine, ganciclovir, foscarnet and steroids also may cause psychiatric symptoms. Reactions of anxiety and depression are very frequent among HIV-infected individuals. Reports from Africa have suggested a higher frequency of psychosis among HIV-infected individuals than in the West, but further studies are needed to confirm this finding (Howlett *et al.*, 1994).

REFERENCES

Anders KH, Grievra WF, Tomiyasu U *et al.* (1986) The neuropathology of AIDS: UCLA experience and review. *American Journal of Pathology* **124**: 537–558.

Aronow HA, Brew BJ and Price RW (1988) The management of the neurological complications of HIV infection and AIDS. *AIDS* **2** (supplement 1): S151–159.

Baumgarter JE, Rachlin JR, Beckstead JH *et al.* (1990) Primary central nervous system lymphomas: natural history and response to radiation therapy in 655 patients with acquired immunodeficiency syndrome. *Journal of Neurosurgery* **73**: 206–211.

Behar R, Wilef C and McCutchan JA (1987) Cytomegalovirus polyradiculoneuropathy in acquired immune deficiency syndrome. *Neurology* **37**: 557–561.

Belec L, Testa J, Vohito MD *et al.* (1989a) Virologie: manifestations neurologiques et psychiatriques du SIDA en République Centrafricaine. *Bulletin de la Societé de Pathologie Exotique* **82**: 97–307.

Belec L, Gherardi R, Goerges AJ *et al.* (1989b) Peripheral facial paralysis and HIV infection: report of four African cases and review of the literature. *Journal of Neurology* **236**: 411–414.

Berger JR and Mucke L (1988) Prolonged survival and partial recovery in AIDS-associated progressive multifocal leukoencephalopathy. *Neurology* **38**: 1060–1065.

Berger JR, Sheramata WA, Resnick L *et al.* (1989) Multiple sclerosis-like illness occurring with human immunodeficiency virus infection. *Neurology* **39**: 324–329.

Berger JR, Harris J, Gregorios J *et al.* (1990) Cerebrovascular disease in AIDS: a case-control study. *AIDS* **4**: 239–244.

Bishburg E, Sunderam G, Reichman LB *et al.* (1986) Central nervous system tuberculosis with the acquired immunodeficiency syndrome and its related complex. *Annals of Internal Medicine* **105**: 210–213.

Budka H (1991) Neuropathogy of human immunodeficiency virus infection. *Brain Pathology* **1**: 163–175.

Buskila D and Gladman D (1990) Musculoskeletal manifestations of infection with human immunodeficiency virus. *Reviews of Infectious Diseases* **12**(2): 223–235.

Carne CA, Tedder RS, Smith A *et al.* (1985) Acute encephalopathy coincident with seroconversion for anti-HTLV-III. *Lancet* **ii**: 1206–1208.

Conlon CP (1989) HIV infection presenting as Guillain–Barré syndrome in Lusaka, Zambia. *Transactions of the Royal Society of Tropical Medicine and Hygiene* **83**: 109.

Cornblath DR *et al.* (1991) Research criteria for diagnosis of chronic inflammatory demyelinating polyneuropathy (CIDP). *Neurology* **41**: 617–618.

De Gans J, Portegies P, Tiessens G *et al.* (1990) Therapy for cytomegalovirus poly-radiculomyelitis in patients with AIDS: treatment with ganciclovir. *AIDS* **4**: 421–425.

Desmet P, Kayembe K and De Vroey C (1989) The value of cryptococcal serum antigen screening among HIV positive/AIDS patients in Kinshasa, Zaire *AIDS* **3**: 77–78.

Dix RD, Waitzman DM, Follansbee S *et al.* (1985) Herpes simplex virus type 2 encephalitis in two homosexual men with persistent lymphadenopathy. *Annals of Neurology* **17**: 203–206.

Fischl MA, Olson RM, Follansbee SE *et al.* (1993) Zalcitabine compared with zidovudine in patients with advanced HIV-1 infection who received previous zidovudine therapy. *Annals of Internal Medicine* **118**(10): 762–769.

Fuller GN, Jacobs JM and Guiloff RJ (1989) Association of painful peripheral neuropathy in AIDS with cytomegalovirus infection. *Lancet*, 937–940.

Hicks CB, Benson PM, Lupton GP *et al.* (1987) Seronegative secondary syphilis in a patient infected with the human immunodeficiency virus with Kaposi sarcoma. *Annals of Internal Medicine* **107**: 492–495.

Howlett WP, Kya WM, Mmuni KA *et al.* (1989) Neurological disorders in AIDS and HIV disease in the northern zone of Tanzania. *AIDS* **3**: 289–296.

Howlett WP, Luabeya MK and Kayembe KNT (1994) Neurologic and psychiatric manifestations of HIV infection in Africa. In: *AIDS in Africa* (eds S Mboup, PJ Kani and MR Kalengayi), pp 393–422. New York: Raven Press.

Kovacs JA (1992) Efficacy of Atovaquone in treatment of toxoplasmosis in patients with AIDS. *Lancet* **340**: 637–638.

Lambert JS, Seidlin M, Reichman RC *et al.* (1990) 2', 3'-dideoxyinosine (ddI) in patients with the acquired immunodeficiency syndrome or AIDS-related complex. *New England Journal of Medicine* **322**: 1330–1340.

Leport C, Raffi F, Matheron S *et al.* (1988) Treatment of central nervous system toxoplasmosis with pyrimethamine/sulfadiazine combination in 35 patients with the acquired immunodeficiency syndrome. *American Journal of Medicine* **84**: 94–100.

Lucas SB, Hounnou A, Peacock C *et al.* (1993) The mortality and pathology of HIV infection in a West African city. *AIDS* **7**: 1569–1579.

Luft GJ and Remington JS (1988) Toxoplasmic encephalitis. *Journal of Infectious Diseases* **157**(1): 1–6.

Maj M (1990) Organic mental disorders in HIV-1 infection. *AIDS* **4**: 831–840.

Masden JC, Small CB, Weiss L *et al.* (1988) Multifocal cytomegalovirus encephalitis in AIDS. *Annals of Neurology* **23**: 97–99.

Miller D and Riccio M (1990) Non-organic psychiatric and psychosocial syndromes associated with HIV-1 infection and disease. *AIDS* **4**: 381–388.

Morgello S, Block GA, Price RW *et al.* (1988) Varicella–zoster virus leukoencephalitis and cerebral vasculopathy. *Archives of Pathology and Laboratory Medicine* **112**: 173–177.

Pallangyo K, Hakanson A, Lema L *et al.* (1992) High HIV seroprevalence and increased HIV-associated mortality among hospitalized patients with deep bacterial infections in Dar es Salaam, Tanzania. *AIDS* **6**: 971–976.

Perriens JH, Mussa M, Luabeya MK *et al.* (1992) Neurological complications of HIV-1 seropositive internal medicine inpatients in Kinshasa, Zaire. *AIDS* **5**: 333–340.

Portegies P and Brew BJ (1992) Update on HIV-related neurological illness. *AIDS* **5** (supplement 2): S211–S217.

Portegies P, de Gans J, Lange JMA *et al.* (1989) Declining incidence of AIDS dementia complex after introduction of zidovudine treatment. *British Medical Journal* **299**: 819–821.

Powderly WG (1993) Cryptococcal meningitis and AIDS. *Clinical Infectious diseases* **17**: 837–842.

Price RW and Brew BJ (1988) The AIDS dementia complex. *Journal of Infectious Diseases* **158**(5): 1079–1083.

Ramiandrisoa H, Dumas M, Giordano D *et al.* (1991) Human retroviruses HTLV-I, HIV-1, HIV-2 and neurological diseases in West Africa. *Journal of Tropical and Geographical Neurology* **1**: 39–44.

Simpson DM and Wolfe DE (1991) Neuromuscular complications of HIV infection and its treatment. *AIDS* **5**: 917–926.

So Yt, Holtzman DM, Abrams DI *et al.* (1988) Peripheral neuropathy associated with AIDS. *Archives of Neurology* **45**: 945–948.

Welby SB, Rogerson SJ and Beeching NJ (1991) Autonomic neuropathy is common in human immunodeficiency virus infection. *Journal of Infection* **23**: 123–128.

Wong MC, Suite NA and Labar DR (1990) Seizures in human immunodeficiency virus infection. *Archives of Neurology* **47**: 640–642.

World Health Organization, Global programme on AIDS (1990) Report of the second consultation on the neuropsychiatric aspects of HIV-1 infection. *WHO document: WHO/GPA/MNH/90.1.*

World Health Organization (1994) Acquired immunodeficiency syndrome (AIDS) – Data as at 31 December 1993. *Weekly Epidemiological Record* **69**: 5–12.

5

Rabies

David A. Warrell and Margaret J. Warrell

The Centre for Tropical Medicine, University of Oxford, John Radcliffe Hospital, Headington, Oxford

RABIES VIRUS

Rabies virus and four genotypes of rabies-related viruses capable of causing disease in humans form part of the genus *Lyssavirus* of the family Rhabdoviridae – rod- or bullet-shaped RNA viruses (Table 5.1) (Francki *et al.*, 1991). Virus isolated from naturally infected animals is known as 'street' virus. Repeated intracerebral passage in rabbits produces a 'fixed' virus, with a shortened incubation period and reduced pathogenicity for other species, which is used for vaccine production. Nucleotide sequencing of the glycoprotein, nucleoprotein and pseudogene regions of the viral genome (Tordo and Poch, 1988; Tordo *et al.*, 1988) allows the identification of strains of rabies and rabies-related viruses and has revealed their geographical and vector-related diversity (Smith *et al.*, 1991, 1992; Bourhy *et al.*, 1993; Smith and Seidel, 1993).

Mokola virus, Duvenhage virus and European bat lyssavirus have also been responsible for human infections. Mokola virus (genotype 3) (Bourhy *et al.*, 1989), found in shrews (*Crocidura* species), rodents and domestic cats and

TABLE 5.1 Lyssaviruses infecting humans

Serogroup	Vector species
1 Rabies	Mammals
3 Mokola	Shrews, cats, dogs, rodents (Africa)
4 Duvenhage	Bats (Africa)
5 European bat Lyssavirus	
Biotype 1	Insectivorous bats, principally *Eptesicus serotinus*
6 European bat Lyssavirus	
Biotype 2	*Myotis dasycneme, M. daubentoni*
	Unknown bat (Finland)

dogs in West and Southern Africa (Swanepoel *et al.*, 1993), caused a febrile illness with respiratory tract symptoms in a child who recovered (Familusi and Moore, 1972) and a fatal encephalitis in another (Familusi *et al.*, 1972). Duvenhage virus (genotype 4) (Swanepoel *et al.*, 1993) caused a fatal illness indistinguishable from furious rabies, in a South African who was bitten by a bat but had received a full postexposure course of rabies vaccine (Meredith *et al.*, 1971). Routine rabies fluorescent antibody tests were negative in the Duvenhage case and weakly positive in the Mokola cases. Tissue culture rabies vaccines have not protected animals against challenge with Mokola virus and their effect against Duvenhage virus is uncertain (Wiktor *et al.*, 1984; Fekado *et al.*, 1988; Lafon *et al.*, 1990). European bat lyssaviruses (genotype 5 and 6) have been found in several species of insectivorous bats (e.g. *Eptesicus serotinus*, *Myotis* species) in Denmark, Germany, the Netherlands, Russia, Poland, Spain, Switzerland and France (King and Turner, 1993). Two Russian girls (Selimov *et al.*, 1989) and a zoologist in Finland died of rabies following bat bites (Lumio *et al.*, 1986).

EPIDEMIOLOGY

Rabies is a zoonosis endemic throughout the world save for the British Isles, Iceland, mainland Norway, Sweden, Spain (except Ceuta in North Africa), Portugal, Cyprus and other Mediterranean islands, Australia, New Guinea, Bali, New Zealand, Antarctica, Oceania, parts of Malaysia, Singapore, Japan, South Korea, Taiwan, Hong Kong islands (but not the New Territories) and some of the Caribbean islands.

Rabies is primarily an infection of wild mammals spread by bites (rarely by inhalation of aerosols in bat caves and by ingestion of infected prey). The ecology of rabies virus can be divided into urban and sylvatic phases which may overlap. Important wild mammal reservoir species include skunks, foxes, raccoons and insectivorous bats in the United States; foxes in the Arctic; mongooses in Grenada and Puerto Rico; vampire bats in Middle and South America; wolves, jackals and small carnivores in Africa and Asia; and foxes, wolves, raccoon dogs and insectivorous bats in Europe.

Transmission occurs predominantly within a single species. In many parts of Africa and Asia, in urban areas of Latin America and elsewhere (including Britain and Japan before the disease was eradicated), domestic dogs are the principal reservoir of rabies. Humans are occasionally infected by wild mammals, but domestic dogs and cats, the principal vectors in the urban phase of rabies, are responsible for more than 90% of human cases world-wide.

Vampire bats (Desmodontinae) occur only in Mexico, Latin America, Trinidad and Isla de Margarita. Between 500 000 and 1 000 000 head of cattle are lost each year from vampire bat-transmitted paralytic rabies ('derriengue'), at a cost of more than US$100 million. More than 150 humans are known to have died from vampire bat-transmitted rabies since 1980 (Baer, 1975a; Lopez *et al.*,

1992). Non-haematophagous bats have been responsible for a few cases of human rabies in North America, India, Europe and South Africa (Baer, 1975b).

Cyclical epizootics of rabies, such as the current fox epizootic in Europe, result from an uncontrolled increase in the population of the key reservoir species.

Incidence of Human Rabies

The true incidence of human rabies throughout the world is not reflected in official figures. In India alone, the estimated mortality is between 30 000 and 50 000 per year (Steele, 1988). Other countries with a high incidence of human rabies are shown in Table 5.2. In the United States there have been 20 cases of human rabies since 1980, 10 of which were probably contracted outside the country (Centers for Disease Control, 1994) eight of the indigenous cases were attributable to rabies virus of insectivorous bat origin. Rabies was eradicated from Britain by 1903 and the last two patients to be infected in this country, died in 1902, but there had been 173 deaths in England and Wales in the preceding 15 years. In the last 20 years, 11 people have died of rabies in England (Gardner, 1991). Nine were infected in the Indian subcontinent, and two in Africa.

TRANSMISSION

Virus can penetrate broken skin and intact mucosae. In humans, infection is usually by inoculation of virus-laden saliva through the skin by the bite of a rabid dog or other mammal (Figure 5.1). Even without a bite, saliva from a rabid animal can infect if the skin is abraded by a scratch. There is no good evidence that humans can be infected by ingesting the flesh of rabid animals, although this was described by Charles Darwin in Patagonia.

Inhalation of rabies virus is an important route of transmission among

TABLE 5.2 Estimated human mortality from rabies 1992 (WHO, 1994)

Country	Deaths per year		Deaths/10^6 population
India	30 000 (50 000)*		35.5
Pakistan		(6 500)*	
Bangladesh	2 000		18
China	1 024		
Indonesia	1 070		11.6
Nepal	200		11
Sri Lanka	112		6.4
Philippines	300	(500)*	6
Vietnam	309	(2 000)*	4.7

Sudan (128), Laos (242) and Thailand (115) also have high reported human rabies mortalities.
* Other estimates.

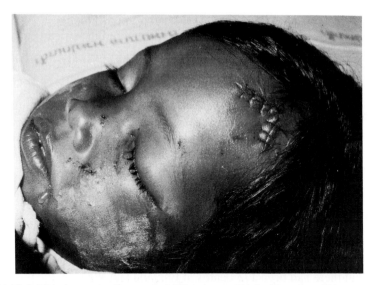

Figure 5.1 Thai child who received severe facial bites by a rabid dog. Suturing of bite wounds is not recommended as it may inoculate virus deeper into the wound. Copyright D.A. Warrell.

gregarious cave-dwelling bats. Two men died of rabies after visiting caves in Texas inhabited by millions of bats, many of which were rabid (Winkler, 1975). They are thought to have inhaled an aerosol of the bats' infected nasal secretions. Two laboratory workers in the United States contracted rabies after inhaling 'fixed' rabies virus while preparing vaccines (Winkler *et al.*, 1973; Centers for Disease Control, 1991). 'Rage de laboratoire' resulted from the accidental use of vaccine containing live virus; for example, in Fortaleza, Brazil, in 1960, 18 people developed paralytic rabies 4–13 days after their first injection of vaccine (Pará, 1965).

Person-to-person transmission of rabies has been proven in four recipients of infected corneal grafts and suspected in others (Helmick *et al.*, 1987; Sureau *et al.*, 1981). The donors had died of undiagnosed neurological diseases, such as Guillain–Barré syndrome and flaccid quadriplegia. Saliva, respiratory secretions, tears and urine of rabies patients contain virus but there are no virologically proven cases of spread to other people. Transplacental infection has been reported in animals and, very rarely, in humans (Sipahioglu and Alpant, 1985). Several women with rabies encephalitis have been delivered of healthy babies. The transmission of rabies from mother to suckling infant via the breast milk has been suspected in at least one human case and occurs in animals.

PATHOGENESIS

After inoculation, rabies virus may replicate locally in muscle cells and gains access to peripheral nerves, probably mainly by attaching to acetylcholine receptors at the neuromuscular junction (Murphy, 1977; Conlon *et al.*, 1989; Tsiang, 1993). It then travels centripetally in a subviral form, perhaps as infectious naked nucleocapsid, within the axoplasm. In the central nervous system, there is massive viral replication on membranes within neurones and intercellular transmission across synapses. Centrifugal spread follows, in the axoplasm of efferent nerves, including those of the autonomic nervous system, to many organs and tissues (Wunner, 1987). There is replication and shedding of virus from salivary glands so that, in animals, the virus can be transmitted to another host by bites. In humans, virus is shed from salivary and lacrimal glands, taste buds, respiratory tract and into milk and urine. Viraemia has not been detected in humans. In the central nervous system, the characteristic clinical features may be the result of localization in the brainstem and limbic system in furious rabies, and in the spinal cord in paralytic rabies. There is alteration in the activity of neurotransmitters such as 5-hydroxytryptamine (5HT), *N*-methyl-D-aspartate (NMDA) and γ-amino-*n*-butyric acid (GABA) (Tsiang, 1993; Ladogana, 1994), impaired nerve excitability suggesting a primitive axonal neuropathy (Maton *et al.*, 1976; Prier *et al.*, 1979) and electroencephalographic abnormalities (Maton *et al.*, 1976; Tsiang *et al.*, 1989; Gourmelon *et al.*, 1991; Hantson *et al.*, 1993).

IMMUNOLOGICAL RESPONSES

Human Rabies Encephalitis

There is no detectable immune response until symptoms develop, suggesting that rabies virus evades or suppresses the immune system. Neutralizing and other antibodies become detectable in serum after about 7 days and in cerebrospinal fluid (CSF) a little later, rising to high titres in patients whose lives are prolonged by intensive care (Hattwick, 1974; Anderson *et al.*, 1984). There is little evidence of a cell-mediated immune response (Wiktor *et al.*, 1977). Peripheral blood lymphocyte transformation has been shown in some patients with furious rabies, but not in those with paralytic disease (Hemachudha *et al.*, 1988). Very low levels of interferon are induced in human patients (Merigan *et al.*, 1984). In animals, latent infections can be reactivated by corticosteroids and stress, providing a possible explanation for the very long incubation periods reported in some human cases (Smith *et al.*, 1991).

Rabies Vaccination

Neutralizing antibody is not found until 7–14 days or more after the first dose of vaccine (Turner, 1985). Only viral surface glycoprotein can induce neutralizing antibody, which protects against subsequent challenge with rabies virus in animals (Dietzschold and Ertl, 1991). Cell-mediated immunity is also important (Dietzschold and Ertl, 1991). Neutralizing antibody titre is the best available measure of immune response and protection. In experimental animals a very low level of rabies antibody accelerates the terminal phase of the encephalitis ('early death' phenomenon) perhaps by enhancing viral replication (Prabhakar and Nathanson, 1981). Transient low levels of interferon may be induced by the first dose of rabies vaccine (Nicholson *et al.*, 1979). In animals, interferon induced by viruses or synthetic inducers, or the administration of exogenous interferon, was effective postexposure prophylaxis against rabies.

ANIMAL RABIES

Mammals and birds are susceptible to rabies in the following decreasing order: foxes and other wild Canidae, skunks, Felidae, Viverridae, rodents, lagomorphs, humans, domestic dogs, herbivores, chickens and opossums.

In dogs the incubation period is usually between 3 and 12 weeks (extreme range 5 days to 14 months). The first symptom is scratching or biting at the site of the infection. 'Furious' and 'dumb' patterns of symptoms are seen. Clinical features include early change in behaviour, dysphagia, ptosis, altered bark, paralysis of the jaw, neck and hind limbs (Figure 5.2), hypersalivation, congested conjunctivae, pruritis, shivering, trembling, snapping at imaginary objects, pica and extreme restlessness, causing the animal to wander miles

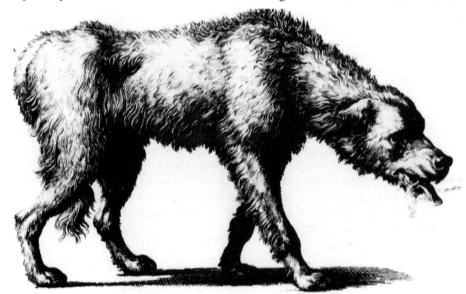

Figure 5.2 French print of rabid dog published in 1800 showing the characteristically paralysed hind quarters, neck and jaw muscles and hypersalivation. (By courtesy of the Wellcome Institute for the History of Medicine Library).

from home. Dogs with furious rabies attack humans, other dogs/animals and inanimate objects. Virus may be excreted in the saliva 3 days before symptoms appear, and the animal usually dies within the next 7 days. This is the basis for the traditional 10-day observation period for dogs that have bitten humans. There are rare reports, from India, Ethiopia and elsewhere, of chronic excretion of virus in the saliva of apparently healthy dogs (Fekadu, 1993).

Rabid foxes lose their fear of humans and the majority develop the paralytic form of the disease. An extreme degree of furious rabies is seen in 75% of infected cats. Cattle and other domestic ungulates usually show paralytic signs with dysphagia, hypersalivation, groaning, trembling, colic, diarrhoea, tenesmus and rectal prolapse. Horses often show furious features with sexual excitement (Kaplan *et al.*, 1986).

HUMAN RABIES ENCEPHALITIS: CLINICAL FEATURES

The incubation period is usually between 20 and 90 days (extreme range 4 days to many years) and tends to be shorter after facial bites (average 35 days) than bites on the limbs (average 52 days) (Hattwick, 1974; Editorial, 1991; Smith *et al.*, 1991).

Prodromal Symptoms

The first symptom is usually itching, pain or paraesthesia at the site of the healed bite wound (Figure 5.3) (Kaplan *et al.*, 1986). Other symptoms may include fever, chills, malaise, weakness, tiredness, headache, photophobia, myalgia, anxiety, depression, irritability and symptoms of upper respiratory tract and

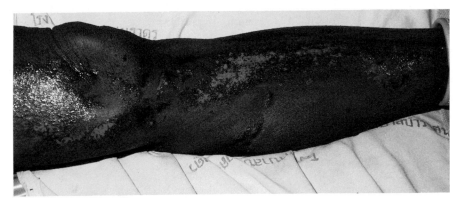

Figure 5.3 Excoriation by scratching, a prodromal symptom of rabies. This patient developed itching of the left leg 2 months after being bitten on the calf by a mad dog (note pigmented healed bite wounds). Overt signs of furious rabies developed a few days later. Copyright D.A. Warrell.

gastrointestinal infections. After a few days, symptoms of either furious or paralytic rabies will appear, depending on whether the spinal cord or brain are predominantly infected.

Furious Rabies

Furious rabies is the commoner presentation. Most patients develop hydrophobia, the pathognomonic symptom/sign of rabies (Warrell, 1976; Kaplan *et al.*, 1986). This reflex response consists of violent and jerky inspiratory spasms during which the neck and back are extended as in opisthotonos and the arms are thrown up. The episode may end in generalized convulsions with cardiac or respiratory arrest. There is associated terror which patients are unable to explain (Warrell *et al.*, 1976). Pain in the throat and chest, laryngopharyngeal spasms, choking and fear of aspiration are not consistent features. Initially, hydrophobia may be provoked by attempts to drink water (Figure 5.4), but can be excited by a variety of stimuli including a draught of air on the skin ('aerophobia') (Figure 5.5), water splashed on the skin, irritation of the respiratory tract or, ultimately, the sight, sound or even mention of water.

Patients experience hyperaesthesia and at times generalized arousal, during which they become wild, hallucinated, fugitive and sometimes aggressive. Between these episodes there are lucid intervals. Despite these dramatic symptoms, attributable to brainstem encephalitis, conventional neurological examination may prove surprisingly normal, but if the patient is asked to swallow their accumulated saliva, or a draught of air is blown on the skin (by a fan or opening a window), a diagnostic hydrophobic spasm may be provoked. Reported neurological abnormalities include meningism, cranial nerve lesions (especially III, VI, VII, IX, X, XI and XII), upper motor neurone lesions, fasciculation and involuntary movements. Disturbances of the hypothalamus or autonomic nervous system include hypersalivation (Figure 5.6), lacrimation (Figure 5.7), sweating, hypertension or hypotension, hyperthermia or hypothermia, inappropriate secretion of ADH, or diabetes insipidus and, rarely, priapism with spontaneous orgasms (Talaulicar, 1977; Udwadia *et al.*, 1988).

Without supportive treatment, about one-third of the patients will die during a hydrophobic spasm in the first few days (Dupont and Earle, 1966). The rest lapse into coma and generalized flaccid paralysis and rarely survive for more than a week without intensive care.

Illustrative Case History 1 (Warrell *et al.*, 1976; Kaplan *et al.*, 1986)

A 20-year-old Nigerian rural health inspector was bitten by a dog on his ankle while riding his motorbike. The wounds were cleaned with iodine at a local dispensary but since there was nothing remarkable about the dog's appearance or behaviour (dogs often chase bicycles) and the dog ran off after the incident, the

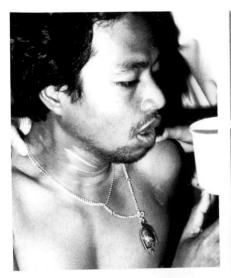
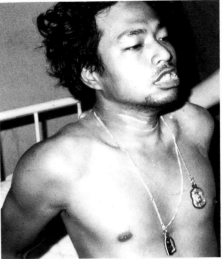
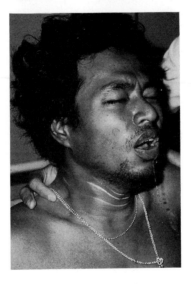

Figure 5.4 Hydrophobic spasm in a Thai man showing inspiratory spasm provoked by sipping water and associated terror. Copyright D.A. Warrell.

possibility of rabies was dismissed. The bite wounds healed but, 36 days after the incident, the man noticed pain and numbness around the scars. These feelings continued and, 3 days later, he had fever and headache. Suspecting malaria, he took chloroquine. He put the tablets on his tongue and took a sip of water, but as the water entered his mouth there was a violent involuntary gasp and he choked. At the same moment he experienced an inexplicable and overwhelming feeling of terror. So vivid and frightening was this experience that he dared not eat or

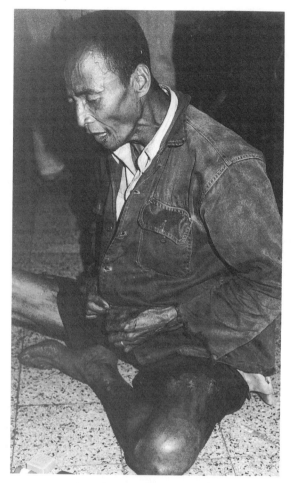

Figure 5.5 Aerophobia. Hydrophobic spasm (note powerful contraction of sternocleidomastoid) provoked by a draught of air in a Thai patient waiting in a hospital corridor. Note also scratch marks on both thighs, the result of prodromal itching. Copyright D.A. Warrell.

drink for the next 2 days for fear that the terror would return. He was admitted to a mission hospital where he was given intravenous fluids and was then transferred to the university hospital. On examination he was found to be an alert, intelligent man who spoke English fluently. Apart from loss of sensation on the fauces and around the bite wound, there was no neurological abnormality. However, when he was asked to swallow or was exposed to a draught, his body was racked by jerky spasms involving the inspiratory muscles and limbs, he looked terrified and cowered beneath the bedclothes. He described the attacks as being like electric shocks causing confusion. He denied pain in the throat but feared that drinking water might cause him to choke.

Since intensive care was not feasible, the patient was made comfortable with

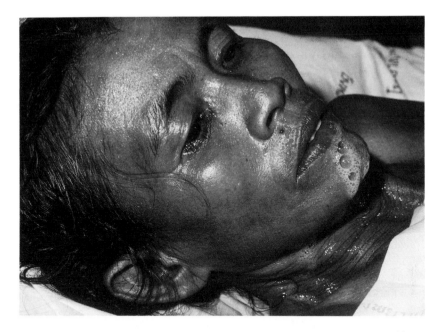

Figure 5.6 Hyperpyrexia (sweating) and hypersalivation in a Thai woman with furious rabies. Copyright D.A. Warrell.

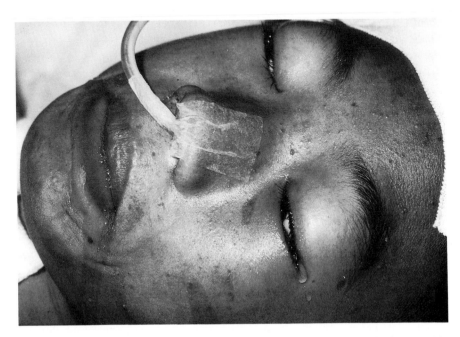

Figure 5.7 Lacrimation and hypersalivation in a Thai patient under intensive care for furious rabies. Copyright D.A. Warrell.

sedatives and analgesics. Calm reassurance persuaded him to swallow porridge and even liquids. He slept peacefully after being given the drugs but always awoke frightened, confused and hallucinating. During the next 36 hours he became increasingly excitable and required frequent doses of the drugs. At times he was very confused and wild, knocking over the bedside table and shouting that he was dying. He then lapsed into coma. His respiration was irregular, with pauses of several minutes between groups of breaths. He sweated profusely and tears ran from his eyes continuously. Although by this time all treatment had been stopped, he remained comatose, unresponsive and generally flaccid and died 7 days after his first symptom.

Illustrative Case History 2 (Kaplan *et al.*, 1986)

A 23-year-old English woman was bitten on the leg by a neighbour's pet dog in the Himalayan foothills of Himachal Pradesh. The wound was cleaned, using whisky as an antiseptic, and the village doctor was consulted. He cleaned the wound with iodine and dressed it with antiseptic powder. It was not thought that the dog was rabid because it was a pet defending its territory. The woman was treated with vitamins, antibiotic capsules and a homoeopathic remedy, but no tetanus toxoid was available in that village or in the Red Cross hospital in a large local town. The bite wound finally healed after she returned to England a month later. Two months after the bite, the woman felt unusually tired for 3 days and noticed aching and shooting pains in the waist and small of her back. She had missed two periods and wondered if she were pregnant. She became anxious and depressed and seemed to catch her breath when she tried to drink. Her general practitioner thought that these symptoms were related to anxiety about the possible pregnancy, but it soon became impossible for her to drink more than small sips of liquid. When she rode on her husband's motorbike, the wind made her catch her breath and when she lay in bed the feeling of her hair against her face was unbearable. She sat up in bed frequently, apparently terrified. The next day her legs felt heavy, painful and so tender that she could not bear the weight of her cat sitting on her lap. That night she was confused, hallucinated and incontinent of urine and on the next day was unable to eat or drink. On the way to the doctor's surgery even the draught through a crack in the car window was intolerable. At the surgery, she was incontinent of urine, was intermittently hallucinating and screaming with terror. At this stage she was considered to be suffering from hysteria and was given an injection of tranquillizer. A psychiatric consultation was arranged. By the evening she was wild and agitated, awoke just before midnight in a terrified state and collapsed. She continued in a state of terror, hallucination and pain throughout the night and, early next morning, her pulse seemed to stop and, when the emergency services arrived, she had a cardiac arrest from which she was resuscitated. She was admitted to the intensive care unit of the local hospital but died there less than 48 hours later without recovering consciousness.

Paralytic or Dumb Rabies

This is the clinical pattern in less than a fifth of human cases except in cases of vampire bat-transmitted rabies which is paralytic in type (Kaplan *et al.*, 1986). After the usual prodromal symptoms, especially fever, headache and local paraesthesiae, flaccid paralysis is first noticeable in the bitten limb, and ascends symmetrically or asymmetrically with pain, fasciculation (Phuapradit *et al.*, 1985) and sometimes myoedema (Hemachudha *et al.*, 1987a) in the affected muscles and mild sensory disturbances. Seizures have been reported as the presenting feature (Hemachudha, 1989; Hemachudha *et al.*, 1989). Paraplegia and sphincter involvement then develop and finally fatal paralysis of deglutitive and respiratory muscles. Hydrophobia is unusual, but may be represented by a few pharyngeal spasms in the terminal phase of the illness (Warrell, 1976; Kaplan *et al.*, 1986). Even without intensive care, patients with paralytic rabies have survived for up to 30 days.

Other Manifestations and Complications (Hattwick *et al.*, 1972; Emmons *et al.*, 1973; Hattwick and Gregg, 1975)

In patients whose lives are prolonged by intensive care, a variety of complications may develop. In the respiratory system, asphyxiation and respiratory arrest may complicate the hydrophobic spasms or generalized convulsions of furious rabies and the bulbar and respiratory paralysis of dumb rabies. Aspiration pneumonia and a primary rabies pneumonitis have been described. Respiratory arrhythmias include cluster, 'Biot's breathing' and apneustic breathing. There are some similarities to respiratory myoclonus (Warrell *et al.*, 1976). Pneumothorax may complicate inspiratory spasms. In the cardiovascular system, life-threatening cardiac arrhythmias can occur including supraventricular tachycardias (Figure 5.8), sinus bradycardia, atrioventricular block and sinus arrest. Hypotension, pulmonary oedema and congestive cardiac failure are attributable

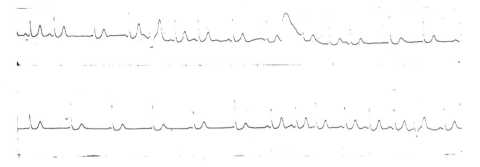

Figure 5.8 Supraventricular tachycardia in a Nigerian patient with furious rabies. Copyright D.A. Warrell.

to myocarditis (Warrell, 1976; Warrell *et al.*, 1976). In the nervous system, raised intracranial pressure resulting from cerebral oedema or internal hydrocephalus has been reported in a few cases (Hattwick *et al.*, 1972), but cerebrospinal fluid opening pressure is usually normal and papilloedema rarely found (Warrell, 1976). Electrophysiological evidence of diffuse axonal neuropathy is consistent with histological appearances of degeneration of peripheral nerve ganglia and axons (Maton *et al.*, 1976; Prier *et al.*, 1979). In the gastrointestinal system, haematemesis may be caused by 'stress' ulcers or Mallory–Weiss syndrome.

Differential Diagnosis (Warrell, 1976; Kaplan *et al.*, 1986)

Rabies should be suspected in patients who develop neurological symptoms after being bitten by a mammal in a rabies-endemic area and in patients with bizarre neurological symptoms (especially agitation and inspiratory spasms) who are immigrants from or have travelled to rabies-endemic countries. Patients may forget that they have been bitten. Hydrophobia is diagnostic of furious rabies and is unlikely to be mimicked accurately by someone with hysterical rabies. Patients with unsuspected rabies have been referred to otolaryngologists or psychiatrists (Anderson *et al.*, 1984).

Tetanus can also follow an animal bite. The pharyngeal form of cephalic tetanus ('hydrophobic tetanus') can, in particular, resemble rabies, but its incubation period is shorter (usually less than 15 days) and unlike rabies there is trismus, the muscle rigidity persists between spasms, the CSF is universally normal and the prognosis is better. Hydrophobia does not occur in other encephalitides: the combination of intense brainstem encephalitis and furious behaviour in a conscious patient would be most unlikely, except in rabies. Delirium tremens and intoxication by plants (e.g. *Datura fastuosa*) and drugs (phenothiazines and amphetamines) may enter the differential diagnosis.

Paralytic rabies can be confused with other causes of ascending (Landry-type) paralysis. Postvaccinal encephalomyelitis caused by nervous tissue and suckling mouse brain vaccines usually develops within 2 weeks of starting vaccination. In poliomyelitis objective sensory disturbances are absent and fever rarely persists after paralysis has developed. Examination of CSF may help to distinguish acute inflammatory polyneuropathy (Guillain–Barré syndrome). *Herpes simiae* (B virus) encephalomyelitis is transmitted by monkey bites, but its incubation period (3–4 days) is shorter than in rabies. Vesicles may be found in the monkey's mouth and at the site of the bite. The diagnosis can be confirmed by viral culture and serology. Treatment is with acyclovir.

PATHOLOGY

In the brain, spinal cord and peripheral nerves there is ganglion cell degeneration, perineural and perivascular mononuclear cell infiltration, neuronophagia and formation of glial (Babès) nodules (Tangchai *et al.*, 1970; Perl, 1975). Inflammatory changes are most marked in the midbrain and medulla in furious rabies and in the spinal cord in paralytic rabies (Tangchai and Vejjajiva, 1971; Chopra *et al.*, 1980). Negri bodies (Figure 5.9) are virtually diagnostic eosinophilic intracytoplasmic inclusions which consist of masses of viral ribonucleoprotein, with a basophilic inner body, containing fragments of cellular organelles including ribosomes and occasional virions. They can be demonstrated by Sellar's H&E or Schleiften' stains in smears or histological sections of grey matter in up to 75% of human cases, especially in hippocampal pyramidal cells and cerebellar Purkinje cells. Neuronolysis is surprisingly mild and patchy, and there may be no detectable inflammatory response. The brainstem, limbic system and hypothalamus appear to be most severely affected.

There is diffuse axonal degeneration of peripheral nerves in patients who survive for several days (Tangchai and Vejjajiva, 1971). There is focal degeneration of salivary and lacrimal glands, pancreas, adrenal medulla and lymph nodes and, in about 25% of cases, an interstitial myocarditis, with round cell infiltration (Warrell, 1976; Warrell *et al.*, 1976).

LABORATORY DIAGNOSIS (Kaplan and Koprowski, 1973)

A sick animal which has bitten a patient should be killed and its brain examined without delay, by direct immunofluorescent antibody test (Trimarchi and Debbie, 1991) or rapid enzyme immunodiagnosis (WHO Expert Committee on Rabies, 1992). In some countries, staining for Negri bodies by Sellar's method (Figure 5.9), which is less specific, is the only method available. Virus can be isolated in mice (3 weeks) or in murine neuroblastoma cell culture (about 4 days) (Rudd and Trimarchi, 1989).

Human rabies encephalitis can be confirmed during life by demonstration of viral antigen by immunofluorescence in nerve twiglets in skin biopsies (Figure 5.10). (Bryceson *et al.*, 1975; Warrell *et al.*, 1988). Newer techniques to identify rabies antigen, e.g. in CSF by PCR, are being evaluated.

During the first week of illness virus may be isolated from saliva, brain, CSF and rarely urine. Rabies antibodies are not usually detectable in serum or CSF before the eighth day of illness but their presence is diagnostic in unvaccinated patients. Rabies neutralizing antibody may leak into the CSF in patients with postvaccinal encephalomyelitis, but a very high titre suggests a diagnosis of rabies.

A mild lymphocytic pleocytosis (average 75×10^3 mm^{-1}) occurs in 60% of patients (Warrell, 1976; Anderson *et al.*, 1984). A peripheral neutrophil leukocytosis is common in the early stages of the disease.

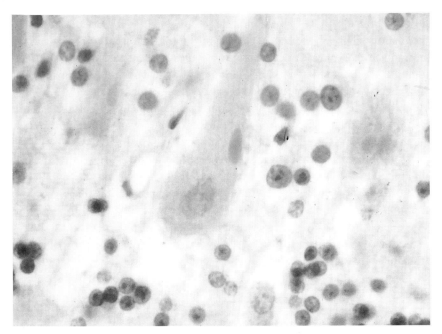

Figure 5.9 Negri bodies. In this section of cerebellum stained with H&E, the Purkinje cell in the centre contains one elongated intracytoplasmic Negri body while the indistinct cell on the right contains two. Armed Forces Institute of Pathology, Photograph AFIP73-12330, with permission.

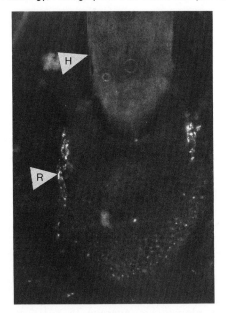

Figure 5.10 Diagnosis of human rabies during life. Vertical section through a hair follicle and shaft (H) showing brilliant fluorescence (R) of nerve cells around the follicle indicating the presence of rabies antigen. Copyright M.J. Warrell.

TREATMENT OF RABIES ENCEPHALITIS

Patients with rabies must be given large doses of sedatives and analgesia to relieve their pain and terror. Rabies is virtually always fatal, but there have been four well-documented cases of survival after intensive care (Hattwick *et al.*, 1972; Porras *et al.*, 1976; Centers for Disease Control, 1991; Alvarez *et al.*, 1994). Two of these patients recovered completely. If the patient's life is prolonged by intensive care, complications such as cardiac arrhythmias, cardiac and respiratory failure, raised intracranial pressure, convulsions, fluid and electrolyte disturbances including diabetes insipidus and inappropriate secretion of antidiuretic hormone and hyperpyrexia must be prevented or treated. Hyperimmune serum (Hattwick *et al.*, 1976), antiviral agents (Warrell *et al.*, 1989), alpha interferon (Merigan *et al.*, 1984; Warrell *et al.*, 1989), corticosteroid and other immunosuppressants have proved useless (Cifuentes *et al.*, 1971).

PROGNOSIS

Rabies encephalitis is fatal but, at the time of the bite, before virus has invaded the nervous system, wound cleaning and postexposure immunization reduces the risk of rabies developing from about 35–67% in untreated cases to almost zero. The risk depends on the biting species and the site and severity of the bites. It is highest following head bites by proved rabid wolves, when the mortality in unvaccinated people may exceed 80% (Babès, 1912).

PREVENTION AND CONTROL

In Rabies-endemic Areas

The design of an appropriate control strategy depends on surveillance to determine the principal wild and domestic animal reservoir species. Laboratory facilities are required to confirm the diagnosis.

Owned animals can be protected by vaccination. Dogs should be muzzled and kept off the streets. In areas where the domestic dog is the main reservoir, such as in the large cities in Latin America, the incidence of canine and hence human rabies can be dramatically reduced through mass vaccination campaigns (Larghi *et al.*, 1988). In most parts of the world, 80–90% of domestic dogs are owned and therefore accessible to vaccination (Wandeler *et al.*, 1993). However, in areas such as Africa and India, stray domestic dogs are an important problem. Attempts to reduce their numbers by catching, poisoning or shooting are relatively ineffective and often excite great hostility among the dog-loving human population. A possibility of immunizing stray dogs by distributing oral vaccine in suitable baits is currently being explored (Perry and Wandeler, 1993). Where wild mammals are the main reservoir, attempts to produce a sustained reduction in the numbers of key species have failed, whereas the distribution of live oral vaccine in suitable baits has been very effective in foxes in Europe and is planned for other species such as raccoons in North America and jackals in Southern Africa (Wandeler, 1991; Bingham *et al.*, 1992; Thomson and King, 1993).

Humans particularly at risk, such as vets and dog catchers, can be given pre-exposure vaccination. Clinics and dispensaries must be supplied with vaccine and antiserum for postexposure prophylaxis of animal bite victims. However, in the developing countries where rabies is most prevalent, control of the disease in domestic dogs may be more cost-effective in saving human lives (Bogel and Meslin, 1990). The public must be educated to recognize the danger of rabies after animal bites and to encourage bite victims to seek treatment as soon as possible.

In Non-endemic Areas

Importation of potential vectors, especially domestic dogs and cats and wild bats and carnivores, should be strictly controlled and, where feasible, imported mammals should be vaccinated against rabies and, in some countries such as Britain and Hawaii, kept in quarantine for a period exceeding the usual incubation period.

Pre-exposure vaccination is needed only by those who handle imported animals, work with rabies virus in laboratories and travellers to rabies-endemic areas whose activities put them at particular risk (e.g. vets, field zoologists and cave explorers).

Postexposure prophylaxis will be needed for people who were exposed to the risk of rabies while abroad.

Pre-exposure Prophylaxis

Three doses of tissue culture rabies vaccine (e.g. Pasteur–Mérieux human diploid cell vaccine – HDCV; Behring purified chick embryo cell vaccine – PCEC; Pasteur–Mérieux purified vero cell vaccine – PVRV) are given on days 0, 3 and 28 (or 21) intramuscularly (i.m.) into the deltoid or anterior aspect of the thigh. Alternatively, 0.1 ml can be injected intradermally (i.d.) at the same intervals unless immunosuppression (e.g. by chloroquine antimalarial chemoprophylaxis) is suspected, in which case the i.m. route must be used. Booster doses may be given i.m. or i.d., or the antibody level checked (minimum 0.5 international units ml^{-1}), at intervals depending on the risk of infection.

Postexposure Prophylaxis (Table 5.3)

Wound Cleaning

Wound cleaning is effective in killing virus in superficial wounds. The wound should be scrubbed with soap/detergent and water under a running tap for at least

TABLE 5.3 Specific postexposure prophylaxis for use in a rabies-endemic area following contact with a domestic or wild rabies vector species, whether or not the animal is available for observation or diagnostic tests

	Treatment
Minor exposure (including licks of broken skin, scratches or abrasions without bleeding)	• start vaccine immediately • stop treatment if dog or cat remains healthy for 10 days • stop treatment if animal's brain proves negative for rabies by appropriate laboratory tests
Major exposure (including licks of mucosa, minor bites on arms, trunk or legs, or major bites – multiple or on face, head, fingers or neck)	• immediate rabies immune globulin vaccine • stop treatment if domestic cat or dog remains healthy for 10 days • stop treatment if animal's brain proves negative for rabies by appropriate laboratory tests

This scheme is a simplification of the recommendations of the WHO Expert Committee on Rabies (1992).

5 min. Debris should be removed, the wound rinsed with plain water and a viricidal agent applied (e.g. 40–70% alcohol (Kaplan and Cohen, 1962), povidone iodine or 0.01% aqueous iodine). Severe wounds may need to be explored under anaesthesia. Suturing should be avoided or delayed and the wound should be left without occlusive dressings (WHO Expert Committee on Rabies, 1992). Tetanus prophylaxis and antimicrobial treatment for bacterial pathogens such as *Pasteurella multocida* may be needed (e.g. amoxicillin/clavulanic acid, cephoxitin or tetracycline).

Active Immunization

Tissue culture vaccines. HDCV, PCEC and PVRV, are the vaccines of choice for postexposure immunization. The recommended postexposure course of these vaccines is a total of 5 doses [1 ml i.m. doses on days 0, 3, 7, 14, 30 (0.5 ml doses for PVRV)] (WHO Expert Committee on Rabies, 1992). An effective but economical regimen of HDCV consists of eight intradermal injections of 0.1 ml (deltoids, suprascapular, lower quadrant abdominal wall and thighs) on day 0, four i.d. injections of 0.1 ml (deltoids and thighs) on day 7 and a single i.d. dose of 0.1 ml on days 28 and 91 (Warrell *et al.*, 1983, 1984, 1985; Suntharasami *et al.*, 1987; Dutta *et al.*, 1994).

Nervous tissue vaccines. Semple type vaccines are still the most widely used in Africa and Asia. Subcutaneous injections of 2 or 5 ml of 5% brain suspension are given on 14 or 21 consecutive days followed by booster doses, the abdomen often being used as a suitable target for these numerous subcutaneous injections. Postvaccinal neurological reactions are not uncommon. In Latin America, suckling mouse brain (Fuenzalida) vaccine is the most widely used, but neuroparalytic reactions occur despite reduced contamination by myelin protein in the immature brains of the young mice used in its production.

Neurological reactions to nervous tissue vaccines. These occur in up to 1 in 220 courses of Semple type with a 3% mortality (Swaddiwuthipong *et al.*, 1987). They are allergic responses to myelin and related neural proteins in the vaccine (Hemachudha *et al.*, 1987b). In Latin America, neuroparalytic reactions complicated 1:7865 to 1:27 000 courses of suckling mouse brain vaccine with a 22% mortality (Held *et al.*, 1972). Most reactions to Semple vaccine affect the central nervous system, whereas at least 70% of those following suckling mouse brain vaccine involved the peripheral nervous system (Warrell and Warrell, 1995).

The usual incubation period is 7–14 days (extreme range 3–35 days) after the first injection of vaccine. Clinical forms include a rapidly reversible mononeuritis multiplex involving particularly the facial nerve but also the oculomotor, vagus, radial, brachial and sciatic nerves, a dorsolumbar transverse myelitis with fever, paralysis and sensory loss in the lower limbs with sphincter involvement, loss of tendon reflexes, extensor plantar responses and severe girdle and thoracic pain, an ascending paralysis (Landry type) which ends in fatal bulbar paralysis in a third of cases and meningoencephalitic and meningoencephalomyelitic reactions. The overall mortality of these reactions is 15–20%. Most survivors make a complete recovery in 2–3 weeks, but a few are left with permanent neurological sequelae. As a differential diagnosis, paralytic rabies must be excluded (Warrell *et al.*, 1988).

A moderate lymphocyte pleocytosis and elevated CSF protein is usual. Pathological changes consist of swelling and chromatolysis of neurones with extensive perivascular demyelination and lymphocytic infiltration in the spinal cord. These features resemble experimental allergic encephalitis, postvaccinal encephalomyelitis of smallpox, postinfectious encephalomyelitis and acute multiple sclerosis. Corticosteroids, for example, prednisolone 40–60 mg day^{-1}, are thought to be helpful (Vejjajiva, 1967), and the use of cyclophosphamide has been suggested. Vaccination should be stopped as soon as symptoms appear and the course continued with a tissue culture vaccine.

Passive Immunization

Rabies immune globulin (RIG) has proved valuable in protection (Baltazard and Bahmanyar, 1955; Fathi *et al.*, 1970; Fang-Tao *et al.*, 1986), presumably by neutralizing rabies virus during the first week after initial vaccination, before neutralizing antibody has appeared, and by enhancing the T lymphocyte response to vaccine (Celis *et al.*, 1985). Its use is recommended at the start of all primary postexposure courses of rabies vaccine, especially after severe bites (on the head, neck, hands and multiple or deep bites). Unfortunately, it is too expensive and in too short supply to be used in most postexposure treatments in tropical developing countries.

The dose of equine RIG is 40 units kg^{-1} body weight. Anaphylactic reactions, which occur in 1–6% of those treated (Wilde *et al.*, 1989), are not reliably predicted by skin testing. Human rabies immune globulin (HRIG) is given in a dose of 20 units kg^{-1} body weight. RIG is infiltrated round the bite wound if anatomically feasible and the remainder is given intramuscularly at a site distant from the vaccine (WHO Expert Committee on Rabies, 1992).

Postexposure Prophylaxis in People Who Have Received Previous Vaccination

If a complete pre- or post-exposure course of a potent tissue culture vaccine has been given, or if the neutralizing antibody level exceeds 0.5 international units ml^{-1}, only two doses of tissue culture vaccine need be given on days 0 and 3, with a third dose on day 7 for severe bites. Passive immunization is not required. Otherwise full postexposure treatment must be given.

REFERENCES

Alvarez L, Fajardo R, Lopez E *et al.* (1994) Partial recovery from rabies in a nine-year-old boy. *Paediatric Infectious Disease Journal* **13** (12): 1154–1155.

Anderson LJ, Nicholson KG, Tauxe RV and Winkler WG (1984) Human rabies in the United States, 1960 to 1979: epidemiology, diagnosis and prevention. *Annals of Internal Medicine* **100**: 728–735.

Babès V (1912) *Traité de la Rage*. Paris: JB Baillière et fils.

Baer GM (1975a) Bovine paralytic rabies and rabies in the vampire bat. In: *The Natural History of Rabies*, vol. II (ed. GM Baer), pp 155–175. New York: Academic Press.

Baer GM (1975b) Rabies in non-hematophagous bats. In: *The Natural History of Rabies* (ed. GM Baer), pp. 79–97. New York: Academic Press.

Baltazard M and Bahmanyar M (1955) Practical trial of antirabies serum in people bitten by rabid wolves. *Bulletin of the World Health Organization* **13**: 747–772.

Bingham J, Foggin CM, Gerber H, Hill FW, Kappeler A, King AA, Perry BD and Wandeler AI (1992) Pathogenicity of SAD rabies vaccine given orally in chacina baboons (*Papio ursinus*). *Veterinary Record* **131**(3): 55–56.

Bogel K and Meslin F-X (1990) Economics of human and canine rabies elimination: guidelines for programme orientation. *Bulletin of the World Health Organization* **68**(3): 281–291.

Bourhy H, Tordo N, Lafon M and Sureau P (1989) Complete cloning and molecular organization of a rabies-related virus: Mokola virus. *Journal of General Virology* **70**: 2063–2074.

Bourhy H, Kissi B and Tordo N (1993) Molecular diversity of the *Lyssavirus* genus. *Virology* **194**(9): 70–81.

Bryceson ADM, Greenwood BM, Warrell DA, Davidson NMcD, Pope HM, Lawrie JH, Barnes HJ, Bailie WE and Wilcox GE (1975) Demonstration during life of rabies antigen in humans. *Journal of Infectious Diseases* **131**(1): 71–74.

Celis E, Wiktor TJ, Dietzschold B and Koprowski H (1985) Amplification of rabies-virus induced stimulation of human T-cell lines and clones by antigen-specific antibodies. *Journal of Virology* **56**(2): 426–433.

Centers for Disease Control (1991) Rabies prevention – United States 1991: recommendations of the Immunization Practices Advisory Committee (ACIP). MMWR. *Morbidity and Mortality Weekly Report* (RR-3) **40**.

Centers for Disease Control (1994) Human rabies Miami 1994. MMWR. *Morbidity and Mortality Weekly Report* **43**(42): 773–775.

Chopra JS, Banerjee AK, Murthy JMK and Pal SR (1980) Paralytic rabies. A clinicopathological study. *Brain* **103**: 789–802.

Cifuentes E, Calderon E and Bijlenga G (1971) Rabies in a child diagnosed by a new intra-vitam method. The cornea test. *Journal of Tropical Medicine and Hygiene* **74**(1): 23–25.

Coulon P, Derbin C, Kucera P, Lafay F, Prehaud C and Flamand A (1989) Invasion of the peripheral nervous systems of adult mice by the CVS strain of rabies virus and its avirulent derivative AV01. *Journal of Virology* **63**(8): 3550–3554.

Dietzschold B and Ertl HCJ (1991) New developments in the pre- and post-exposure treatment of rabies. *Immunology* **10**(5): 427–439.

Dupont JR and Earle KM (1966) Human rabies encephalitis. A study of forty-nine fatal cases with a review of the literature. *Neurology* (Minneas) **15**: 1023–1034.

Dutta JK, Warrell MJ and Dutta TK (1994) Intradermal rabies immunization for pre- and post-exposure prophylaxis. *National Medical Journal of India* **7**(3): 119–122.

Editorial (1991) Human rabies: strain identification reveals lengthy incubation. *Lancet* **337**: 822–823.

Emmons RW, Leonard LL, de Genaro F, Protas ES, Bazeley PL, Giammona ST and Sturckow K (1973) A case of human rabies with prolonged survival. *Intervirology* **1**: 60–72.

Familusi JB and Moore DL (1972) Isolation of a rabies-related virus from the cerebrospinal fluid of a child with 'aseptic meningitis'. *African Journal of Medical Science* **3**: 93–96.

Familusi JB, Osunkoya BO, Moore DL, Kemp GE and Fabiyi A (1972) A fatal human infection with Mokola virus. *American Journal of Tropical Medicine and Hygiene* **21**: 959–963.

Fang-Tao L, Shu-Beng C, Guan-Fu W, Fan-Zhen Z, Nai-Min C and Ji-Zui F (1986) Study of the protective effect of the primary hamster kidney cell rabies vaccine. *Journal of Infectious Diseases* **154**(6): 1047–1048.

Fathi M, Sabeti A and Bahmanyar M (1970) Séroprophylaxie antirabique chez les sujets mordus par loups enragés en Iran. *Acta Medica Iran* **13**(1–2): 5–9.

Fekadu M (1993) Canine rabies. *Onderstepoort Journal of Veterinary Research* **60**: 421–427.

Fekadu M, Shaddock JH, Sanderlin DW and Smith JS (1988) Efficacy of rabies vaccines against Duvenhage virus isolated from European house bats (*Eptesicus serotinus*), classic rabies and rabies-related viruses. *Vaccine* **6**: 533–539.

Francki RIB, Fauquet CM, Knudson DL and Brown F (eds) (1991) Classification and nomenclature of viruses. *Fifth Report of the International Committee on Taxonomy of Viruses*. Vienna: Springer Verlag.

Gardner SD and King AA (1991) Rabies – recent developments in research and human prophylaxis. In: *Current Topics in Clinical Virology* (ed. P Morgan-Capner) pp 141–163. Public Health Laboratory Service.

Gourmelon P, Briet D, Clarenclon D, Court L and Tsiang H (1991) Sleep alterations in experimental street rabies virus infection occur in the absence of major EEG abnormalities. *Brain Research* **554**(1–2): 159–165.

Hantson P, Guerit JM, de Touretchaninoff M, Deconinck B, Mahieu P, Dooms G, Aubert-Tulkens G and Brucher JM (1993) Rabies encephalitis mimicking the electrophysiological pattern of brain death. A case report. *European Neurology* **33**(3): 212–217.

Hattwick MAW (1974) Human rabies. *Public Health Review* **3**(3): 229–274.

Hattwick MAW and Gregg MB (1975) The disease in man. In: *The Natural History of Rabies*, vol. II (ed. GM Baer), pp 281–304. New York: Academic Press.

Hattwick MAW, Weis TT, Stechschulte CJ, Baer GM and Gregg MB (1972) Recovery from rabies: a case report. *Annals of Internal Medicine* **76**: 931–942.

Hattwick MAW, Corey L and Creech WB (1976) Clinical use of human globulin immune to rabies virus. *Journal of Infectious Diseases* **133** (supplement) A266–272.

Held JR and Lopez Adaros H (1972) Neurological disease in man following administration of suckling mouse brain antirabies vaccine. *Bulletin of the World Health Organization* **46**: 321–327.

Helmick CG, Tauxe RV and Vernon AA (1987) Is there a risk to contacts of patients with rabies? *Reviews of Infectious Diseases* **9**(3): 511–518.

Hemachudha T (1989) Rabies. In: *Viral Disease. Handbook of Clinical Neurology*, vol. 12 (ed. RR McKendall), pp 383–404. Amsterdam: Elsevier.

Hemachudha T, Tirawatnpong S and Phanthumchinda K (1989) Seizures as the initial manifestation of paralytic rabies. *Journal of Neurology, Neurosurgery and Psychiatry* **52**(6): 808–810 (letter).

Hemachudha T, Phanthumchinda K, Phanuphak P and Manutsathit S (1987a) Myoedema as a clinical sign in paralytic rabies. *Lancet* **i**: 1210 (letter).

Hemachudha T, Griffin DE, Giffels JJ, Johnson RT, Moser AB and Phanuphak P (1987b) Myelin basic protein as an encephalitogen in encephalomyelitis and polyneuritis following rabies vaccination. *New England Journal of Medicine* **316**(7): 369–374.

Hemachudha T, Phanuphak P, Sriwanthana B, Manutsathit S, Phanthumchinda K, Siriprasomsup W, Ukachoke C, Rasameechan S and Kaoroptham S (1988) Immunologic study of human encephalitic and paralytic rabies. Preliminary report of 16 patients. *American Journal of Medicine* **84**(4): 673–677.

Kaplan C, Turner GS, Warrell DA (1986) *Rabies the Facts*, 2nd edn, pp 21–67. Oxford: Oxford University Press.

Kaplan MM and Cohen D (1962) Studies on the local treatment of wounds for the prevention of rabies. *Bulletin of the World Health Organization* **26**: 765–775.

Kaplan MM and Koprowski H (1973) *Laboratory Technique in Rabies*, 3rd edn. Geneva: WHO.

King AA and Turner GS (1993) Rabies: a review. *Journal of Comparative Pathology* **108**: 1–39.

Ladogana A, Bouzamondo E, Pocchiari M and Tsiang H (1994) Modification of tritiated gamma-amino-n-butyric acid transport in rabies virus-infected primary cortical cultures. *Journal of General Virology* **75**(3): 623–627.

Lafon M, Edelman L, Bouvet JP, Lafage M and Montchatre E (1990) Human monoclonal antibodies specific for the rabies virus glycoprotein and N protein. *Journal of General Virology* **71**(8): 1689–1696.

Larghi OP, Arrosi JC, Nakajata-AJ and Villa-Nova A (1988) Control of urban rabies. In: *Rabies* (eds JB Campbell and KM Charlton), pp 407–422. Boston: Kluwer Academic.

Lopez A, Miranda P, Tejada E and Fishbein DB (1992) Outbreak of human rabies in the Peruvian jungle. *Lancet* **339**: 408–411.

Lumio J, Hillbom M, Roine R, Ketonen L, Haltia M, Valle M, Neuvonen E and Lähdevirta J (1986) Human rabies of bat origin in Europe. *Lancet* **i**: 378.

Maton PN, Pollard JD and Newsom-Davis J (1976) Human rabies encephalomyelitis. *British Medical Journal* **1**: 1038–1040.

Meredith CD, Rossouw AP and van Praag Koch H (1971) An unusual case of human rabies thought to be of chiropteran origin. *South African Medical Journal* **45**(28): 767–769.

Merigan TC, Baer GM, Winkler WG, Bernard KW, Gibert CG, Chany C, Veronesi R *et al.* (1984) *Annals of Neurology* **16**(1): 82–87.

Murphy FA (1977) Rabies pathogenesis. Brief review. *Archives of Virology* **54**(4): 279–297.

Nicholson KG, Kuwert EK, Werner J and Harrison P (1979) Interferon response to human diploid cell strain rabies vaccines in man. *Archives of Virology* **61**: 35–39.

Pará M (1965) An outbreak of post-vaccinal rabies (Rage de laboratoire) in Fortaleza, Brazil in 1960. Resistant fixed virus as the etiological agent. *Bulletin of the World Health Organization* **33**: 172–182.

Perl DP (1975) The pathology of rabies in the central nervous system. In: *The Natural History of Rabies*, vol. I (ed. GM Baer), pp 235–272. New York: Academic Press.

Perry BD and Wandeler AI (1993) The delivery of oral rabies vaccines to dogs: an African perspective. *Onderstepoort Journal of Veterinary Research* **60**: 451–457.

Phuapradit P, Manatsathit S, Warrell MJ and Warrell DA (1985) Paralytic rabies: some unusual clinical presentations. *Journal of the Medical Association of Thailand* **68**(2): 106–110.

Porras C, Barboza JJ, Fuenzalida E, Adaros HL, Oviedo de Diaz AM and Durst J (1976) Recovery from rabies in man. *Annals of Internal Medicine* **85**: 44–48.

Prabhakar BS and Nathanson N (1981) Acute rabies death mediated by antibody. *Nature* **290**: 590–591.

Prier S, Gibert C, Bodros A, Vachon F, Atanasiu D and Masson M (1979) Les neuropathies de la rage humaine. Etude clinique et électrophysiologique de deux cas. *Revue Neurologique (Paris)* **135**(2): 161–168.

Rudd RJ and Trimarchi CV (1989) Development and evaluation of an in vitro virus isolation procedure as a replacement for the mouse inoculation test in rabies diagnosis. *Journal of Clinical Microbiology* **27**(11): 2522–2528.

Selimov MA, Tatarov AG, Botvinkin AD, Klueva EV, Kulikova LG and Khismatullina NA (1989) Rabies related Yuli virus: identification with a panel of monoclonal antibodies. *Acta Virologica* (Praha) **33**(6): 542–546.

Sipahioglu U and Alpaut S (1985) Transplacental rabies in humans. *Mikrobiyoloji Bülteni* **19**(2): 95–99.

Smith JS and Seidel HD (1993) Rabies: a new look at an old disease. *Progress in Medical Virology* **40**: 82–106.

Smith JS, Fishbein DB, Rupprecht CE and Clark K (1991) Unexplained rabies in three immigrants in the United States. A virologic investigation. *New England Journal of Medicine* **324**(4): 205–211.

Smith JS, Orciari LA, Yager PA, Seidel HD and Warner CK (1992) Epidemiologic and historical relationships among 87 rabies virus isolates as determined by limited sequence analysis. *Journal of Infectious Diseases* **166**(2): 296–307.

Steele JH (1988) Rabies in the Americas and remarks on global aspects. *Reviews of Infectious Diseases* **10** (supplement): S585–S597.

Suntharasamai P, Warrell MJ, Warrell DA, Chanthavanich P *et al.* (1987) Early antibody responses to rabies post-exposure vaccine regimens. *American Journal of Tropical Medicine and Hygiene* **36**(1): 160–165.

Sureau P, Portnoi D, Rollin P, Lapresle C, Lapresle C, Chaouni-Berbich A and Gros F (1981) Prévention de la transmission inter-humaine de la rage après greffe de cornée. *Comptes Rendus de l' Academie des Sciences Paris.* Serie III **293**: 689–692.

Swaddiwuthipong W, Prayoonwiwat N, Kunasol P and Choomkasien P (1987) A high incidence of neurological complications following sample anti-rabies vaccine. *SE Asian Journal of Tropical Medicine and Public Health* **18**(4): 526–531.

Swanepoel R, Barnard BJH, Meredith CD, Bishop GC, Brückner GK, Foggin CM and Hüdschle OJB (1993) Rabies in southern Africa. *Onderstepoort Journal of Veterinary Research* **60**: 325–346.

Talaulicar PM (1977) Persistent priapism in rabies. *British Journal of Urology* **49**(6): 462.

Tangchai P and Vejjajiva A (1971) Pathology of the peripheral nervous system in human rabies. A study of nine autopsy cases. *Brain* **94**: 299–306.

Tangchai P, Yenbutr D and Vejjajiva A (1970) Central nervous system lesions in human rabies. A study of twenty-four cases. *Journal of the Medical Association of Thailand* **53**(7): 471–486.

Thomson G and King A (eds) (1993) Rabies in Southern and Eastern Africa. Proceedings of a workshop held at the Faculty of Veterinary Science, University of Pretoria, Onderstepoort, South Africa 3–5 May 1993. *Onderstepoort Journal of Veterinary Research* **60**(4): 263–512.

Tordo N and Poch O (1988) Structure of rabies virus. In: *Rabies* (eds JB Campbell and KM Charlton), pp 25–45. Boston: Kluwer Academic.

Tordo N, Poch O, Ermine A, Keith G and Rougeon F (1988) Completion of the rabies virus genome sequence determination: highly conserved domains among the L(polymerase) proteins of unsegmented negative-strand RNA viruses. *Virology* **165**: 565–576.

Trimarchi CV and Debbie JG (1991) The fluorescent antibody in rabies. In: *The Natural History of Rabies*, 2nd edn (ed. GM Baer), pp 219–233. Boca Raton, FL: CRC Press.

Tsiang H (1993) Pathophysiology of rabies virus infection of the nervous system. *Advances in Virus Research* **42**: 375–412.

Tsiang H, Gourmelon P, Briet D and Court L (1989) Functional alterations in rabies virus infection. In *Progress in Rabies Control* (eds O Thraenhart, H Koprowski, K Bögel, P Sureau), pp 43–47. Royal Tunbridge Wells: Wells Medical.

Turner GS (1985) Immune response after rabies vaccination: basic aspects. *Annales de l'Institute Pasteur. Virology* **136E**: 435–460.

Udwadia ZF, Udwadia FE, Rao PP and Kapadia F (1988) Penile hyperexcitability with recurrent ejaculations as the presenting manifestation of a case of rabies. *Postgraduate Medical Journal* **64**: 85–86.

Vejjajiva A (1967) Neurological sequelae of anti-rabies inoculation. *Journal of the Medical Association of Thailand* **50**: 806–811.

Wandeler AI (1991) Oral immunization of wildlife. In: *The Natural History of Rabies*, 2nd edn (ed. GM Baer), pp 485–503. Boca Raton, FL: CRC Press.

Wandeler AI, Matter HC, Kappeler A and Budde A (1993) The ecology of dogs and canine rabies: a selective review. *Review of Scientific Technology* **12**(1): 51–71.

Warrell DA (1976) The clinical picture of rabies in man. *Transactions of the Royal Society of Tropical Medicine and Hygiene* **70**(3): 188–195.

Warrell DA, Davidson NMcD, Pope HM, Bailie WE, Lawrie JH, Ormerod LD, Kertesz A and Lewis P (1976) Pathophysiologic studies in human rabies. *American Journal of Medicine* **60**: 180–190.

Warrell MJ and Warrell DA (1995) Rhabdovirus infections of humans. In: *Exotic Viral Infections. Handbook of Infectious Diseases*, vol. 3 (eds. JS Porterfield and DAJ Tyrrell), pp 343–383. London: Chapman & Hall.

Warrell MJ, Warrell DA, Suntharasamai P and Viravan C *et al.* (1983) An economical regimen of human diploid cell strain anti-rabies vaccine for post-exposure prophylaxis. *Lancet* **ii**: 301–304.

Warrell MJ, Suntharasamai P, Nicholson KG, Warrell DA *et al.* (1984) Multi-site intradermal and multi-site subcutaneous rabies vaccination: improved economical regimens. *Lancet* **i**: 874–876.

Warrell MJ, Nicholson KG, Warrell DA, Suntharasamai P *et al.* (1985) Economical multiple site intradermal immunisation with human diploid-cell-strain vaccine is effective for post-exposure rabies prophylaxis. *Lancet* **i**: 1059–1062.

Warrell MJ, Looareeswuan S, Manatsathit S, White NJ, Phuapradit P, Vejjajiva A, Hoke CH, Burke DS and Warrell DA (1988) Rapid diagnosis of rabies and post-vaccinal encephalitides. *Clinical and Experimental Immunology* **71**: 229–234.

Warrell MJ, White NJ, Looareesauwan S, Phillips RE *et al.* (1989) Failure of interferon alfa and tribavirin in rabies encephalitis. *British Medical Journal* **299**: 830–833.

WHO (1994) World survey of rabies 28 for year 1992. *WHO/Rabies/94.210.*

WHO Expert Committee on Rabies (1992) *WHO Technical Report Series* **824**: 1–84.

Wiktor TJ, Doherty PC and Koprowski H (1977) Suppression of cell-mediated immunity by street rabies virus. *Journal of Experimental Medicine* **145**(6): 1617–1622.

Wiktor TJ, Macfarlan RI, Fuggin CM and Koprowski H (1984) Antigenic analysis of rabies and Mokola virus from Zimbabwe using monoclonal antibodies. *Developments in Biological Standardization* **47**: 199–211.

Wilde H, Chomchey P, Prakongsri S, Puyaratabandhu P and Chutivongse S (1989) Adverse effects of equine rabies immune globulin. *Vaccine* **7**: 10–11.

Winkler WG (1975) Airborne rabies. In: *The Natural History of Rabies*, vol. II (ed. GM Baer), pp 115–121. New York: Academic Press.

Winkler WG, Fashinell TR, Leffingwell L, Howard P and Conomy JP (1973) Airborne rabies transmission in a laboratory worker. *Journal of the American Medical Association* **226**: 1219–1221.

Wunner WH (1987) Rabies viruses – pathogenesis and immunity. In: *The Rhabdoviruses* (ed. RR Wagner), pp 361–426. New York: Plenum Press.

6

Subacute Sclerosing Panencephalitis

Subhashini Prabhakar and Mathew Alexander

Department of Neurological Sciences, Christian Medical College Hospital, Vellore 632004, India

INTRODUCTION

Subacute sclerosing panencephalitis is a slowly progressive disorder typically seen in childhood and adolescence with an invariably fatal outcome. It is a unique slow viral disorder in that the aetiological agent, the measles virus, has been isolated and identified.

HISTORICAL PERSPECTIVE

The first two cases of subacute sclerosing panencephalitis (SSPE) termed as 'inclusion encephalitis' by Dawson (1934), were characterized by subacute progression of behavioural abnormalities, mental regression and involuntary jerking of extremities. The unique features in these cases were an acute neuronal degeneration, Cowdry type A inclusion bodies and perivascular inflammatory infiltrates, as well as areas of intense gliosis in white matter, indicative of a chronic process. In 1945, Van Bogaert reported three similar cases of 'leuco-encephalite sclerosante' in whom gliosis and inflammation of white matter was predominant. Greenfield in 1950, recognizing the similarity between the 'inclusion body encephalitis', the 'panencephalitis' of Pette and Doring, and the 'leuco-encephalite sclerosante' of Van Bogaert, proposed the term 'subacute sclerosing panencephalitis' (Poser, 1983).

Intranuclear inclusion bodies suggested an underlying viral aetiology although Dawson and others were unable to transmit the disease to laboratory animals. Three decades later a causal link between the measles virus and SSPE was considered, when Bouteille *et al.* (1965) and Tellez and Harter (1966) demonstrated paramyxovirus-like tubular filaments in the brain biopsy of a patient with SSPE. This was confirmed by Connolly *et al.* (1967) who reported marked elevations of measles antibody titres in sera and cerebrospinal fluid (CSF) of patients, and the presence of measles antigens by immunofluorescence in the brains of three patients with SSPE. Viral isolation and culture was achieved when the measles virus was isolated from a patient with SSPE by coculturing infected brain cells with permissive HeLa cells (Horta-Barbosa *et al.*, 1969; Payne *et al.*, 1969). Recovery of the virus was limited even with this technique, and unlike wild-type measles virus the SSPE virus seemed to be a defective cell-associated virus in culture. The next significant finding, and pivotal to our understanding of the mechanisms of viral persistence, was the absence or diminished expression of measles virus M proteins in SSPE virus-infected cells (Hall and Choppin, 1979; Hall *et al.*, 1979).

In 1949 Radermacker described distinctive EEG abnormalities that were pathognomonic of SSPE. Changes in CSF, such as elevation in the first zone of colloidal gold curve, raised immunoglobulins and the demonstration of oligoclonal bands in the sera and CSF of patients by Karcher *et al.* (1959) suggested a role for altered immunity in the development or induction of the disease.

Epidemiological reports revealed the world-wide prevalence of this disease. National registries of SSPE were established in the USA (1969), UK (1970) and Lebanon (1974), and the results of these studies have contributed significantly to our understanding of the evolution of this illness (Jabbour *et al.*, 1972; Haddad *et al.*, 1974; Dick and Miller, 1983).

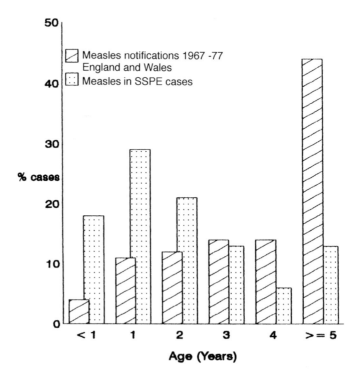

Figure 6.1   Age at measles in SSPE cases and general population. From Miller (1989).

EPIDEMIOLOGY

The annual incidence is < 0.1 to 5–6 cases per million population (Cernercu and Milea, 1983; Hinman *et al.*, 1983; Radhakrishnan *et al.*, 1988) with very high rates up to 21 per million still being reported from India (Saha *et al.*, 1990).

An exposure to measles infection is present in 80–90% of cases and children infected in the first 2 years are at greatest risk (Figure 6.1). In the tropics, where the attack rates are higher during these years a large number of infants (20–40%) possess a passive immunity to measles which prevents overt disease, but probably renders them more susceptible to SSPE (Rammohan *et al.*, 1982). A higher incidence in boys (ratio 3:1) and early age of measles are thought to be related to intensive exposure to the virus (Modlin *et al.*, 1977; Aaby *et al.*, 1984) and predispose to SSPE.

There has been an increase in the mean age of onset for both sexes from 9.5 years to 12 years in recent years. The median interval between measles and the onset of SSPE is about 7 years (range 3 months to 18 years), with a recent trend of longer disease latencies (Figure 6.2). Neither the age of exposure to measles, nor severity of infection, seem to affect the age of onset or course of the illness (Dyken, 1989).

Geographic clustering has been noted in at least ten countries, but does not

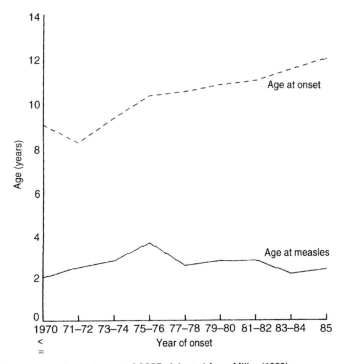

Figure 6.2 Ages at measles and onset of SSPE. Adapted from Miller (1989).

correspond to a high incidence of measles. Earlier studies implicated a possible role of racial and genetic factors for the male preponderance and greater incidence in certain races (Moodie *et al.*, 1980; Dhib-Jhalbut and Haddad, 1983). However, evidence to the contrary is a higher proportion of female patients in the older age groups, and involvement of only one of monozygotic twins following simultaneous exposure to measles, as well as absence of HLA association (Dhib-Jhalbut and Haddad, 1983; Schoub *et al.*, 1992).

Triggering factors like acute febrile illnesses or vaccination preceding the onset of overt symptoms of SSPE have been reported in 16–40% of patients (Baguley and Glasgow, 1973; Risk *et al.*, 1983; Gnanamuthu, 1989), as well as a small epidemic following Salk vaccine (Baguley and Glasgow, 1973). Other suspected risk factors include exposure to birds and sick animals in rural areas (Detels *et al.*, 1973).

Widespread immunization in the developed countries has achieved greater than 90% reduction in the incidence of SSPE (Bloch *et al.*, 1985; Miller *et al.*, 1992). Interestingly, an increase in the age of onset and latency of infection have been observed in vaccinated children who had natural infection while a decrease in latency and severe disease has been observed in children who only had vaccine (Dyken, 1989). There is no evidence that sporadic cases of SSPE following vaccination are related to the attenuated vaccine virus.

CLINICAL FEATURES

The natural history of SSPE is characterized by a highly variable temporal course ranging from an almost acute onset with rapid progression and death within a few months to a protracted course over several years with periods of stabilization and even improvement (Risk and Haddad, 1979). A fully developed case of SSPE can very easily be diagnosed by history and observation. According to the Risk and Haddad classification, the clinical course can be divided into five stages. Onset is usually insidious with behavioural changes, decline in school performance and intellectual skills, impaired memory, visuospatial incapacities and fluctuations in mood which may be very subtle and in many instances recalled only in retrospect (Stage 0–I). This stage may last for several months or years.

The next stage of disease is characterized by developments of myoclonic jerks, increasing motor disability, ataxia and convulsive seizures. Myoclonic jerks which are stereotyped occurring 4–10 per minute synchronous with EEG discharges may involve one or all limbs from the onset. Initially the attacks are mild and the patient does not fall (Stage IIa) but as the illness progresses the jerks become violent and result in falls (Stage IIb) and eventually the patient is bedridden (Stage IIc). Extrapyramidal features such as dyskinesia, chorea, athetosis, dystonic postures, ballismus may occur in about 20–25% of children. Visual loss may be due to involvement of the occipital cortex, chorio-retinitis or optic atrophy. Papilloedema is rare. Patients become progressively uncommunicative probably due to worsening dementia, rather than language disturbances which are uncommon. Dysarthria and dysphagia may be noted during the late second stage. In the final stage of illness (Stage III) the child lapses into a stupor, hypertonia is replaced by hypotonia and autonomic instability with temperature fluctuations; myoclonic jerks diminish in intensity and eventually disappear. The patient may remain in this stage for several years, ultimately succumbing to intercurrent infection. Spontaneous improvement or stabilization (Stage IV) may occur during any of these stages and may last for a variable period of time before eventual relapse occurs (Stage V).

Pathology

Gross examination of brain may reveal mild to moderate atrophy of the cerebral hemispheres. Microscopic examination shows widespread degeneration of neurones and disorganization in the cortex, the parieto-occipital cortex being preferentially involved. Focal or diffuse perivascular infiltrates of lymphocytes, plasma cells and phagocytes are seen in the meninges and in the brain parenchyma. In severely affected areas there is considerable loss of neurones, neuronophagia, microglial and astrocytic hyperplasia. Cowdry type A intranuclear inclusions in the neurones and oligodendroglia (Figure 6.3a,b) are diffuse in rapidly progressive fatal cases while in chronic cases they are

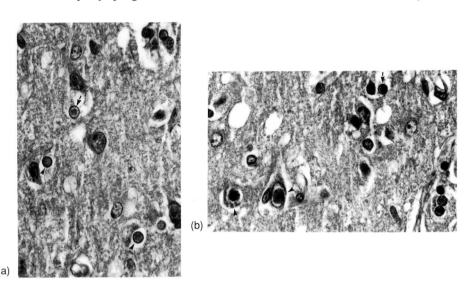

Figure 6.3 (a) Intranuclear inclusions in the neurones (arrow head) and oligodendroglia (arrow) in a case of SSPE (H & E x360). (b) Intranuclear inclusions in oligodendroglia (arrow) occupying the nucleus while an intranuclear inclusion in a small neurone (arrow head) shows a clear halo separating the nuclear membrane and the dense central inclusion (H & E x360). (Courtesy of Dr S Nimhaus, Bangalore.)

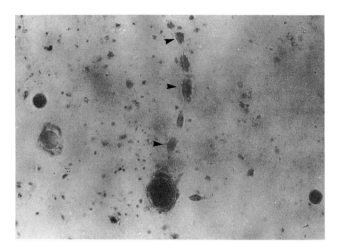

Figure 6.4   Immunocytochemical localization of the measles viral antigen, both in the nucleus and cytoplasm of neurone and the oligodendroglia. The viral antigen is seen spreading along the axon (arrow). PAP technique. Hyperimmune human CSF as polyclonal primary antibody (H & E x440). (Courtesy of Dr S Nimhaus, Bangalore.)

conspicuous in the basis pontis. Immunopathological studies of SSPE brains demonstrate measles virus (MV) antigen in neuronal nuclei, cytoplasm and processes (Figure 6.4) and in oligodendroglia even in areas where myelin is preserved. The white matter abnormalities include perivascular inflammatory infiltrates and focal or diffuse gliosis, and areas of active demyelination particularly in chronic progressive cases (Ohya *et al.*, 1974, Figure 6.5). The age of the patient and duration of illness seem to correlate inversely with the presence and amount of MV antigens in the brain (Budka, 1989; Vani *et al.*, 1994). In situ hybridization studies have confirmed the presence of the genome even in cells negative for MV antigen by immunofluorescence (Haase *et al.*, 1981a,b). By electronmicroscopy viral nucleocapsids can be seen in both the cytoplasm and the intranuclear inclusions (Herndon and Rubenstein, 1967).

PATHOGENESIS

While viral infection with measles virus underlies the pathogenesis of SSPE, what is not known is how and why in a very small proportion of children exposed to such a ubiquitous infection of childhood, the virus persists in a dormant state and reactivates to cause an inexorably progressive illness (Horta-Barbosa *et al.*, 1971). A complex interaction between the host, the infecting virus, as well as undelineated environmental factors are intricately involved in the eventual manifestation of the clinical disease.

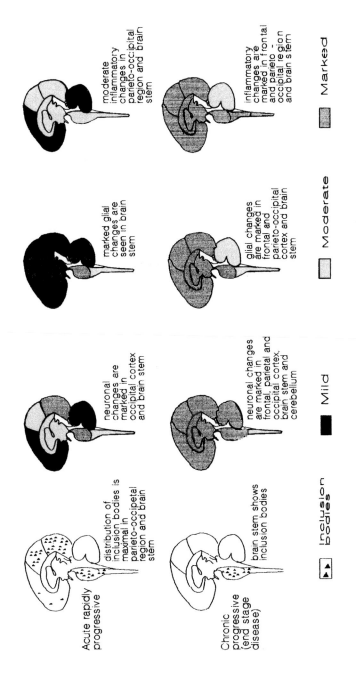

Figure 6.5 Schematic representation of neuropathological findings in SSPE. Modified from Ohya *et al.* (1974).

SSPE Agent

Measles virus is a negative-stranded RNA virus which expresses six major polypeptides, the haemagglutinin (H) and fusion (F) proteins on cell membrane, the nucleocapsid consisting of polypeptide (P), nucleocapside (NP) and large polypeptide L and the M protein which is a membrane protein. M protein plays a major role in replication by stabilizing the envelope and directs subplasmalemmal alignment of nucleocapsids before budding. The SSPE virus is structurally and antigenically similar to measles virus except for minor differences in cross neutralization studies and growth characteristics in vitro. Current perception is that SSPE agent is a natural mutant or a measles virus possibly modified by prolonged passage in the CNS tissue (Carrigan and Knox, 1990). A consistent although not an invariable difference between the measles virus and SSPE virus is the absence of M proteins. Antibodies to M proteins in CSF, as well as measles virus M protein in brain tissues are absent in most SSPE patients and may result in persistent infection (Hall and Choppin, 1979; Hall *et al.*, 1979).

The importance of M protein in experimental SSPE has also been confirmed by elegant small animal models. Chronic subclinical infection with a defective or cell-associated virus was achieved only in weaning animals. Recovery of virus required cocultivation procedures (Johnson and Byington, 1977; Thormar *et al.*, 1978), the disappearance of M protein from brain was coincidental to disappearance of infectious virus and development of cell-associated infection (Johnson *et al.*, 1981). The presence of measles antibodies was necessary for the development of persistent infection in vitro and in vivo.

Recent studies on M protein genes from the wild-type and SSPE viruses have revealed a high degree of conservation of the M proteins; sequencing and cloning experiments of M protein genes from different SSPE patients revealed either several missense mutations, premature stop codons or biased hypermutation events (Cattaneo *et al.*, 1988; Wong *et al.*, 1991). When M gene in the cDNA of an infectious virus was replaced with M genes derived from four patients with SSPE, three of the four SSPE M genes proved non-functional while one was functional (Ballart *et al.*, 1991). This suggests that M protein abnormality need not be an invariable feature of SSPE. Other studies suggest mRNA abnormalities and translational defects resulting in unstable proteins (Carter *et al.*, 1983).

Host Factors

Most cells in the CNS are poor substrates for viral replication (Hasse *et al.*, 1985), but some are relatively permissive. When small amounts of virus are introduced into relatively resistant cells, infection remains confined, the genome persists and goes undetected because of limited replication and synthesis of antigens. Viral gene products accumulate and spread from cell to cell via neuronal processes, and cell fusion (Iwasaki and Kaprowski, 1974). As a consequence low-level sustained antigenic stimulation results in production of virus-specific antibodies distinctive of SSPE. In vitro studies reveal that anti-measles antibodies modulate expression of M, P and F proteins within the cells and on cell membranes and favour survival of infected cells, and facilitate replication of virus which in turn promotes generation of mutant strains (Fujinami and Oldstone, 1980). The role of elevated measles antibodies in patients with SSPE is not known, but the development of SSPE in patients with hypogammaglobulinaemia as well as immunosuppression who have low antibody titres, suggests that it may be an epiphenomenon (Johnson, 1984).

Immune complexes of antigen, complement and immunoglobulins are demonstrated in blood vessels walls and may cause alteration of blood–brain barrier (BBB) permeability and permit access of lymphocytes into the central nervous system, resulting in inflammatory reaction and demyelination (Poser, 1989). Some studies on cellular immune responses indicate that SSPE patients have normal in vitro responses to non-specific mitogens, and allogenic lymphocytes, while others report impaired T cell function. Impaired capacity to generate cytoxic T lymphocyte major histocompatibility class (MHC) II restricted response in vitro was demonstrated (Dhib-Jhalbut *et al.*, 1989). Virus-specific cytoxicity is important for recovery from viral infections and its impairment may explain a mechanism of

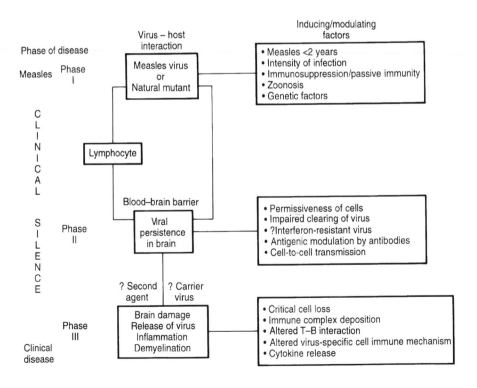

Figure 6.6 Pathogenesis of subacute sclerosing panencephalitis.

measles virus persistence. It is conceivable that presence of viral RNA in lymphocytes (Fournier *et al.*, 1985) alters T and B cell functions. In SSPE brains, analysis of T cell subsets within the perivascular infiltrates reveals mild increase in CD8+ subsets (15%), while total T lymphocytes and CD4+ helper cells are abundant in both perivascular spaces and parenchyma. Cells expressing MHC class II molecules (probably stimulated astrocytes and macrophages) are also abundant (Nagano *et al.*, 1991). These cells are targets of cytotoxic T4 cells and along with activated lymphocytes are involved in inflammatory cytokine secretion. This creates a conducive environment for active immune-mediated tissue injury and lesion development (Figure 6.6).

It is possible that antigenic challenge of a second infection could alter the dormant state of SSPE virus and result in disease expression. In addition there are seroepidemiological data which suggest that an exposure to another virus, such as Epstein–Barr virus or parainfluenza type I virus may transform the measles virus into a defective virus (Scully *et al.*, 1986).

LABORATORY INVESTIGATIONS

When a child presents with typical features, laboratory investigations are merely confirmatory. However, when a child presents in Stage 0 or I or with an atypical presentation then the laboratory investigations aid in establishing the diagnosis.

CSF

Routine analysis of CSF is generally normal except for mild elevation in protein content without pleocytosis. IgG concentration in CSF is in the range $0.1–0.54$ g l^{-1} with mean value 0.18 ± 0.09 g l^{-1}, while IgA and IgM may be detected occasionally. Agar gel isoelectric focusing (IEF) of serum and CSF reveals oligoclonal bands of IgG which represent restricted heterogeneity and are specific for measles proteins (Karcher *et al.*, 1982).

Presence of high titres of measles antibody in CSF is the single most diagnostic feature of SSPE (Karcher *et al.*, 1982). Various serological methods used are complement fixation (CF), haemagglutination inhibition (HAI) and virus neutralization (VN).

Antibody titres may fluctuate during the natural course of illness or as a result of therapeutic modulation. Serum CSF and HAI titres range from 1:40 up to 1:2048 (Salmi *et al.*, 1972; Saha, 1989) and titres in CSF from 1:40 to over 1:512 by complement fixation and HAI methods. The CSF/serum ratio ranges from 1:2 to 1:128. In rare instances, measles antibodies may be undetectable early in the disease, but become positive on subsequent study (Saha, 1989). Indirect immunofluorescence (IF) as well as ELISA for virus-specific IgM and IgG are highly sensitive (Kahane *et al.*, 1979; Chiodi *et al.*, 1986).

EEG

The presence of Raedermaker's periodic complexes is diagnostic of the disease. Early in SSPE, the EEG may be normal or show only moderate non-specific slowing. The onset of myoclonic jerks is associated with episodes of suppression burst pattern in which high amplitude of slow and sharp waves occur at intervals of 3–5 s on a slow background. This EEG pattern, although not unique to SSPE, is characteristic of Stage II disease. An increase in the frequency with shortening of intervals between complexes are seen as the illness progresses (Wulff, 1982). Later in the illness, the EEG becomes disorganized with high-amplitude random dysrrhythmic slowing, and marked reduction in amplitudes in the terminal stages of illness.

In 1950, Cobb proposed the brainstem as the site of origin of periodic events, that they required a relatively preserved functional cortex to manifest, and disappeared with severe cortical damage. More recently, dipole tracing methods used to clarify the origin of periodic synchronous discharges and myoclonus have shown that both source generators were located in the subcortical part of the cerebrum and an area adjacent to the thalamus (Yagi *et al.*, 1992).

Evoked Potentials

Alteration of visual-evoked responses may be detected in the early stages of the disease and correlate with the clinical progression (Trapani *et al.*, 1991). Abnormalities in brainstem auditory-evoked responses, i.e. prolonged III–V interpeak latencies, seem to parallel the clinical course of the disease. Other studies have not shown statistically significant BAER alteration (Markand *et al.*, 1980; Trapani *et al.*, 1991).

CT and MRI Scans

The radiological abnormalities encountered in early stages are few. CT scan may be normal or show signs of mild brain swelling in early stages, followed after a variable period of time by low-attenuation white matter lesions which may or may not enhance with contrast. Cortical atrophy and ventricular dilatation develop during the late stages of disease but do not seem to reflect the neurological or psychological status of the patient (Krawiecki *et al.*, 1984).

MRI scan is more sensitive in detecting abnormalities. The commonest abnormality seen is areas of hyperintensity in the parieto-occipital cortex and white matter in the T2-weighted images (Winer *et al.*, 1990). The evolution of CT and MRI is well shown in Figure 6.7a, b, c.

PET Scan

Serial PET scan studies suggest topographic progression of the disease process. Initial hypermetabolism in the basal ganglia found in early Stage II has been

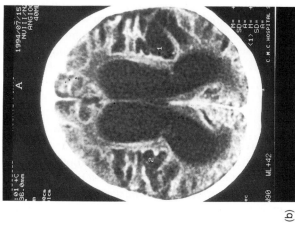

(b)

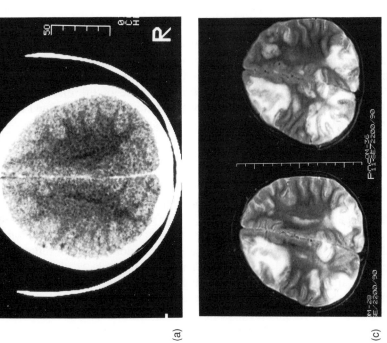

(a)

(c)

Figure 6.7 Eight-year-old boy with acute onset and rapid progression into Stage III within 4 months. (a) CT scan done 2 months after onset of symptoms. Note obliteration of sulci, diffuse hypoattenuation of white matter and small ventricles. (b) CT scan 9 months after onset. Note gross diffuse atrophy, dilation of ventricles, irregular areas of hypoattenuation in white matter and gyral enhancement of parietal cortex. (c) MRI scan 3 weeks following the first CT scan shows hyperintense lesions (T2-weighted images) involving parieto-occipital, frontal cortices and white matter.

proposed to be related to increase in neuronal activity in basal ganglia with resultant functional inhibition of frontal, parietal and temporal cortical areas. As the process spreads, metabolic activity in the basal ganglia decreases, followed by reduction in functional inhibition. It is hypothesized that the clinical symptoms in Stage II are related to the metabolically active inflammatory process in the basal ganglia while the major symptoms of Stage III are related to hypermetabolic inflammation of midline structures and brainstem. Terminally, the basal ganglia structures are hypometabolic as a result of structural and neuronal damage (Huber *et al.*, 1992).

TREATMENT

So far no single drug or combination of drugs has been proven to be of unequivocal benefit. One of the most important impediments in treatment of SSPE is the inability to detect early manifestations of the disease, when presumably the inflammatory changes are still reversible. Once tissue destruction has occurred, a reversal process is not possible.

Of the therapeutic agents that have been tested, Inosiplex (Isoprinosine-a 1:3 complex of inosine and dimethyl amino p73 isopropanol-*p*-acetamido-benzoate) has been associated with higher rates of remission and long-term survival in patients in whom the probability of spontaneous remission is 5%. At a concentration of 50–100 mg ml^{-1} or in vivo doses of 25 mg kg^{-1} day^{-1}, increase in the number of CD4+ lymphocytes, NK cell function and a proliferative response to mitogens occur probably by potentiating interferons and increasing production of IL-1 and IL-2. In doses higher than 50 mg kg^{-1} day^{-1}, it augments the number of CD8+ lymphocytes and inhibits mitogen response and NK cytotoxicity (Anlar *et al.*, 1994). The recommended daily dose is 100 mg kg^{-1} day^{-1} , and is without major side effects.

Interferons (IFN) suppress replication of virus and also influence the immune system. They up-regulate NK cells and MHC expression of target cells for cytotoxic T cells. Intravenous administration of α-interferon has not proved to be useful because of poor penetration of the blood–brain barrier. Modest improvement with intraventricular and intrathecal routes of administration have been reported in a small number of patients (Huttenlocher *et al.*, 1986; Panitch *et al.*, 1986). Prolonged therapy is necessary for sustained response as reported worsening has been documented on discontinuing therapy (Cianchetti *et al.*, 1989). The value of interferons in producing sustained remission or altering survival states remains to be determined.

Cimetidine, an H2 receptor antagonist, was used in SSPE for its immunomodulatory effect (Anlar *et al.*, 1993). There was no worsening in the cimetidine-treated group during the study period whereas the placebo group worsened. However, there were no differences in the immunological studies, CSF measles antibody titres and IgG index of the two groups. Antiviral agents have not been used successfully in SSPE.

In summary, no agent has yet been convincingly shown to have sustained benefit in the condition.

REFERENCES

Aaby P, Bukh J, Lisse JM *et al.* (1984) Risk factors in subacute sclerosing panencephalitis: age and sex dependent host reactions or intensive exposure? *Reviews of Infectious Diseases* **6**: 239–250.

Anlar B, Gucuyener K, Imir T *et al.* (1993) Cimetidine as an immunomodulator in subacute sclerosing panencephalitis: a double blind, placebo-controlled study. *Paediatric Infectious Disease Journal* **12**: 578–581.

Anlar B, Yalaz K, Imir T *et al.* (1994) The effect of Inosiplex in subacute sclerosing panencephalitis: a clinical and laboratory study. *European Neurology* **34**: 44–47.

Baguley DM and Glasgow GL (1973) Subacute sclerosing panencephalitis and Salk vaccine. *Lancet* **ii**: 763.

Ballart I, Huber M, Schmid A *et al.* (1991) Functional and nonfunctional measles virus matrix genes from lethal human brain infection. *Journal of Virology* **65(6)**: 3161–3166.

Bloch AB, Orenstein WA, Stetler HC *et al.* (1985) Health impact of measles vaccination in the United States. *Pediatrics* **76**: 524–532.

Bouteille M, Fontaine C, Vedrenne C *et al.* (1965) Sur un cas d'encephalite subaigue a inclusions: etude anatomo-clinique et ultrastructurale. *Revue Neurologie* **133**: 454–458.

Budka H (1989) Neuropathology of SSPE. *Proceedings of the Third International Symposium on SSPE*. Vellore, India, pp 123–136.

Carrigan DR and Knox KK (1990) Identification of interferon-resistant subpopulations in several strains of measles virus: positive selection by growth of the virus in brain tissue. *Journal of Virology* **64(4)**: 1600–1615.

Carter MJ, Wilcocks MM, ter Meulen V *et al.* (1983) Defective translation of measles virus matrix protein in a subacute sclerosing panencephalitis cell line. *Nature* **305**: 153–155.

Cattaneo R, Schmid A, Eschle D *et al.* (1988) Biased hypermutation and other genetic changes in defective measles virus in human brain infections. *Cell* **155**: 255–265.

Cernescu C and Milea S (1983) Epidemiology of subacute sclerosing panencephalitis in Romania between 1976-1982. *Virologie* **34**: 239–250.

Chiodi F, Sundqvist V and Norrbye E (1986) Measles IgM antibodies in cerebrospinal fluid and serum in subacute sclerosing panencephalitis. *Journal of Medical Virology* **18**: 149–158.

Cianchetti C, Muntoni F, Fratta A *et al.* (1989) Intraventricular alpha-interferon treatment of subacute sclerosing panencephalitis. *Proceedings of the Third International Symposium on SSPE*. Vellore, India, pp 203–209.

Connolly JH, Allen JV, Hurwitz LJ *et al.* (1967) Measles virus antibody and antigen in subacute sclerosing panencephalitis. *Lancet* **i**: 542–544.

Dawson JR (1934) Cellular inclusions in cerebral lesions of epidemic encephalitis. *Archives of Neurology and Psychiatry* **31**: 685.

Detels R, Broad JA, McNew J *et al.* (1973) Further epidemiological studies of subacute sclerosing panencephalitis. *Lancet* **ii**: 11.

Dhib-Jalbut S and Haddad FS (1983) An epidemiologic review on SSPE. *Proceedings of the First International Symposium on SSPE*, Beirut, 1983, pp 245–261.

Dhib-Jalbut S, Jacobson S and McFarlin D (1989) Impaired human studies of subacute sclerosing panencephalitis. *Annals of Neurology* **25**: 272–280.

Dick G (1973) Register of cases of subacute sclerosing panencephalitis. *British Medical Journal* **3**: 359.

Dick G and Miller C (1983) Register of cases of subacute sclerosing panencephalitis in England and Wales. *Proceedings of the First International Symposium on SSPE, Beirut, 1983*, pp 217–225.

Dyken PR (1989) The changing pattern of SSPE, USA. *Proceedings of the Third International Symposium on SSPE*. Vellore, India, pp 39–43.

Fournier JG, Tardieu M, Lebon P *et al.* (1985) Localization of measles virus nucleic acid sequence in infected cells by hybridization in situ. *New England Journal of Medicine* **313**: 910–915.

Fujinami RS and Oldstone MB (1980) Alterations in expression of measles virus polypeptides by antibody: molecular events in antibody-induced antigenic modulation. *Journal of Immunology* **125**: 78–85.

Gnanamuthu C (1989) SSPE in Vellore. *Proceedings of the Third International Symposium on SSPE*. Vellore, India, pp 77–84.

Haase AT, Ventura P, Gibbs CJ *et al.* (1981a) Measles virus nucleotide sequences: detection by hybridization in situ. *Science* **212**: 672–675.

Haase AT, Swowloand P, Stowring L *et al.* (1981b) Measles virus genome in infections of the central nervous system. *Journal of Infectious Diseases* **44**: 154–160.

Haase H, Gantz D, Eble B *et al.* (1985) Natural history of restricted synthesis and expression of measles virus genes in subacute sclerosing panencephalitis. *Proceedings of the National Academy of Sciences, USA* **82**: 3020–3024.

Haddad F, Risk W and Jabbour J (1974) Subacute sclerosing panencephalitis in the Middle East. *Lancet* **ii**: 1025.

Hall WW and Choppin PW (1979) Evidence for the lack of synthesis of the M polypeptide of measles virus in brain cells in subacute sclerosing panencephalitis. *Virology* **99**: 443–447.

Hall WW, Lamb RA and Choppin PW (1979) Measles and subacute sclerosing panencephalitis virus proteins: lack of antibodies to the M protein in patients with subacute sclerosing panencephalitis. *Proceedings of the National Academy of Sciences, USA* **76**: 2047–2051.

Herndon RM and Rubinstein W (1967) Light and electron microscopy observation on the development at viral particles in the inducers of Dawson's encephalitis (subacute sclerosing panencephalitis) *Neurology* **18**: 8–20.

Hinman AR, Orenstein WA, Bloch AB *et al.* (1983) Impact of measles in the United States. *Reviews of Infectious Diseases* **5**: 439–444.

Horta-Barbosa L, Fucillo DA, Sever JL *et al.* (1969) Subacute sclerosing panencephalitis: isolation of measles virus from a brain biopsy. *Nature* **221**: 974.

Horta-Barbosa L, Hamilton R, Witti B *et al.* (1971) Subacute sclerosing panencephalitis: isolation of measles virus from lymph node biopsies. *Science* **173**: 840–841.

Huttenlocher PR, Picchietti DL, Roos RP *et al.* (1986) Intrathecal interferon in subacute sclerosing panencephalitis. *Annals of Neurology* **19**: 303–305.

Huber M, Pawlik G, Banborschkes *et al.* (1992) Changing patterns of glucose metabolism during the course of SSPE as measured with 18 FDG-positron-emission tomography. *Journal of Neurology* **239**: 157–161.

Iwasaki Y and Koprowski H (1974) Cell to cell transmission of virus in the central nervous system: subacute sclerosing panencephalitis. *Laboratory Investigation* **31**: 187–196.

Jabbour JT, Duenas DA, Sever JL *et al.* (1972) Epidemiology of subacute sclerosing panencephalitis: a report of the SSPE Registry. *Journal of American Medical Association* **220**: 959–962.

Johnson KP and Byington DP (1977) Subacute sclerosing panencephalitis: animal models. In: *Microbiology* (ed. D Schlesinger), pp 511–515. Washington DC: American Society for Microbiology.

Johnson KP, Norrby E, Swoveland P and Carrigan D (1981) Experimental sub acute sclerosing panencephalitis: selective disappearance of measles virus matrix protein from the central nervous system. *Journal of Infectious Diseases* **144**: 161–169.

Johnson RT (1984) *Viral infections of the nervous system.* New York: Raven Press, pp 182–185.

Kahane S, Goldstein V and Sarov I (1979) Detection of IgG antibodies specific for measles virus by ELISA. *Intervirology* **12**: 39–46.

Karcher D, van Sande M and Lowenthal A (1959) Micro-electrophoresis in agargel of proteins of the cerebrospinal fluid and central nervous system. *Journal of Neurochemistry* **4**: 135.

Karcher D, Thormar H, Lowenthal A *et al.* (1982) Subacute sclerosing panencephalitis antibodies against measles virus polypeptides. *Journal of Neurology* **227**: 29–34.

Krawiecki NS, Dyken PR, Gammal TE *et al.* (1984) Computed tomography of the brain in subacute sclerosing panencephalitis. *Annals of Neurology* **15**: 489–493.

Markand ON, Ochs R, Worth RM *et al.* (1980) Brainstem auditory evoked potentials in chronic degenerative central nervous system disorders. In: *Evoked Potentials* (ed. C Barber), pp 367–375. Baltimore: University Park Press.

Miller CL (1989) Changes in the epidemiology of SSPE in England and Wales 1970–1988. *Proceedings of the Third International Symposium on SSPE.* Vellore, India, pp 15–23.

Miller C, Farrington CP and Harbert K (1992) The epidemiology of subacute sclerosing panencephalitis in England and Wales 1970–1989. *International Journal of Epidemiology* **21**: 998–1006.

Modlin JF, Jabbour TJ and White JJ (1977) Epidemiologic studies of measles, measles vaccine and subacute sclerosing panencephalitis. *Journal of Pediatrics* **59**: 505–512.

Moodie JW, Mackezie DJ and Kippo A (1980) Subacute sclerosing panencephalitis in Southern Africa: recent additions to the SSPE registry. *South African Medical Journal* **58**: 964–967.

Nagano I, Nakamura S, Yoshioka M *et al.* (1991) Immunocytochemical analysis of the cellular infiltrate in brain lesions in subacute sclerosing panencephalites. *Neurology* **41**: 1639–1642.

Ohya T, Martinez AJ, Jabbour JT *et al.* (1974) Subacute sclerosing panencephalitis: correlation of clinical neurophysiologic and neuropathologic findings. *Neurology* **24**: 211–218.

Panitch HS, Plascencia JG, Norris FH *et al.* (1986) Subacute sclerosing panencephalitis: remission after treatment with intraventricular interferon. *Neurology* **36**: 562–566.

Payne FB, Baublis JV, Itabasi HH *et al.* (1969) Isolation of measles virus from cell cultures of brain from a patient with subacute sclerosing panencephalitis. *New England Journal of Medicine* **281**: 585–589.

Poser CM (1983) Subacute sclerosing panencephalitis: an historical retrospective. *Proceedings of the First International Symposium on SSPE.* Beirut, pp 19–38.

Poser CM (1989) The pathogenesis of demyelination in subacute sclerosing panencephalitis. *Proceedings of the Third International Symposium on SSPE*. Vellore, India, pp 1–6.

Radhakrishnan K, Thakur AK, Maloo JC *et al.* (1988) Descriptive epidemiology of some rare neurological diseases in Benghazi, Libya. *Neuroepidemiology* **72**: 159–164.

Rammohan KW, McFarland HF and McFarlin DE (1982) SSPE after passive immunisation and natural measles infection: role of antibody in persistence of measles virus. *Neurology* **32**: 390–394.

Risk WS and Haddad FS (1979) The variable natural history of subacute sclerosing panencephalitis. *Archives of Neurology* **36**: 610–614.

Risk WR, Haddad FS, Dhib-Jalbut S *et al.* (1983) Epidemiology of SSPE: 136 cases from the Middle East. *Proceedings of the First International Symposium Subacute Sclerosing Panencephalitis*, Beirut, 1983, pp 197–213.

Saha V (1989) Diagnosis of subacute sclerosing panencephalitis. The Vellore Experience. *Proceedings of the Third International Symposium on SSPE*, Vellore, India, pp 137–141.

Saha V, John TJ, Mukundan P *et al.* (1990) High incidence of subacute sclerosing panencephalitis in South India. *Epidemiology and Infection* **104**: 151–156.

Salmi AA, Norrby E and Panelius M (1972) Identification of different measles virus specific antibodies in the serum and cerebrospinal fluid from patients with subacute sclerosing panencephalitis and multiple sclerosis. *Infection and Immunity* **6**: 248–254.

Schoub BD, Johnson S and McAnerney Jo M (1992) Observations of subacute sclerosing panencephalitis in South Africa. *Transactions of The Royal Society of Tropical Medicine and Hygiene* **86**: 550–551.

Scully RE, Mark EJ and McNeely VU (1986) Case records of the Massachusetts General Hospital. *New England Journal of Medicine* **314**: 1689–1700.

Tellez NI and Harter DH (1966) Subacute sclerosing leukoencephalitis: ultrastructure of intranuclear and intracytoplasmic inclusions. *Science* **154**: 899–901.

Thormar H, Mehta PD and Brown HR (1978) Comparison of wild type and subacute sclerosing panencephalitis strains of measles virus: neurovirulence in ferrets and biological properties in cell cultures. *Journal of Experimental Medicine* **148**: 551–556.

Trapani GDi, Mazza S, Tomassetti *et al.* (1991) Clinical-electrophysiological correlations in a long term case of subacute schlerosing panencephalitis with partial clinical improvement. *European Neurology* **31**: 23–29.

Vani KR, Yasha TC, Rao VT *et al.* (1994) Measles virus antigen localisation in the brains of subacute sclerosing panencephalitis – a pathological and immunochemical study. *Neurology India* **42**: 69–75.

Winer JB, Pires M, Kermode A *et al.* (1990) Resolving MRI abnormalities with progression of subacute sclerosing panencephalitis. *Neuroradiology* **33(2)**: 178–180.

Wong TC, Ayata M, Ueda S *et al.* (1991) Role of biased hypermutation in evolution of subacute sclerosing panencephalitis virus from progenitor acute measles virus. *Journal of Virology* **65(5)**: 2191–2199.

Wulff CH (1982) Subacute sclerosing panencephalitis: serial electroencephalographic studies. *Journal of Neurology, Neurosurgery and Psychiatry* **45**: 418–421.

Yagi S, Miura Y, Kataoka N *et al.* (1992) The origin of myoclonus and periodic synchronous discharges in subacute sclerosing panencephalitis. *Acta Paediatrica Juponica* **34**: 310–315.

7

Poliomyelitis and Other Anterior Horn Cell Disorders

M. Gourie-Devi

Department of Neurology, National Institute of Mental Health and Neurosciences, Bangalore, India

INTRODUCTION

In many tropical countries acute paralytic poliomyelitis continues to be the commonest anterior horn cell disorder. The prevalence of chronic degenerative disorders such as amyotrophic lateral sclerosis (ALS) and spinal muscular atrophy is similar to that in more developed countries. Community-based survey of a rural population of 57 660 in Gowribidanur, State of Karnataka, India showed that the prevalence of amyotrophic lateral sclerosis was 4 per 100 000, similar to that in Western countries which varies from 1 to 7 per 100 000 population (Kurtzke, 1982; Gourie-Devi, 1986; Gourie-Devi et al., 1987a). The clinical profile of ALS is, in general, uniform with the exception of lower age of onset in the developing world compared with Western societies, 46 versus 66 years (Juergens et al., 1980; Gourie-Devi et al., 1987b). Motor neurone disease in those 30 years of age or younger accounts for nearly one-third of cases seen in India and Nigeria (Osuntokun et al., 1974; Bharucha et al., 1987; Chopra et al., 1987; Gourie-Devi et al., 1987b).

Atypical and relatively benign forms of chronic anterior horn cell (AHC) disorders, the monomelic amyotrophy and Madras motor neurone disease, which have unique geographic distribution to Asian countries, merit special mention. Both these disorders constituted 12% of 323 chronic AHC disorders in a large series from South India (Gourie-Devi et al., 1987a).

In this chapter, acute poliomyelitis and its late effects, monomelic amyotrophy and Madras motor neurone disease are considered in detail in view of their special relevance to tropical countries.

POLIOMYELITIS

The resolution of the World Health Assembly in 1988 to eradicate poliomyelitis by the year 2000 is a landmark event in the long struggle against this disease (WHO, 1988). The epidemiology of poliomyelitis has changed considerably from what was originally a relatively uncommon disease occurring sporadically, affecting infants and confined to countries with temperate climate, to an epidemic disease affecting older individuals and with rapid spread to tropical countries (Nathanson and Martin, 1979).

In many developed countries, sustained use of polio virus vaccine has led to a decline in the incidence of poliomyelitis and to eventual elimination of wild poliovirus infection (Strebel *et al.*, 1992). Recently, the Pan American Health Organisation announced the elimination of poliomyelitis from Latin America (de Quadros *et al.*, 1991).

Epidemiology

The global incidence of polio has shown a dramatic fall from 66 per 1000 in 1981 to 8 per 1000 in 1993 and the number of countries reporting no cases for the year has steadily increased from 80 in 1985 to 141 in 1993 (WHO, 1994). An efficient surveillance system capable of detecting all cases of poliomyelitis is crucial in determining the incidence. Unfortunately, in countries with high levels of poliomyelitis the efficiency of surveillance is far from satisfactory at less than 10%. Poliomyelitis is widespread in India and continues to be a major public health problem. With enhanced coverage by oral polio vaccine (OPV) there is a decline in reported cases of poliomyelitis (WHO, 1994). Despite this success, it is a matter of serious concern that the Indian subcontinent contributes three of every four poliomyelitis cases reported in the world.

In developing countries, lameness surveys have been used as an alternative method to estimate paralytic poliomyelitis. Prevalence varies from 6.8 per 1000 children 5–9 years old in Nigeria to 8.8 per 1000 children 0–14 years old in India (Parakoyi and Babaniyi, 1990; Kumar *et al.*, 1991). In a community-based neuroepidemiological survey in rural Karnataka in India, the crude prevalence rate of poliomyelitis sequelae was 99 per 100 000 population, ranking fourth among all neurological disorders (Gourie-Devi *et al.*, 1987a). The age-specific rate per 1000 children of 0–5 years was 3.4 and for 6–10 years was 1.5. Another effective approach is the survey of acute flaccid paralysis (AFP) in the Americas (Dietz *et al.*, 1992). While the sensitivity of AFP defined 'as a child less than 15 years of age with acute flaccid paralysis' was high, the specificity for detecting paralytic poliomyelitis was low. Laboratory confirmation of poliomyelitis for all such identified cases is necessary for determining prevalence. Acute-onset flaccid paralysis includes a wide variety of neurological disorders, with geographical differences. For example, in Northern China, acute motor axonal neuropathy, also known as Chinese paralytic syndrome, has emerged as a distinctive clinical entity (McKhann *et al.*, 1993). Recognizing the importance of AFP survey, the World Health Organization recently prepared a document reviewing current information on AFP and formulated diagnostic criteria (WHO, 1993).

In countries considered to be free from indigenous wild poliovirus a small number of imported cases have been reported (Hovi *et al.*, 1983; Sutter *et al.*, 1991; Joce *et al.*, 1992; Strebel *et al.*, 1992). Very recently, poliomyelitis cases have been reported in Netherlands and Canada among members of religious groups that do not accept vaccination (CDC, 1992 and 1993) and others in Malaysia who opted not to vaccinate their children for sociocultural reasons (Ismail and Lal, 1993). Outbreaks of polio can also occur when the herd immunity to the virus strain is poor as was seen in recent years in Finland (Hovi *et al.*, 1986). The frequency of vaccine-associated paralytic poliomyelitis (VAPP) although low with approximately one case per 2.5 million doses of OPV, is causing concern in countries that have almost eliminated wild polio virus (Strebel *et al.*, 1992). Infants receiving first or second dose of OPV, contacts of recipients of OPV and immunocompromised individuals are at risk for developing VAPP.

Poliomyelitis is a seasonal disease occurring usually in hot and rainy seasons and generally affects children under 3 years of age. The disease is more severe when older children and adults are affected. In poliomyelitis and other enterovirus infections males are more frequently affected and suffer from more severe disease than females. Increased incidence of paralysis in those receiving injections within a month of infection with poliovirus is a well-recognized feature. In the recent large outbreak in Oman, immunization with diphtheria and tetanus toxoid and pertussis vaccine injection during the incubation period of polio virus infection was considered to have caused provocative poliomyelitis (Sutter *et al.*, 1992). It has been suggested that injection produces damage to nerve endings allowing easy access of polio virus to the nervous system (Wyatt, 1990) and, by inducing reflex hyperemia in the spinal cord associated with the area injected, leads to localization of the virus (Bodian, 1954). Irrespective of the causal mechanisms, the public health message to avoid unnecessary injections in children, particularly in polio endemic countries emerges quite clearly. Other predisposing factors like tonsillectomy, trauma and physical exertion influence the severity and location of the disease.

Pathogenesis

The poliovirus belongs to the group of human enteroviruses which comprise a genus in the picornavirus family. The usual method of spread from host to host is by faecal contamination and is primarily an enteric infection with the virus replicating in the cells of the oropharynx and intestine and later spreading to lymphatic tissues. This is followed by viraemia and 1–4 weeks later the central nervous system (CNS) is involved. An alternative pathway of virus spread to the nervous system from the intestine is along peripheral nerves (Sabin, 1956). The infection is inapparent without any clinical symptons in 90–95% of infected individuals and the ratio of paralytic to subclinical infection in poliomyelitis is low ranging from 1:100 to 1:1000 (Melnick and Ledinko, 1953).

The selective vulnerability of motor neurones in the anterior horn of the spinal cord has been attributed to the presence of viral receptors on the cell surface or alternatively to the spread of virus along nerve fibres (Brown *et al.*, 1987). Other neurones which may also be involved are intermediate and posterior horn nuclei in the spinal cord, motor nuclei and reticular formation nuclei in the brainstem and Betz cells and neurones in the thalamus and hypothalamus. Lesions in cerebellar vermis and roof nuclei have also been documented.

Clinical Features

The paralytic phase is often preceded by a preparalytic period of 1–2 days, with symptoms of fever, headache, vomiting, diarrhoea, sore throat and muscle pain. Either immediately or within 3–4 days, CNS involvement can occur and non-paralytic poliomyelitis with meningitis, encephalitis or, rarely, acute cerebellar ataxia are seen. The virus may be cleared during any of these stages. Among the three paralytic syndromes of spinal, bulbar and bulbospinal types, the spinal form is by far the commonest. Rapidly progressive asymmetric flaccid paralysis beginning more often in lower than in upper limbs, with hyporeflexia reaching a maximum within 5–6 days, is the typical picture. Bulbar paralysis is known to occur in 8–18% of patients in the tropics (Mahadevan *et al.*, 1989). The observation that the serious forms such as bulbar and bulbospinal occur more in partially immunized than in non-immunized children has not been confirmed in recent studies (Deivanayagam and Nedunchelian, 1991). Facial weakness, dysphagia and dysphonia are common while weakness of muscles innervated by the trigeminal and hypoglossal nerves are much less common and extraocular muscles involvement is rare. Bulbar poliomyelitis is generally associated with spinal involvement, and is infrequently restricted to the bulbar cranial nerves. Sensory loss is rare, although severe muscle pain is seen in the acute phase.

Cerebrospinal fluid shows leukocytosis varying from 30 to 100 mm^{-3}, initially dominated by polymorphs with an early shift within a few hours to 2 days to lymphocytes. Isolation and culture of wild-type poliovirus from the stool provides confirmation. However, in countries where wild virus is widespread, false-positive stool cultures in carriers may confuse the picture and the paralysis may be due to some other agent (Achar, 1973). In such situations, a four-fold rise in antibody titre is a reliable diagnostic parameter. Recently, demonstration of poliovirus-specific IgM antibodies in serum and CSF by mu-capture immuno-assay has been shown to be sensitive and specific (Roivainen *et al.*, 1993). New methods for detection of poliovirus include rapid identification and typing of poliovirus isolates in cell cultures from stool specimen by indirect immunofluor-escence microscopy, identification by polymerase chain reaction (PCR) based on the nucleotide sequence of their RNA genome, and enzyme-linked immuno-sorbent assays (ELISA) using polyclonal and monoclonal antibodies (Novak and Kirkegaard, 1991).

Viruses Other Than Poliovirus Causing 'Poliomyelitis-like Acute Paralysis'

Enteroviruses other than poliovirus, including echovirus-3, coxsackie and entero-virus-71, have been implicated in acute paralytic disorders simulating poliomye-litis (CDC, 1981). Milder forms of the disease commonly without residual deficit are features that differentiate paralysis caused by non-polio enteroviruses from poliovirus. Acute, asymmetric and flaccid paralysis of limbs with or without cranial nerve paralysis appearing a few days to weeks after an episode of acute haemorrhagic conjunctivitis (AHC) due to EV70 occurred in epidemic form in many countries including India, Taiwan, Thailand and Senegal (Wadia *et al.*, 1972; Kono *et al.*, 1976). In a small percentage (less than 10%) when there is no definite history of AHC preceding the neurological disease, the differentiation from poliomyelitis has to be made by serology, since virus isolation from CSF is not successful.

Differential Diagnosis

Acute paralytic poliomyelitis (APP) has to be differentiated from other causes of acute flaccid paralysis, the commonest being Guillain–Barré syndrome (GBS), since identification of even one case of poliomyelitis calls for intense and widespread immunization. Studies by the Pan American Health Organisation of 6859 children with AFP showed that in the majority (75–80%) no virus was isolated from stool culture, wild polio virus in 6%, vaccine-related poliovirus in 5% and other enteroviruses in 15% (Sabin, 1991). Many of the children were therefore considered to have GBS. The presence of bilateral facial weakness, normal cell count and elevated protein in CSF and electrophysiological evidence of abnormal conduction support the diagnosis of GBS. In acute motor axonal neuropathy (AMAN), seasonal occurrence, bilateral facial weakness, frequent involvement of tongue and normal CSF cell count are distinctive features (McKhann *et al.*, 1993). Nerve conduction and electromyographic findings are similar in AMAN and poliomyelitis. In the interesting disorder of 'acute oculobulbar palsy with flaccid paralysis' (AOBP) the features of acute onset of ptosis, external ophthalmoplegia and bulbar paralysis with mild to moderate weakness of limbs are distinctive enough to differentiate it from poliomyelitis (Saini *et al.*, 1986; Gourie-Devi, 1993). Although similar cases have been reported following snake bite, the absence of snake bite in patients with AOBP, spontaneous and dramatic recovery with little or no residual deficit are other characteristic features. Differentiation of cerebral diplegia from poliomye-litis may pose special problems in infants up to the age of 18 months since the presence of extensor plantars may be seen in normal infants and spasticity may not become obvious until 10–18 months of age (Crawford and Hobbs, 1991). Late acquisition of developmental milestones, persistence of primitive responses such as Moro response, palmar grasp, automatic walking, tonic neck reflexes and brisk tendon jerks distinguish it from poliomyelitis.

Treatment and Prevention

In the acute stage, analgesics and hot packs should be given for relief of muscle pain and overstretching of muscles should be prevented by proper positioning and splints to prevent contractures. Gentle passive movement of the limbs in the active stage of the disease and active physiotherapy in the convalescent phase prevent contractures and facilitate recovery. Ventilatory support is necessary for a few patients who have severe bulbar or combination of bulbar and spinal forms. Non-invasive ventilatory support alternatives have been found to result in greater life satisfaction than ventilation through a tracheostomy, for those requiring long-term ventilatory support (Bach and Campagnolo, 1992). In the later stage, after maximum recovery is attained, surgical correction of deformities can be considered to improve mobility and quality of life.

Prevention of poliomyelitis is by immunization with inactivated (Salk) poliovirus vaccine (IPV) and live (Sabin) oral poliovirus vaccine (OPV). IPV-E indicating enhanced potency is also in use currently. Controversy and conflicting opinions on the efficacy of immunization with IPV and OPV continue (Patriarca *et al.*, 1993). In developed countries, using a three-dose schedule of OPV with a coverage of 65% in children 1–4 years of age, the circulation of wild poliovirus was eliminated due to 'herd' immunity (Nathanson, 1982). Unfortunately, in developing countries, several large-scale epidemics occurred despite apparent adequate coverage (Sutter *et al.*, 1991; Otten *et al.*, 1992; John, 1993). This was attributed to short-lived gut immunity due to OPV which was overcome by wild poliovirus type I. This relatively lower susceptibility of children in developing countries to gut infection, illustrates the geographic differences in immunogenic efficacy of OPV between developed and developing countries (John, 1975; Ramia and Arif, 1991). A five-dose OPV schedule has been suggested to overcome this problem (Balraj *et al.*, 1990). IPV has also been effectively used in many developed and developing countries, and has the additional advantage of being a component of routine immunization schedule by combining the diphtheria–pertusis–tetanus (DPT) vaccine. Further, it is completely safe, unlike OPV which carries a risk of paralytic illness. However, the cost is higher than OPV. Sequential use of IPV and OPV in some countries has led to effective elimination of wild poliovirus and decreased the risk of VAPP (McBean and Modlin, 1987; Strebel *et al.*, 1992). In addition to routine immunization schedules, supplementation with a mass campaign like annual national immunization days has been found to be effective (Kumar *et al.*,

1991). The ease of delivery, acceptability, cost, availability, are some of the issues central to an immunization programme.

Prognosis

Following the acute paralytic phase, improvement usually occurs within the first 3–6 months, and may continue to occur for up to 2 years. Varying degree of residual neurological deficit is often seen with significant disability and eventually reaches a plateau in three-quarters of poliomyelitis survivors while the remaining 25% go on to develop postpoliomyelitis syndrome when new symptoms of fatigue, muscle pain, weakness and atrophy develop two or more decades later (Figure 7.1). Chronic persistence of poliovirus leading to chronic CNS infection is extremely rare and has been reported only in those who are immunodeficient (Wyatt, 1973).

A multipronged approach by strengthening of surveillance of AFP, establishing well-equipped laboratories for confirmation of diagnosis, ensuring adequate supplies of vaccine, public health education, active community participation and support from governmental and non-governmental organizations will facilitate

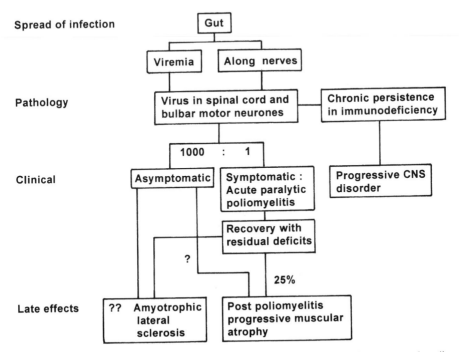

Figure 7.1 Schematic depiction of natural history of poliomyelitis. (Concept of asymptomatic polio leading to postpoliomyelitis progressive muscular atrophy (PPMA) and role of poliovirus in amyotrophic lateral sclerosis (ALS) have to be confirmed.)

the expanded programme on immunization and eventually lead to global eradication of poliomyelitis.

LATE EFFECTS OF POLIOMYELITIS (POSTPOLIO SYNDROME)

Although it was recognized more than 100 years ago that survivors of APP may develop new symptoms years later, this problem has attracted increasing attention only in the last two decades. The entity of postpolio syndrome (PPS) broadly includes a spectrum of clinical features some of which can be attributed to increasing joint instability due to physical effort over a number of years and gain in weight, neuromuscular symptoms due to root, plexus or nerve compression as a result of long-term use of orthotic appliances, wheelchair, etc., and progressive increase in scoliosis, due to unequal limb length and leading to respiratory problems. A distinct clinical syndrome 'postpoliomyelitis progressive muscular atrophy' (PPMA) comprising new weakness and atrophy starting decades after APP, has been attributed to ongoing dynamic changes in the motor units (Dalakas et al., 1984). Specific criteria laid down by Mulder et al. (1972) for the diagnosis of late progression of poliomyelitis include: a credible history of poliomyelitis, partial recovery of function, a minimum 10-year period of stabilization of this recovery from acute poliomyelitis, and the subsequent development of progressive muscular weakness.

Incidence

There are no exact estimates of the frequency of PPMA in different countries, except for a few studies which showed that 25–80% of polio survivors are likely to develop new weakness (Cood et al., 1984; Windebank et al., 1987). In developing countries, the burden of acute poliomyelitis is quite enormous with high numbers of survivors and, therefore, the incidence is also likely to be considerable. No accurate figures exist.

The interval between the onset of APP and the development of new symptoms has ranged from 28.8 to 42.8 years with a mean of 36 years in more developed countries (Halstead et al., 1985; Jubelt and Cashman, 1987; Dalakas and Illa, 1991). In our series from India, in 13 patients seen during a period of 15 years, the interval ranged from 14 to 37 years, with a mean of 23.2 years (Gourie-Devi et al., unpublished observation), a decade earlier than in the more developed countries. A significant observation by Halstead et al. (1985) is that in the patients the interval of occurrence of PPMA (34.4 years median) was shorter by two decades in those with severe initial disease compared with less severe disease (55.8 years median). Risk factors associated with PPMA are onset of poliomyelitis after the age of 10 years, paralysis of all four limbs and requirement of a ventilator (Halstead et al., 1985). All these factors suggest a severe disease. Occurrence of polio at an early age (mean age in our series was 2.4

years), generally below 3 years in developing countries, may be one of the reasons for the lack of reports of many patients with PPMA from these countries. The degree of functional recovery from the initial weakness has also been observed to be an important predictor (Klingman *et al.*, 1988). Recovery from APP has been attributed to reinnervation of muscle fibres with resultant large motor units which are at greater risk of metabolic stress and thus susceptible to delayed dysfunction and death. A definite preponderance of PPMA in men has been observed. The association of minor trauma to the onset of symptoms in PPMA is controversial.

Clinical Features

The chief clinical features of PPMA are muscle weakness, atrophy and pain, cramps and fasciculations. The new weakness and atrophy can involve the muscles affected in the acute paralytic episode which have fully or partially recovered or remained the same (Figure 7.2). Even previously unaffected

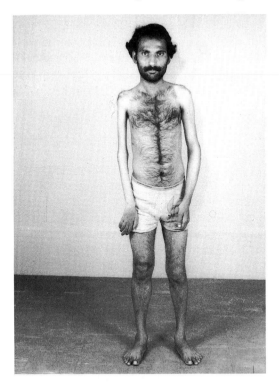

Figure 7.2 A 24-year-old male patient with postpoliomyelitis progressive muscular atrophy. Polio at 3 years of age with involvement of all four limbs; residual deficit of atrophy and weakness of right upper limb; new weakness and atrophy of both upper limbs and left lower limb at 18 years of age.

muscles can be involved. Increasing difficulty in activities that earlier could be satisfactorily performed despite the residual deficit after APP, may result in considerable disability necessitating modification or cessation of the particular activity. More serious consequences, like swallowing difficulty and hypoventilation, may appear due to new weakness of bulbar and intercostal muscles respectively. Muscle pain and cramps are disturbing symptoms interfering with sleep. Recent increase in fasciculations, which were previously present intermittently or continuously over long periods of time, are reported in some patients. The tendon reflexes are sluggish or absent and signs of involvement of upper motor neurone are usually absent, but brisk tendon reflexes without or with extensor plantar response are seen in a few patients (Mulder *et al.*, 1982). The illness progresses slowly with an estimated deterioration of neuromuscular function of 1% per year (Dalakas *et al.*, 1986).

Conventional electromyography findings suggest an ongoing chronic denervation with large motor units providing evidence of coexistent reinnervation and evidence of active, recent denervation by the presence of increased jitter on single fibre EMG (Dalakas *et al.*, 1986; Cashman *et al.*, 1987). Muscle biopsy provides confirmatory evidence for reinnervation (type grouping) and denervation (scattered atrophic angulated fibres) (Dalakas *et al.*, 1986). Unfortunately, neither EMG nor muscle biopsy abnormalities convincingly distinguish PPMA from poliomyelitis with stable residual neurological deficit (Cashman *et al.*, 1987). Interestingly, sparse inflammatory infiltrates in muscle and spinal cord have been observed in poliomyelitis many years after the acute episode and also in those with PPMA (Dalakas *et al.*, 1986; Pezeshkpour and Dalakas, 1988).

Pathogenesis

There is diversity of opinion concerning the aetiology of PPMA. Virologic studies have not provided convincing proof of persistence or reactivation of poliovirus and similarly there is no supportive evidence for immune-mediated mechanisms being responsible (Kurent *et al.*, 1979; Dalakas *et al.*, 1986). However, a recent study has shown increased intrathecal synthesis of IgM antibodies to poliovirus (Sharief *et al.*, 1991). Earlier, it was speculated that loss of unaffected motor neurones with ageing may be responsible for the new weakness and atrophy, but careful studies have shown that decrease in number of motor neurones occurs only after the age of 60 years and therefore the occurrence of PPMA in the fourth decade cannot be explained (Tomlinson and Irving, 1977). The widely accepted hypothesis is that on a background of reduced number of anterior horn cells following poliomyelitis, recovery occurs due to reinnervation of muscles by collateral sprouting with development of large motor units. Over a number of years, as a result of ageing the ability of axons to sprout may decline or the expanded motor units may not be able to sustain the excessive metabolic stress and undergo 'metabolic fatigue' leading to degeneration of collateral or terminal sprouts or even to loss of anterior horn cells

(Pestronk *et al.*, 1980). It is possible that PPMA may also develop in patients who fully recover from the APP since recovery has been attributed to enlarged motor units and these are expected to be larger than in patients with partial recovery (Klingman *et al.*, 1988). Extending this logic to poliovirus infection without clinical paralysis is also plausible (Figure 7.1) since it has been shown that invasion and destruction of 50% of motor neurones by poliovirus is necessary for manifest paralysis (Sharrad, 1953).

Management

Careful assessment of physical ability without fatigue helps in giving appropriate advice for daily activities within the limits of muscle weakness and disability. Careful programmed exercises are found to be beneficial (Owen, 1985). Use of brace, orthotic appliances, wheelchair and ventilator may be necessary along with general measures of weight reduction and corrective surgery. Psychosocial problems seen in many patients need to be resolved by counselling and enhancing social support systems.

POLIOMYELITIS AND AMYOTROPHIC LATERAL SCLEROSIS

A causal relationship between APP and ALS (Figure 7.1) had been suggested based on epidemiological data of higher frequency of poliomyelitis in ALS patients (Zilkha, 1962; Poskanzer *et al.*, 1979). The recent evidence of similar geographic distribution of both the disorders in England and Wales also supports the association (Martyn *et al.*, 1988). These views have, however, been strongly refuted by others (Alter *et al.*, 1982). Virological and immunological studies have yielded conflicting and contradictory evidence and further studies are necessary to resolve the issue (Antel *et al.*, 1976; Kott *et al.*, 1978; Kascsak *et al.*, 1982).

MONOMELIC AMYOTROPHY

Monomelic amyotrophy (MMA) with the characteristic features of wasting and weakness of muscles is usually restricted to a single upper or lower limb. It generally occurs in young males, and has a benign outcome with evidence of anterior horn cell involvement (Gourie-Devi *et al.*, 1984). Hirayama *et al.* (1959) first described young men with atrophy of one upper limb and used the term 'juvenile muscular atrophy of unilateral upper extremity'. From India, since Gourie-Devi *et al.* (1984) observed patients with atrophy of one upper or lower limb, the label of 'monomelic amyotrophy' was proposed to describe the disorder. 'Benign focal amyotrophy', 'wasted leg syndrome' and 'non-familial juvenile spinal muscular atrophy of upper extremity' are some of the other eponyms for this disorder (Prabhakar *et al.*, 1981; Riggs *et al.*, 1984; Peiris *et al.*, 1989). More than 500 patients have been reported, predominantly from countries in Asia which include Japan, India, Hong Kong, Malaysia, Sri Lanka and Taiwan (Hirayama *et al.*, 1959, 1963; Sobue *et al.*, 1978; Singh *et al.*, 1980; Prabhakar *et al.*, 1981; Gourie-Devi *et al.*, 1984, 1987b; Tan *et al.*, 1985; Peiris *et al.*, 1989; Chan *et al.*, 1991; Kao *et al.*, 1993a). Surprisingly, very few similar cases have been reported from Western countries (Pilgaard, 1968; Compernolle, 1973; Riggs *et al.*, 1984; Serratrice *et al.*, 1987). In all reports, unilateral upper limb involvement was commoner than lower limb involvement, and interestingly while upper and lower limb involvement have been reported from India, no cases with lower limb involvement have been observed in Japan. The proportion of single limb atrophy in motor neurone disease is not generally known; data from one centre in South India show that monomelic amyotrophy constituted 8% of all types of chronic anterior horn cell disease (Gourie-Devi *et al.*, 1987b).

Clinical Features

The clinical features are described under two groups: upper limb atrophy and lower limb atrophy.

Upper Limb Atrophy

In the majority, the age of onset ranges from 15 to 36 years (mean 20 years) with very few developing symptoms below the age of 15 years. Men far outnumber women with a ratio of 3.7:1 to 4:1. Right upper limb appears to have a greater predilection than left upper limb. In the vast majority of cases, the atrophy is confined to a single upper limb, but in a few, evidence of contralateral limb affection can be observed during the course of the illness. Except for a few familial cases, almost all are sporadic (Sobue *et al.*, 1978). The onset is insidious with initial symptoms of impairment of skilled finger movements, tremors, atrophy of hand and forearm and worsening of symptoms on exposure to cold. The muscular atrophy has a characteristic pattern with involvement of muscles innervated by C8–T1 roots, i.e. the small muscles of hand and flexors and extensors of the wrist with conspicuous sparing of the brachioradialis (Figure 7.3a, b). In a few patients, the biceps and triceps muscles may also be affected, in others the proximal muscles of the shoulder girdle may be involved and in the majority, fasciculations are seen in atrophied muscles. Minipolymyoclonus observed in outstretched hands is a striking feature and often attracts the attention of the patient. Another noteworthy feature is aggravation of symptoms and weakness and appearance of pain and stiffness on exposure to cold weather or on dipping the hands in cold water. Other autonomic features in the form of sweating disturbances, coldness of hands and cyanosis may be present in a few patients. The tendon reflexes in the affected limb are generally sluggish or absent; in some they are normal and only in a few patients one or more reflexes may be brisk (Sobue *et al.*, 1978; Gourie-Devi *et al.*, 1984). The reflexes in the unaffected upper limb and both lower limbs remain normal. Rarely they may be hyperactive with flexor plantar responses.

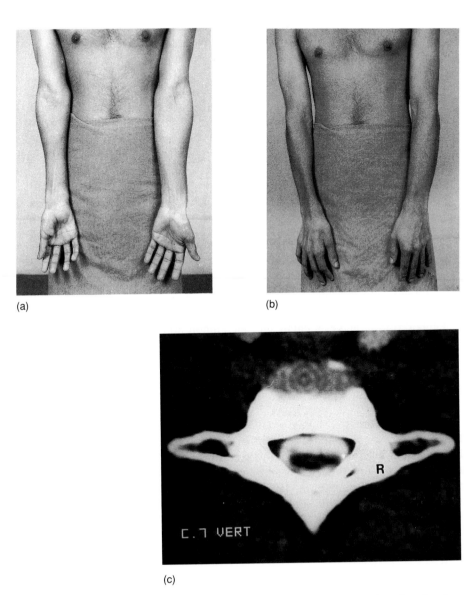

(a)

(b)

(c)

Figure 7.3 Monomelic amyotrophy of right upper limb in a 22-year-old male patient. Atrophy of muscles of hand and forearm: (a) palmar view and (b) dorsal view. Relative sparing of brachioradialis is clearly seen. (c) Metrizamide CT shows focal atrophy of cervical spinal cord on right side at C7 level.

Lower Limb Atrophy

In this group, male preponderance is also seen with a ratio of 20:1. All cases are sporadic with a mean age of onset of 25 years (range 11–36 years), few developing symptoms beyond the age of 30 years. The right lower limb is affected three times as frequently as the left. Unlike in upper limb atrophy, in many, it is difficult to determine exactly the onset since the atrophy is brought to the notice of the patient accidentally by observers. The duration of illness from the time of noticing wasting to first examination ranged from a few weeks to as long as 15 years, the average being 3 years. Pain on walking is an initial symptom in some and, interestingly, very few complain of weakness. The calf muscles are the commonest group to be atrophied, followed in order of frequency by anterior tibial and quadriceps muscles and, in some, atrophy extends proximally to involve gluteii and distally to affect intrinsic muscles of the foot (Figure 7.4a, b). Uniform wasting of the entire extremity is a feature in nearly one-half of the patients. Rarely, the thigh muscles alone are atrophied. Shortening of the limb has not been observed, indicating that the disease did not start in infancy or early childhood. Fasciculations are present in at least one-third of patients, and foot deformity is seen in a few patients. The weakness is mild compared with the degree of atrophy. Tendon reflexes as a rule are sluggish in the atrophied limb and normal in other limbs. Pyramidal signs are absent.

In both groups, hypertrophy of muscles has not been recorded in any patient. Except for mild impairment of sensation reported in a few with upper limb atrophy, other parts of the nervous system are not involved. Skeletal defects such as kyphoscoliosis and pes cavus are uncommon and seen in less than 10% of patients.

Course

The disease progresses slowly over 2–4 years followed by a stationary phase. Even in patients with long duration of illness extending up to 20 years, the disease is confined to one limb in many, while in 13–37%, particularly in cases with upper limb involvement, it may spread to the other upper limb but never to the lower limbs (Sobue *et al.*, 1978; Singh *et al.*, 1980). In patients with lower limb atrophy, the opposite limb has never been found to be affected.

Investigations

Electromyography shows a neurogenic pattern in the atrophied muscles and may also show abnormalities in clinically normal muscles of the affected limb. The clinical symptoms of stiffness of the hand on exposure to cold are not substantiated by EMG evidence of myotonic discharges. In the clinically unaffected

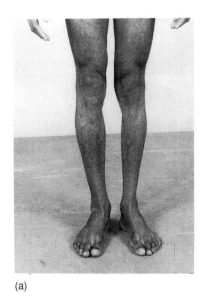

(a)

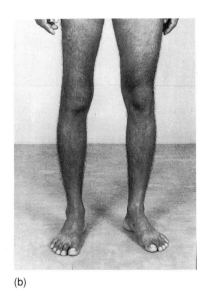

(b)

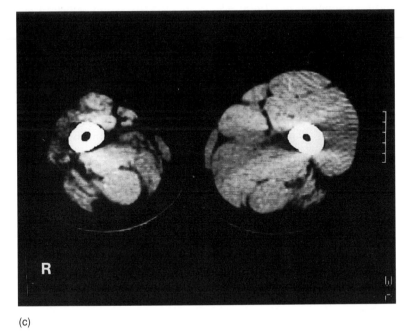

(c)

Figure 7.4 Monomelic amyotrophy of lower limb. (a) Atrophy of muscles of left leg and foot in a 25-year-old male patient. (b) In a 28-year-old male patient, atrophy of muscles of right thigh and slight atrophy of right leg muscles is shown. (c) CT shows gross atrophy of quadriceps femoris and moderate atrophy of posterior femoral muscles.

upper limb, electromyographic abnormalities may be detected in a few cases. In the group with lower limb amyotrophy the changes are less frequent in the unaffected lower limb. Unaffected lower limbs in upper limb atrophy group and upper limbs in lower limb atrophy group do not show electromyographic abnormalities. The motor nerve conduction is normal or shows a mild reduction due to drop out of motor units. Conduction block has not been reported (Gourie-Devi et al., 1987b). Muscle biopsy provides confirmatory evidence of chronic partial denervation with reinnervation. Combination of neurogenic atrophy and myopathic changes has also been observed (Prabhakar et al., 1981; Gourie-Devi et al., 1984).

Metrizamide computerized tomography (CT) myelography and magnetic resonance imaging (MRI) may demonstrate localized spinal cord atrophy in the lower cervical segments which is unilateral or asymmetrical (Figure 7.3c) with more change on the side of the muscular atrophy (Metcalf et al., 1987; Mukai et al., 1987; Gourie-Devi et al., 1992). Additional findings in some cases are stretching and ventral shifting of the cord in the ventroflexed position of the neck, increased signal intensity in the posterior epidural space representing congestion of the internal vertebral venous plexus (Mukai et al., 1987). Studies to look for evidence of viral infection have not shown antibodies for polio, cox sackie B group, Echo group, influenza A and B, adenogroup and herpes simplex viruses (Sobue et al., 1978; Kao et al., 1993b). No evidence of hexosaminidase deficiency has been detected (personal unpublished observations).

Pathological study, based on a single autopsy of a patient who had one upper limb atrophy from the age of 15 years and died of lung cancer at 38 years, showed a decrease in the number of both large and small anterior horn cells at the level of the lower cervical segments, particularly C7 and C8, and chromatolysis with lipofuchsin accumulation (Hirayama et al., 1987). There were no changes in the blood vessels, the posterior horns and white matter.

Upper limb atrophy has to be distinguished from intrinsic spinal cord lesions, root, brachial plexus and peripheral nerve disorders. The characteristic pattern of muscle weakness and wasting, absence of sensory abnormalities, electrophysiological tests and CT myelography or MRI help in excluding other disorders. In countries where leprosy is endemic, unusual forms of leprous neuropathy presenting with pure motor features of wasting and weakness of small muscles of the hand need particular mention. The lack of past history of poliomyelitis in childhood with residual deficit differentiates MMA from PPMA. In distal chronic spinal muscular atrophy, the wasting and weakness may be confined to one hand and these cases resemble the present condition. However, in most of these patients, EMG abnormalities are seen in both upper and in some lower limbs as well, indicating that the disease process is more diffuse than MMA. In rare instances when the atrophy is confined to quadriceps femoris muscle the possibility of femoral neuropathy or myopathy have to be considered. Electromyography, nerve conduction and muscle biopsy will clarify the matter. It is noteworthy that in MMA isolated atrophy of quadriceps muscle has not been seen without associated wasting of leg or foot muscles. Polymyositis, although usually symmetric, in rare instances can manifest with involvement of one limb, remaining either confined to the limb, or extending years later to involve the other limbs. The schematic approach to single limb atrophy in the young shown in Figure 7.5 may be useful in analysing the problem of wasting and weakness confined to a single limb.

Aetiopathogenesis

The possible aetiological considerations include viral infections and vascular insufficiency of the spinal cord. The studies done so far do not provide supportive evidence for past infection with polio or other viruses (Sobue *et al.*, 1978; Kao *et al.*, 1993b). Since the criteria laid down by Mulder *et al.* (1972) are not satisfied, MMA stands out quite distinctly from PPMA. However, latent infection with poliovirus causing slow loss of anterior horn cells remains a possibility and further studies are necessary to address this issue.

It has been suggested that there might be progressive anterior horn cell degeneration due to a vascular lesion with the associated factors of handedness and strenuous exercises such as sports, precipitating the symptoms (Hirayama *et al.*, 1959). Based on the recent observations on CT myelography and MRI of focal cord atrophy and stretching of cervical cord during flexion of the neck with forward movement of dural canal resulting in traction, compression and vascular insufficiency in the anterior spinal artery territory may be implicated in the pathogenesis (Mukai *et al.*, 1987; Gourie-Devi *et al.*, 1992). In a case control study of 21 patients and 63 control subjects to identify the risk factors associated with MMA, among a number of factors examined, heavy physical activity emerged as the only significant factor, providing further support to the hypothesis of vascular insufficiency (Gourie-Devi *et al.*, 1993). The autopsy findings in one case also suggest vascular insufficiency (Hirayama *et al.*, 1987).

Prognosis

Monomelic amyotrophy is a benign disease with mild disability. The disability is more obvious in patients with upper limb atrophy as some of the critical activities like eating or writing may be partially affected. In individuals with more severe degree of wasting and weakness of hand muscles, training to acquire skilled movements with the other hand may be needed. In those with lower limb involvement there is almost no disability as individuals can take part in almost all daily activities, including walking and running. Reassurance to the patient and the family that the disease does not carry a gloomy prognosis helps restore confidence.

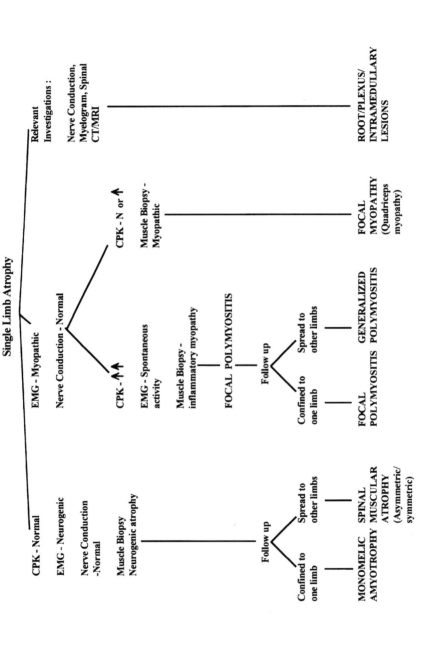

Figure 7.5 Scheme for approach to single liimb atrophy in the young.

MADRAS PATTERN OF MOTOR NEURONE DISEASE

A slow progressive type of sporadic motor neurone disease in the young was recognized in 1970 in Madras, Tamil Nadu, South India, with the special features of deafness and bulbar cranial nerve involvement in more than half the patients (Meenakshisundaram *et al.*, 1970). It is surprising that from the rest of the Indian subcontinent only a few patients have been reported from South India outside Tamil Nadu, West and North India (Wadia *et al.*, 1987; Gourie-Devi and Suresh, 1988). From the other countries in Asia and Africa there are no reports of similar cases.

Clinical Features

The condition (MMND) is sporadic in occurrence, with insidious onset and a slow progression. The age at onset is in the second or the third decade (range 7–30 years, mean 15 years), although in a few patients the illness can start in the first decade (Jagannathan and Kumaresan, 1987; Gourie-Devi and Suresh, 1988).

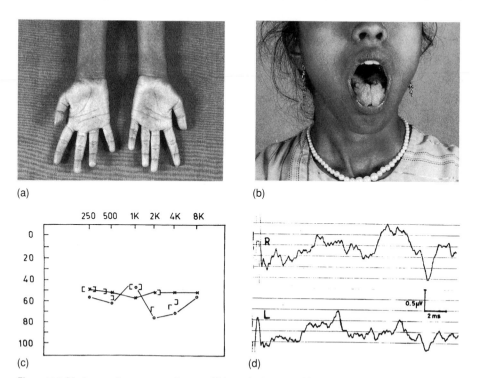

(a)

(b)

(c)

(d)

Figure 7.6 Madras motor neurone disease. Girl aged 17 years with (a) atrophy of intrinsic muscles of both hands; (b) gross atrophy of tongue. (c) Audiogram showing bilateral moderate sensorineural loss (O – right; X – left) and (d) brainstem auditory evoked responses showing absence of all waves (R – right; L – left).

Males are twice as frequently affected as females. The duration of the illness at presentation varies from a few months to 20 years with a mean of 4 years. The most common initial symptoms are atrophy and weakness in the distal muscles of the upper limbs, dysarthria, dysphagia and progressive hearing loss (Figure 7.6a). Mild gait disturbance is also a common complaint and is often due to spasticity but in a few bilateral foot drop causing high steppage gait can also occur. As the illness progresses there is evidence of extension to the proximal muscles of the arms and shoulder girdle. In many the atrophy is asymmetric and continues to be so even after years of the illness. Fasciculations are commonly seen in the affected muscles and in some cases minipolymyoclonus of fingers is quite prominent. Tendon reflexes are usually brisk in all limbs, although occasionally the reflexes are sluggish in upper limbs when wasting of muscles is severe. Extensor plantar response is invariably present. Superficial reflexes, abdominal and cremasteric, are preserved. Bulbar cranial nerve involvement is seen in nearly 75% of the subjects, the most common being atrophy, weakness and fasciculations of the tongue (Figure 7.6b). Slurred speech, dysphagia, nasal regurgitation, hoarseness, nasal intonation of voice and sluggish palatal move-ment are seen. Trapezius and sternomastoid muscles are less frequently involved. In nearly a third, bilateral asymmetric facial palsy of peripheral type is noted. Deafness may appear either as an initial symptom along with motor symptoms or with bulbar cranial nerve involvement, or may follow them after an interval. In rare instances, deafness may even precede other neurological symptoms. Sensorineural deafness is an unique feature of this disorder and is observed in more than half the affected individuals. The hearing impairment is characteristically bilateral and progresses slowly over a few months to years leading to deafness.

Electromyography and muscle biopsy show evidence of chronic partial denervation with reinnervation. Active denervation is seen in limb muscles in a few patients. Abnormalities of carbohydrate metabolism with high plasma pyruvate and low citrate levels are significant findings (Valmikinathan *et al.*, 1973). No abnormalities of hexosaminidase levels have been demonstrated (personal unpublished observations). Cranial CT done in a few patients has not shown any evidence of atrophy of the brainstem. Audiometry shows sensori-neural deafness varying from moderate to complete (Figure 7.6c). Electro-cochleography shows preservation of cochlear microphonics (Wadia *et al.*, 1987) and brainstem auditory evoked responses (BAER) show absence of all waves (Figure 7.6d). These abnormalities are invariably present in symptomatic subjects but may also be detected in the absence of impairment of hearing. Caloric tests are normal, indicating intact vestibular function.

Pathogenesis

MMND is restricted to the Indian subcontinent, particularly affecting South Indians who are of Dravidan origin. There is no clue that this could be a genetic disorder, as all the reported cases have been non-familial (Jagannathan and Kumaresan, 1987; Gourie-Devi and Suresh, 1988). Similarly it is unlikely that environmental factors are responsible, since there was no history of exposure to any particular type of toxin or environmental pollutant. There are no significant antecedent events to implicate viral infection like poliomyelitis, trauma, electric shock or vaccination in the causation of the disease (Jagannathan and Kumaresan, 1987). Neuroaudiological tests showing sensorineural loss on audiometry, preservation of cochlear microphonics and absence of all waves of BAER, localize the site of the lesion in the cochlear nerve or in the spinal ganglion (Wadia *et al.*, 1987). The main brunt is clearly on the motor nuclei of cranial nerves and anterior horn cells in cervical spinal cord as well as corticospinal tracts. In the absence of autopsy studies, it is not known whether there is involvement of other tracts.

Prognosis

The muscle wasting and weakness in the limbs progresses slowly over years, yet does not lead to significant disability. The tongue also atrophies slowly but the bulbar palsy is not severe enough to necessitate nasogastric tube feeding even in patients with many years of progression, as long as 20 years (Gourie-Devi and Suresh, 1988). The hearing impairment, however, progresses in many to almost total deafness and constitutes a serious handicap. There is no documented case of a patient having died due to the illness.

CONCLUSION

This chapter reviews the current global status of poliomyelitis with respect to incidence, immunization and strategy adopted towards eradication. Increasing awareness of postpoliomyelitis progressive muscular atrophy and the physical, emotional and social consequences of new weakness and its pathogenesis are highlighted. In view of the unique geographic distribution of the two benign forms of motor neurone disease, monomelic amyotrophy and Madras motor neurone disease, to Asian countries, the clinical and epidemiological data of these disorders are reviewed.

ACKNOWLEDGEMENTS

The author is grateful to Dr T.G. Suresh, who was earlier associated with the work on monomelic amyotrophy, Madras motor neurone disease and postpoliomyelitis progressive muscular atrophy. The help of Mr H. Nagaraj in preparation of the manuscript is also acknowledged.

REFERENCES

Achar ST (1973) Acute infectious diseases. In: *Pediatrics in Developing Tropical Countries* (ed. J Viswannathan), pp 228–268. New Delhi: Orient Longman.

Alter M, Kurland LT and Molgaard CA (1982) Late progressive muscular atrophy and antecedent poliomyelitis. In: *Human Motor Neurone Diseases* (ed. LP Rowland), pp 303–309, New York: Raven Press.

Antel JP, Arnason BGW, Fuller TC and Lehrich JR (1976) Histocompatibility typing in amyotrophic lateral sclerosis. *Archives of Neurology* **33**: 423–425.

Bach JR and Campagnolo DI (1992) Psychosocial adjustment of post-poliomyelitis ventilator assisted individuals. *Archives of Physical Medicine and Rehabilitation* **73**: 934–939.

Balraj V, John TJ, Thomas M and Mukundan S (1990) Efficacy of oral poliovirus vaccine in rural communities of North Arcot district, India. *International Journal of Epidemiology* **19**: 711–714.

Bharucha EP, Bharucha NE and Bhandari SN (1987) Motor neurone disease in West India. In: *Motor Neurone Disease: Global Clinical Patterns and International Research* (ed. M. Gourie-Devi), pp 165–170. New Delhi: Oxford & IBH.

Bodian D (1954) Viremia in experimental poliomyelitis II. Viremia and the mechanism of the 'provoking' effect of injections or trauma. *American Journal of Hygiene* **60**: 358–370.

Brown Jr RH, Johnson D, Ogonowski M and Weiner HL (1987) Type I human poliovirus binds to human synaptosomes. *Annals of Neurology* **21**: 64–70.

Cashman NR, Maselli R and Wollmann RL (1987) Late denervation in patients with antecedent paralytic poliomyelitis. *New England Journal of Medicine* **317**: 7–12.

CDC (1981) Enterovirus surveillance report. 1970–1979.

CDC (1992) Poliomyelitis outbreak – Netherlands, 1992. *Morbidity and Mortality Weekly Report* **41**: 979–999.

CDC (1993) Isolation of wild poliovirus type 3 among members of a religious community objecting to vaccination – Alberta, Canada. *Journal of the American Medical Association* **269**: 3104.

Chan YW, Kay R and Schwartz MS (1991) Juvenile distal spinal muscular atrophy of upper extremities in Chinese males: single fiber electromyographic study of arms and legs. *Journal of Neurology, Neurosurgery and Psychiatry* **54**: 165–166.

Chopra JS, Prabhakar S, Singh AP and Banerjee AK (1987) Pattern of motor neurone disease in North India and wasted leg syndrome. In: *Motor Neurone Disease: Global Clinical Patterns and International Research* (ed. M Gourie-Devi), pp 147–163. New Delhi: Oxford & IBH.

Compernolle T (1973) A case of juvenile muscular atrophy confined to one upper limb. *European Neurology* **10**: 237–242.

Cood MB, Mulder DW, Kurland LT, Beard CH and O'Fallon WM (1984) Poliomyelitis in Rochester Minnesota 1935–1955. Epidemiology and long-term sequelae: a preliminary report. In: *Late Effects of Poliomyelitis* (eds LS Halstead and DO Wiechers), pp 121–134, Miami, Symposia Foundation.

Crawford CL and Hobbs MJ (1991) Infantile paralysis in developing countries: is it poliomyelitis or diplegia? *Lancet* **337**: 284–286.

Dalakas M and Illa I (1991) Post-polio syndrome: concepts in clinical diagnosis, pathogenesis, and etiology. In: *Advances in Neurology. Vol. 56: Amyotrophic Lateral*

Sclerosis and Other Motor Neurone Disease (ed. LP Rowland), pp 495–511. New York: Raven Press.

Dalakas MC, Sever JL, Madden DL *et al.* (1984) Late post-poliomyelitis muscular atrophy: clinical, virological, and immunological studies. *Reviews of Infectious Diseases* **6**: S562–567.

Dalakas MC, Elder G, Hallett M *et al.* (1986) A long term follow-up study of patients with post-poliomyelitis neuro-muscular symptoms. *New England Journal of Medicine* **314**: 959–963.

de Quadros CA, Andrus JK, Olive JM *et al.* (1991) Eradication of poliomyelitis; progress in the Americas. *Pediatric Infectious Disease* **10**: 222–229.

Deivanayagam N and Nedunchelian K (1991) Acute poliomyelitis in children: comparison of epidemiological and clinical features among immunised, partially immunised and unimmunised. *Indian Paediatrics* **28**: 609–613.

Dietz V, Lezana M, Sancho CG and Montesano R (1992) Predictors of poliomyelitis case confirmation at initial clinical evaluation: implications for poliomyelitis eradication in the Americas. *International Journal of Epidemiology* **21**: 800–806.

Gourie-Devi M (1986) Discussions on epidemiology of motor neurone disease. In: *Neurology* (eds K Poeck, HJ Freund, H Ganshirt), pp 300–303. Heidelberg: Springer-Verlag.

Gourie-Devi M (1993) Acute onset flaccid paralysis in selected countries of the World: India. In: *Acute Onset Flaccid Paralysis*, pp 23–37. Geneva: World Health Organization (WHO/MNH/EPL/93.3)

Gourie-Devi M, Suresh TG and Shankar SK (1984) Monomelic amyotrophy. *Archives of Neurology* **41**: 388–394.

Gourie-Devi M, Rao VN and Prakashi R (1987a) Neuroepidemiological study in semi-urban and rural areas in South India: pattern of neurological disorders including motor neurone disease. In: *Motor Neurone Disease: Global Clinical Patterns and International Research* (ed. M Gourie-Devi), pp 11–21. New Delhi: Oxford & IBH.

Gourie-Devi M, Suresh TG and Shankar SK (1987b) Pattern of motor neurone disease in South India and monomelic amyotrophy (a benign atypical form). In: *Motor Neurone Disease: Global Clinical Patterns and International Research* (ed. M Gourie-Devi), pp 171–190. New Delhi: Oxford & IBH.

Gourie-Devi M and Suresh TG (1988) Madras pattern of motor neurone disease in South India. *Journal of Neurology, Neurosurgery and Psychiatry* **5**: 773–777.

Gourie-Devi M, Rao CJ and Suresh TG (1992) Computed tomographic myelography in monomelic amyotrophy. *Journal of Tropical and Geographical Neurology* **2**: 32–37.

Gourie-Devi M, Gururaj G, Vasisth S and Subbakrishna DK (1993) Risk factors in monomelic amyotrophy – a case control study. *National Institute of Mental Health & Neuro Sciences Journal* **11**: 79–87.

Halstead LS, Wiechers D and Rossi CD (1985) Late effects of poliomyelitis: A national survey. In: *Late Effects of Poliomyelitis* (eds LS Halstead and DO Wiechers), pp 11–39, Miami, Symposia Foundation.

Hirayama K, Toyokura Y and Tsubaki T (1959) Juvenile muscular atrophy of unilateral upper extremity – a new clinical entity. *Psychiatry Neurology (Jap)* **61**: 2190–2197.

Hirayama K, Tomonaga M, Kitano K *et al.* (1987) Focal cervical poliopathy causing juvenile muscular atrophy of distal upper extremity: a pathological study. *Journal of Neurology, Neurosurgery and Psychiatry* **50**: 285–290.

Hovi T, Cantell K, Huovilainen A *et al.* (1986) Outbreak of paralytic poliomyelitis in

Finland: widespread circulation of antigenically altered poliovirus type 3 in a vaccinated population. *Lancet* **i**: 1427–1432.

Ismail HI and Lal M (1993) Poliomyelitis in Malaysia : two confirmed cases after 6 years without polio. *Annals of Tropical Paediatrics* **13**: 339–343.

Jagannathan K and Kumaresan G (1987) Madras pattern of motor neurone disease. In: *Motor Neurone Disease Global Clinical Patterns and International Research* (ed. M Gourie-Devi), pp 191–193. New Delhi: Oxford & IBH.

Joce R, Wood D, Brown D and Begg N (1992) Paralytic poliomyelitis in England and Wales, 1985-91. *British Medical Journal* **305**: 79–82.

John TJ (1975) Oral poliovaccination of children in the tropics, 2. Antibody response in relation to vaccine virus infection. *American Journal of Epidemiology* **102**: 414–421.

John TJ (1993) Immunisation against polioviruses in developing countries. *Medical Virology* **3**: 149–160.

Jubelt B and Cashman NR (1987) Neurological manifestations of the post-polio syndrome. In : *CRC Critical Reviews in Neurobiology*, vol.3, pp 199–220, Boston: CRC Press.

Juergens MS, Kurland LT, Okazaki PHH and Mulder DW (1980) ALS in Rochester, Minnesota 1925–1977. *Neurology (NY)* **30**: 463–470.

Kao KP, Wu ZA and Chern CM (1993a) Juvenile lower cervical spinal muscular atrophy in Taiwan: report of 27 Chinese cases. *Neuroepidemiology* **12**: 331–335.

Kao KP, Liu WT, Wang SJ and Chern CM (1993b) Lack of serum neutralizing antibody against poliovirus in patients with juvenile distal spinal muscular atrophy of upper extremities. *Brain and Development* **15**: 219–221.

Kascsak RJ, Carp RI, Vilcek JT, Donnenfeld H and Bartfelt H (1982) Virologic studies in amyotrophic lateral sclerosis. *Muscle and Nerve* **5**: 93–101.

Klingman J, Chui H, Corgiat M and Perry J (1988) Functional recovery. A major risk factor for the development of postpoliomyelitis muscular atrophy. *Archives of Neurology* **45**: 645–647.

Kono R, Miyamura K, Tajiri E, Robin Y and Girard P (1976) Outbreak of acute hemorrhagic conjunctivitis in Senegal in 1970. *Japanese Journal of Medical Science, Biology* **29**: 91–94.

Kott E, Livini E, Zamir R and Kuritzky A (1979) Cell-mediated immunity to polio and HLA antigens in amyotrophic lateral sclerosis. *Neurology* **29**: 1040–1044.

Kumar R, Singh A and Kumar V (1991) Survey of village informants – an alternate method to estimate paralytic poliomyelitis prevalence in rural area. *Indian Journal of Paediatrics* **58**: 239–243.

Kurent JE, Brooks BR, Madden DL, Sever JL and Engel WK (1979) CSF viral antibodies. Evaluation in amyotrophic lateral sclerosis and late-onset postpoliomyelitis progressive muscular atrophy. *Archives of Neurology* **36**: 269–273.

Kurtzke JF (1982) Epidemiology of amyotrophic lateral sclerosis. In: *Human Motor Neurone Disease* (ed. LP Rowland), pp 281–302. New York: Raven Press.

Mahadevan S, Ananthakrishnan S, Srinivasan S *et al.*, (1989) Poliomyelitis: 20 years – the Pondicherry experience. *Journal of Tropical Medicine and Hygiene* **92**: 416–421.

Martyn CN, Barken DJP and Osmond C (1988) Motoneurone disease and post poliomyelitis in England and Wales. *Lancet*: **1**: 1319–1322.

McBean AM and Modlin JF (1987) Rationale for the sequential use of inactivated poliovirus vaccine and live attenuated poliovirus vaccine for routine poliomyelitis immunisation in the United States. *Paediatric Infectious Disease Journal* **6**: 881–887.

McKhann GM, Cornblath DR, Griffin JW, *et al.* (1993) Acute motor axonal neuropathy; a frequent cause of acute flaccid paralysis in China. *Annals of Neurology* **33**: 333–342.

Meenakashisundaram E, Jagannathan K and Ramamurthy B (1970) Clinical pattern of motor neurone disease seen in younger age groups in Madras. *Neurology (India)* 18 (supplement I): 109–112.

Melnick JL and Ledinko N (1953) Development of neutralizing antibodies against the three types of poliomyelitis virus during an epidemic period; the ratio of inapparent infections to clinical poliomyelitis. *American Journal of Hygiene* **58**: 207–222.

Metcalf JC, Wood JB and Bertorini TE (1987) Benign focal amyotrophy; metrizamide CT evidence of cord atrophy. Case report. *Muscle Nerve* **10**: 338–345.

Mukai E, Matsuo T, Muto T, Takahashi A and Sobue I (1987) Magnetic resonance imaging of juvenile-type distal and segmental muscular atrophy of upper extremities. *Clinical Neurology (Jap)* **27**: 99–107.

Mulder DW, Rosenbaum RA and Layton DO Jr (1972) Late progression of poliomyelitis or forme fruste amyotrophic lateral sclerosis. *Mayo Clinic Proceedings* **47**: 756–761.

Nathanson N (1982) Eradication of poliomyelitis in the United States. *Reviews of Infectious Diseases* **4**: 940–945.

Nathanson N and Martin JR (1979) The epidemiology of poliomyelitis: Enigmas surrounding its appearance, epidemiology and disappearance. *American Journal of Epidemiology* **110**: 672–692.

Novak JE and Kirkegaard K (1991) Improved method for detecting poliovirus negative strands used to demonstrate specificity of positive-strand encapsidation and the ratio of positive to negative strands in infected cells. *Journal of Virology* **65**: 3384–3387.

Osuntokun BO, Adeuja AOG and Bademosi A (1974) The prognosis of motor neurone disease in Nigerian Africans – A prospective study of 92 patients. *Brain* **97**: 385–394.

Otten MW, Deming MS, Jaiteh KO *et al.* (1992) Epidemic poliomyelitis in the Gambia following the control of poliomyelitis as an endemic disease; I. Descriptive findings. *American Journal of Epidemiology* **135**: 381–392.

Owen RR (1985) Polio residuals clinic and exercise protocol: research implications. In: *Late Effects of Poliomyelitis* (eds LS Halstead and DO Wiechers), pp 207–219. Miami: Symposia Foundation.

Parakoyi B and Babaniyi OA (1990) Prevalence of paralytic poliomyelitis in children of Kwara State, Nigeria: report of a house-to-house survey. *East African Medical Journal* **67**: 545–549.

Patriarca PA, Foege WH and Swartz TA (1993) Progress in polio eradication. *Lancet* **342**: 1461–1464.

Peiris JB, Seneviratne KN, Wickremasinghe HR, Gunatilake SB and Gamage R (1989) Non-familial juvenile distal spinal muscular atrophy of upper extremity. *Journal of Neurology, Neurosurgery and Psychiatry* **52**: 314–319.

Pestronk A, Drachman DB and Griffin JW (1980) Effects of aging on nerve sprouting and regeneration. *Experimental Neurology* **70**: 65–82.

Pezeshkpour GH and Dalakas MC (1988) Long-term changes in the spinal cords of patients with old poliomyelitis. Signs of continuous disease activity. *Archives of Neurology* **45**: 505–508.

Pilgaard S (1968) Unilateral juvenile muscular atrophy of upper limbs. *Acta Orthopaedia Scandinavica* **39**: 327–331.

Poskanzer DC, Cantor HM and Kaplan GS (1969) The frequency of preceding poliomyelitis in amyotrophic lateral sclerosis. In: *Motor Neurone Diseases: Research on*

Amyotrophic Lateral Sclerosis and Related Disorders (eds FH Norris Jr and LT Kurland), pp 286–290. New York: Grune & Stratton.

Prabhakar S, Chopra JS, Banerjee AK and Rana PVS (1981) Wasted leg syndrome; a clinical, electrophysiological and histopathological study. *Clinical Neurology and Neurosurgery* **83:** 19–28.

Ramia S and Arif M (1991) Paralytic poliomyelitis outbreak in Gizan, Saudi Arabia. *Journal of Tropical Pediatrics (London)* **37:** 202–204.

Riggs JE, Schochet SS and Gutmann L (1984) Benign focal amyotrophy. Variant of chronic spinal muscular atrophy. *Archives of Neurology* **41:** 678–679.

Roivainen M, Agboatwalla M and Stenvik M *et al.* (1993) Intrathecal immune response and virus-specific immunoglobulin M antibodies in laboratory diagnosis of acute poliomyelitis. *Journal of Clinical Microbiology* **31:** 2427–2432.

Sabin AB (1956) Pathogenesis of poliomyelitis. Reappraisal in the light of new data. *Science* **123:** 1151–1157.

Sabin AB (1991) Perspectives on rapid elimination and ultimate global eradication of paralytic poliomyelitis caused by polioviruses. *European Journal of Epidemiology* **7:** 95–120.

Saini RK, Singh S, Sharma S *et al.* (1986) Snake bite poisoning presenting as early morning neuroparalytic syndrome in jhuggi dwellers. *Journal of Association of Physicians of India* **34:** 415–417.

Serratrice G, Pellissier JP and Pouget J (1987) Etude nosologique de 25 cas d'amyotrophie monomelique chronique. *Reviews of Neurology (Paris)* **143:** 201–210.

Sharief MK, Hentges R and Ciardi M (1991) Intrathecal immune response in patients with the post-polio syndrome. *New England Journal of Medicine* **325:** 749–755.

Sharrad WJW (1953) Correlation between the changes in the spinal cord and muscular paralysis in poliomyelitis. *Proceedings of the Royal Society of Medicine* **46:** 346–349.

Singh N, Sachdev KK and Susheela AK (1980) Juvenile muscular atrophy localised to arms. *Archives of Neurology* **37:** 297–299.

Sobue I, Saito N, Iida M and Ando K (1978) Juvenile type of distal and segmental muscular atrophy of upper extremities. *Annals of Neurology* **3:** 429–432.

Strebel PM, Sutter RW, Cochi SL *et al.* (1992) Epidemiology of poliomyelitis in the United States one decade after the last reported case of indigenous wild virus-associated disease. *Clinical Infectious Diseases* **14:** 568–579.

Sutter RW, Patriarca PA, Brogan S *et al.* (1991) Outbreak of paralytic poliomyelitis in Oman. Evidence for widespread transmission among fully vaccinated children. *Lancet* **338:** 715–720.

Sutter RW, Patriarca PA, Suleiman AJ *et al.* (1992) Attributable risk of DTP (diphtheria and tetanus toxoids and pertussis vaccine) injection in provoking paralytic poliomyelitis during a large outbreak in Oman. *Journal of Infectious Diseases* **165:** 444–449.

Tan CT (1985) Juvenile muscular atrophy of distal upper extremitis. *Journal of Neurology, Neurosurgery and Psychiatry* **48:** 285–286.

Tomlinson BE and Irving D (1977) The numbers of limb motor neurones in the human lumbosacral cord throughout life. *Journal of the Neurological Sciences* **34:** 213–219.

Valmikinathan K, Mascreen M, Meenakshisundaram E and Snehalatha C (1973) Biochemical aspects of motor neurone disease – Madras pattern. *Journal of Neurology, Neurosurgery and Psychiatry* **36:** 753–756.

Wadia NH, Irani PF and Katrak SM (1972) Neurological complications of a new conjunctivitis. *Lancet* **2:** 970–971.

Wadia PN, Bhatt MH and Misra VP (1987) Clinical neurophysiological examination of deafness associated with juvenile motor neurone disease. *Journal of Neurological Sciences* **78**: 29–33.

Windebank AJ, Daube JR, Litchy WJ *et al.* (1987) Late sequelae of paralytic poliomyelitis in Olmstead County. Minnesota. In: *Research and Clinical Aspects of the Late Effects of Poliomyelitis*, vol. 23 (eds LS Halstead and DO Wiechers), pp 27–38. New York, White Plains: March of Dimes.

WHO (1988) Global eradication of poliomyelitis by the year 2000. In: *Forty-first World Health Assembly*, Geneva, 2–13 May 1988. Resolutions and decisions annexes. (Resolution WHA 41,2,8) Geneva: WHO.

WHO (1993) Acute Onset Flaccid Paralysis. Geneva: WHO (WHO/MNH/EP1/93.3).

WHO (1994) Progress towards the global eradication of poliomyelitis. *Status Report* (WHO/GPV/Polio/94.1), Geneva: WHO

Wyatt HV (1973) Poliomyelitis in hypogammaglobulinemics. *Journal of Infectious Diseases* **128**: 802–806.

Wyatt HV (1990) Incubation of poliomyelitis as calculated from the time of entry into the central nervous system via the peripheral nerve pathways. *Reviews of Infectious Diseases* **12**: 547–556.

Zilkha KH (1962) Discussion on motor neurone disease. *Proceedings of the Royal Society of Medicine* **55**: 1028–1029.

Section 2
BACTERIAL AND FUNGAL CONDITIONS

8

Bacterial Meningitis

Ammar Mubaidin and Milne Anderson

Midland Centre for Neurosurgery and Neurology, Holly Lane, Smethwick, West Midlands, UK

INTRODUCTION

Since earliest times bacterial meningitis has been a major cause of death and disability affecting mankind. Descriptions of disease which we can recognize as meningitis are to be found in sixteenth century writings. That meningitis could exist in epidemic form became recognized in Europe and North America towards the beginning of the nineteenth century and it has been argued that because the clinical syndrome was so distinctive it would not have been ignored by prior writers and therefore represented a new development. Whatever the truth of this, causative organisms were recognized only towards the end of the nineteenth century and attempts to treat the disease with contemporary medications invariably resulted in failure – once established, bacterial meningitis carried a mortality rate of 100%.

Improvement in these figures came about as recently as the late 1930s and 1940s with the discovery and application first of sulphonamides, then of penicillin and thereafter streptomycin and chloramphenicol (Anderson, 1984). Many other antibiotics have been developed since but they unfortunately did not significantly improve mortality or morbidity until the third-generation cephalosporins were introduced in the 1980s which brought about substantial improvement in the treatment of Gram-negative aerobic bacillary meningitis and hope for similar results in other forms of meningitis. Simultaneously our understanding of the pathogenesis of bacterial invasion of the neuraxis and onward dissemination of infection and attendant changes within the brain has opened up the prospect of adjunctive therapy with drugs such as steroids and regimens designed to reduce raised intracranial pressure and protect cerebral perfusion: preliminary results are already very encouraging (Lebel *et al.*, 1988; Quagliarello and Scheld, 1992).

Bacterial meningitis is not a static disease. Whilst the clinical manifestations do not alter significantly, it is becoming evident that the epidemiology and probably the virulence of some bacterial forms are changing. As new antibiotics and vaccines are developed the organisms develop new resistant strains. The immune status of populations and of individuals may vary because of the acquisition of disease such as AIDS or the appearance of famine and malnutrition consequent upon war or political upheaval.

EPIDEMIOLOGY

The major organisms which cause meningitis differ between countries, races and populations, show predilection for particular age groups and change with time (see Tables 8.1 and 8.2). Because notification procedures are much better in some countries than in others it can be difficult to obtain adequate data for comparison. If circumstances are favourable, any bacterium can induce meningitis. Usually, meningitis follows infection by an organism which has specific virulence for the central nervous system (CNS), though in some cases the disease occurs as part of a general infection or as a complication of local infection elsewhere. From those countries with adequate epidemiological data it is evident that approximately 70% of cases occur in children less than 5 years old, and 70% of cases (not the same 70%) are caused by *Haemophilus influenzae*, *Streptococcus pneumoniae* or *Neisseria meningitidis*. In children less than one month old any organism may be

TABLE 8.1 Bacterial meningitis: causal organisms and age

Neonates
Gram-negative bacilli
Listeria
Streptococci (group B)

Infants and preschool children
Haemophilus
Meningococcus

School children and adolescents
Meningococcus
Pneumococcus

Young adults
Pneumococcus
Meningococcus

Adults
Pneumococcus
Meningococcus
Staphylococcus
Streptococcus
Listeria

Elderly
Pneumococcus
Gram-negative bacilli

TABLE 8.2 Predisposing cause and organism in bacterial meningitis

Predisposition	Organism
Sickle cell disease/hyposplenism	Pneumococcus
Malaria	Gram-negative bacilli
Pregnancy/childbirth	Listeria Streptococcus
Alcohol	Pneumococcus
Skull fracture	Staphylococcus Gram-negative bacillus
Diabetes	Pneumococcus Staphylococcus Gram-negative bacillus
Dural fistula	Pneumococcus Gram-negative bacillus
Immune defect – cellular	Listeria
Immune defect – neutropenia	Pseudomonas
Immune defect – humoral	Pneumococcus Haemophilus Meningococcus
CNS shunt	*Staphyglococcus epidermidis*

implicated, Gram-negative bacilli, commonly *Escherichia coli* K1, enteric bacilli, group B streptococci and *Pseudomonas* predominate. *H. influenzae* affects children of less than 5 years old in the main but may rarely occur at other ages when a source of entry of infection such as a cerebrospinal fluid (CSF) leak or otitis media, or immunodeficiency should be sought. The meningococcus affects children and adults and the pneumococcus chiefly affects adults. Meningitis due to Gram-negative bacilli may complicate head injuries, neurosurgery and immune compromise which may attract staphylococci. Streptococcus and *Listeria* infect pregnant women and the immune suppressed. The elderly are at risk of infection from Gram-negative bacilli, *Listeria* and streptococci. Infection with anaerobic organisms and with more than one organism occur in approximately 1% of cases, each as a complication of skull fracture, neurosurgery, paranasal sinus infection or immune suppression. In the USA, *H. influenzae* type b is the commonest form of meningitis, while in the UK the meningococcus and pneumococcus predominate (Roos *et al.*, 1991). Following the introduction of HIB vaccine, the incidence of *Haemophilus* meningitis is falling. To counter this, the incidence of infection acquired in hospital is rising (Durand *et al.*, 1993). The incidence of bacterial meningitis approximates to 3–5 cases per 100 000 population per annum in the USA and Europe with higher figures in less well developed countries – a recent figure for Brazil is 45.8 cases per 100 000 population annually (Bryan *et al.*, 1990) and higher figures have been reported in local outbreaks in several countries. World-wide tuberculosis remains a significant cause of meningitis, not only in countries with poor socioeconomic circumstances.

Meningococcal meningitis is the only significant cause of epidemic meningitis. Epidemics have been reported from countries in most of the continents of the world in the last 20 years. It is endemic in the Sub-Saharan belt of Africa from the Gambia to Ethiopia, where outbreaks tend to occur from March to May. In industrialized countries there is a tendency for outbreaks to occur in late winter and early spring, but localized epidemics may occur at any time. Factors which favour the onset of epidemics include poor hygiene, overcrowding, malnutrition, respiratory disease, low population carrier rates and diminution of herd immunity, and infection with particular meningococcal subgroups – A in Africa, B and C elsewhere. In Africa, such epidemics occur at 8–12 year intervals. Children are most at risk, 5–9 year olds in Africa, under 5s in USA and Europe, yet as many as 10% of an infected population can be more than 45 years old (Schwartz *et al.*, 1989).

PATHOGENESIS

Until relatively recently our understanding of the mechanisms by which bacteria caused meningitis was sketchy. In the last decade an increasing amount of work using animal models and observations in human patients has shed considerable light on the pathogenic processes. While much remains to be explained, sufficient information now exists to suggest that new treatment modalities will soon be available – witness the use of dexamethasone (Lebel *et al.*, 1988). Bacteria that cause meningitis possess neurotropic properties which overcome defence mechanisms surrounding the brain and spinal cord. Usually such organisms colonize the upper respiratory tract. Exceptionally, the portal of entry may be directly into the skull through a fracture or by haematogenous spread. Many of the major meningitis bacteria possess surface characteristics, fimbriae, which aid colonization of mucosa by boosting adherence to epithelial cells. Nasal epithelium secretes IgA and it is necessary for an organism to neutralize this by secreting IgA protease. The possession of a polysaccharide capsule is an important virulence factor which protects the organism against circulating complement after it has gained entry to the bloodstream, and the variation in its molecular makeup explains the difference in pathogenicity between bacteria.

Mechanisms by which the blood–brain barrier is penetrated are not yet worked out. Blood–brain barrier permeability increases perhaps by loosening intercellular junctions and increased pinocytosis. Once within the subarachnoid space there is virtually no immunoglobulin and complement activity so opsonization cannot take place (Simberkoff *et al.*, 1980). A hallmark of bacterial meningitis is a neutrophil response within the CSF. It is still not understood how this comes about. Bacterial cell wall components released into CSF stimulate the production of inflammatory cytokines including interleukins 1 and 6, prostaglandins, and tumour necrosis factor and these probably induce inflammation and blood–brain barrier disruption. By a further series of interactions, cerebral blood flow increases and together with blood–brain barrier breakdown, vasogenic cerebral oedema raises intracranial pressure. Cytotoxic oedema from the products of inflammation from neutrophils and bacteria further raises the pressure causing interstitial oedema by obstructing the flow of CSF from subarachnoid space to blood. Cerebral blood flow drops, vasculitis extends, cerebral autoregulation becomes unreliable and there is a risk of further brain damage from cerebral over- or under-perfusion (Tunkel *et al.*, 1990; Tureen *et al.*, 1990; Ashwal *et al.*, 1992; Quagliarello and Scheld, 1992; Tunkel and Scheld, 1993). It is becoming evident that these changes take place early in the evolution of the syndrome and cause much of the morbidity and mortality, and much effort is now being directed to develop measures to anticipate or counter them.

CLINICAL FEATURES

A classical case of meningitis is easy to recognize. In 24–48 hours the patient develops fever, headache, neck stiffness, malaise, irritability, confusion and photophobia. These symptoms are commonly associated with signs of an upper respiratory infection. Unfortunately, in as high a proportion as 20% of cases some of these features are lacking. The onset may be abrupt and catastrophic within hours. If the patient is at the extremes of age, very ill, or immune compromised, there may be no evidence of meningism so that a high index of suspicion is required for the patient who presents with lethargy, altered menta-tion, and reduced conscious level, with or without pyrexia. In young children, the picture may be quite non-specific. Failure to thrive, disturbance of temperature regulation, a full fontanelle, jaundice and hepatosplenomegaly, and septicaemia may all be due to meningitis. Epileptic seizures accompany meningitis in any age group, but more so in the young, when as many as 40% may have fits, and it is important to recognize that they may be the presenting feature. Convulsions occur frequently in febrile children, and potentially each may suffer from meningitis. Should every such patient have a lumbar puncture? Evidence suggests that if the convulsion is brief, if the child regains consciousness rapidly, if there is no other evidence of meningitis and the child does not appear to be ill, if no focal or persisting neurological deficit exists, and epidemic meningitis is unlikely, it is reasonable to postpone CSF examination and observe the child for a few hours instead (Lorber and Sunderland, 1980). Others hold that preschool children in the tropics who present with convulsions and pyrexia should have a lumbar puncture carried out forthwith (Akpede and Sykes, 1992). Skin rashes occur in about 30% of cases and are most commonly, but not invariably associated with meningococcal infection.

Meningitis from staphylococci, pneumococci, *Haemophilus*, *Listeria* and some viruses may also provoke skin eruptions. Shock may accompany any overwhelming infection and is frequently seen in meningococcal meningitis. Where the ambient temperature is high, when no air-conditioning is available, and fluid replacement is inadequate, any patient with an infection may readily become dehydrated and shocked and in such circumstances no diagnostic significance may be attached to the findings. Focal neurological signs occur in about 15% of cases of bacterial meningitis and may be the result of vasculitis of the main cerebral vessels causing brain infarction, evolving space occupation from a cerebral abscess, or damage to cranial nerves from basal meningeal inflammation. It is particularly important to observe and monitor the level of consciousness of the patient, for this correlates closely with survival rates. As consciousness decreases so does recovery – 55% of adults who present in coma do not live (Carpenter and Petersdorf, 1962; Swartz and Dodge, 1965; Geiseler *et al.*, 1980; Klein *et al.*, 1986).

A high index of suspicion is necessary for the timely diagnosis of a case of bacterial meningitis – any delay reduces the chances of a successful outcome, and the one message to be derived from all clinical series is that postponement of treatment is likely to bring about an unsatisfactory outcome. Search must be made for a locus of infection and for any factors which may predispose the patient to suffer from meningitis, or illnesses which may diminish immunity and render the patient vulnerable to challenge from organisms which in other circumstances may not be pathogenic. Certain organisms may be associated with particular conditions. Pneumococcal meningitis is associated with alcoholism, sickle cell disease, hyposplenism, skull fractures and otitis media. Gram-negative infection may complicate cerebral malaria. Listerial infection occurs in neonates, pregnant women and the immune suppressed. TB meningitis may be complicated by the simultaneous occurrence of other bacterial infection. Patients who are immune suppressed by reason of disease or treatment of disease are liable to infection by a diverse range of organisms, many of which would not be pathogenic in normal circumstances. AIDS patients may on occasion develop meningitis from TB or syphilis (Price and Worley, 1995). In our experience, diabetic patients are particularly exposed to misdiagnosis because the confusion and drowsiness of hypoglycaemia or ketoacidosis may mask signs of meningitis, or be attributed to diabetes.

DIAGNOSIS

The diagnosis of a case of meningitis begins with a high index of clinical suspicion which must nowadays be spread over a widening constellation of symptoms and signs, is supported by finding appropriate abnormalities on examination, and confirmed after laboratory study of CSF obtained by lumbar puncture. Characteristically, the CSF is under pressure, looks turbid, has a raised protein content (above 50 mg dl^{-1}), reduced glucose (which should be compared with a specimen of venous blood taken simultaneously: a ratio of less than 0.3 CSF : blood is abnormal and is found in approximately 75% of patients (Marton and Gean, 1986), and contains an increased number of polymorphonuclear leukocytes, usually hundreds, which comprise more than 60% of the cells present. Similar changes may be found in some cases of tuberculous, brucella and viral meningitis, parameningeal pathology and carcinomatosis. The fluid should be examined straight away under the microscope by an experienced observer, after appropriate staining. It should be possible to identify bacteria and confirm their species after culture in 80% of cases – this figure diminishes if the examination is undertaken by inexperienced observers, if antibiotics have been administered beforehand, or if the organism is particularly fastidious. Many tests have been applied to CSF to improve the positive organism identification rate. These include immunological tests to detect bacterial antigen by various techniques – counterimmunoelectrophoresis, latex particle agglutination, radio-immunoassay, enzyme-linked immunosorbent assay and coagglutination – limulus lysate assay for endotoxin, estimation of lactic acid level and C-reactive protein. Unfortunately none combines specificity with adequate sensitivity sufficiently reliably to be useful in the acute situation, or where sophisticated laboratory facilities are lacking (Anderson, 1984). Newer molecular techniques, particularly the polymerase chain reaction, promise much (Eisenstein, 1990; Darnell, 1993), but experience is not yet sufficient to recommend their widespread application. It is likely that expense and the necessity for laboratory sophistication will limit their usefulness.

It has been mentioned earlier that CSF pressure is high in bacterial meningitis and that cerebral oedema occurs. It is also possible to develop intracranial space occupation from infarction or abscess. It follows, therefore, that lumbar puncture may be hazardous, and carries the risk of inducing cerebral and hindbrain herniation with disastrous results (Duffy, 1969; Horwitz *et al.*, 1980; Rennick *et al.*, 1993) This has certainly been our experience and we cannot agree with those who advocate apparently indiscriminate CSF examination in suspected cases of meningitis, neither do we believe that the hazards of lumbar puncture have been exaggerated; indeed it is our suspicion that not a few deaths are wrongly attributed to overwhelming infection or cardiovascular collapse, when they actually result from brain coning. On the other hand, it is necessary to examine the CSF as early as possible because delay in instituting treatment reduces the chances of survival, and how to do this safely in all potential cases of meningitis can be difficult, requiring experience and luck. Unfortunately, the absence of papilloedema does not mean that intracranial pressure is normal. If there is any focal sign or symptom or if the conscious level is depressed, brain imaging should be undertaken first. If there is no evidence of space occupation or brain herniation, lumbar puncture may be undertaken after the patient has been given mannitol and dexamethasone.

If cranial imaging with computed tomography (CT) or magnetic resonance imaging (MRI) is available it should be undertaken. Early in the evolution of disease no abnormality may be seen. It may be possible to visualize meningeal and ependymal enhancement, exudate around the base of the brain, cerebral oedema squashing the ventricles, or hydrocephalus from aqueductal or basal adhesions. Infarction, brain abscess, subdural collection may all be demonstrated and other conditions which give rise to similar clinical syndromes such as subarachnoid haemorrhage and tumour may be excluded (Cabral et al., 1987; Sze and Zimmerman, 1988). It should not be forgotten to look for skull fractures and evidence of paranasal sinus infection such as fluid levels, and for mastoiditis. MRI scanning may be technically difficult if the patient is restless or requires assistance with breathing. It has been reported that CT brain imaging does not influence the management of bacterial meningitis in children (Friedland et al., 1992). We take the view that if it is available and can be undertaken expeditiously then it should be. Away from main centres, skull X-rays can be examined for signs of paranasal sinusitis, fractures and pineal shift to imply space occupation. Meningitis develops too quickly for the radiological signs of raised intracranial pressure to develop.

In all cases, if there is an obvious site of infection, specimens should be taken from it for culture. Blood cultures should be taken if septicaemia or endocarditis is suspected. If there is any doubt about malaria, appropriate examination of thick blood smears must be done. Haemoglobinopathies, particularly sickle cell disease, should be sought. A full blood count, blood glucose and electrolytes and osmolality must be estimated. In tropical countries and in children, dehydration is almost a constant finding and must be corrected. Electrolyte disturbance may be compounded by sodium loss from inappropriate secretion of antidiuretic hormone (Kaplan and Feigin, 1978). Other investigations are undertaken according to clinical need. Electroencephalography is not useful in acute bacterial meningitis.

TREATMENT

Immediately the diagnosis is made, treatment must be given. Vital functions of respiration and perfusion must be supported, fluid replaced and electrolytic disturbance corrected. Antibiotics appropriate to the organism should be administered, in our view, parenterally, in doses sufficiently high to achieve bactericidal levels in CSF which are necessarily 10 to 20 times higher than the in vitro minimal bactericidal concentration for the organism. We do not believe that there is any place for the routine installation of antibiotics intrathecally – every year there are iatrogenically induced fatalities when the wrong dose and preparation is given. An ideal antibiotic would be lipid-soluble to cross into CSF, and active within purulent and acidic CSF. The dose which should be given and the frequency of administration are determined by the rate of metabolism and clearance from the CSF. In practice it does not seem to matter if an antibiotic is bactericidal or bacteriostatic, provided it is given in high enough dose. Penetration to the CSF is facilitated by meningeal inflammation.

In cases where an organism cannot be identified, knowledge of local drug

TABLE 8.3 Empirical treatment of bacterial meningitis

Children	Third-generation cephalosporin Ampicillin and chloramphenicol
Adults	Penicillin and third-generation cephalosporin
Comatose with no history	Penicillin and chloramphenicol, or third-generation cephalosporin with metronidazole and acyclovir

resistance patterns is important and antibiotics are chosen empirically (Table 8.3). Children should be treated with ampicillin and chloramphenicol combined, or with a third-generation cephalosporin (Klein *et al.*, 1992). Adults should be given penicillin or a third-generation cephalosporin. Elderly patients should have a third-generation cephalosporin together with ampicillin. In the immune-compromised the nature of the immune deficit influences the choice of antibiotic – ampicillin to cover *Listeria* should be used for cell-mediated defects, penicillin and a third-generation cephalosporin for humoral defects and a third-generation cephalosporin for neutropenia together with ceftazidime and an aminoglycoside if infection with *Pseudomonas* seems likely (Rubin and Hooper, 1985; Tunkel *et al.*, 1990). If AIDS patients develop meningitis it is most likely due to fungi, but TB and syphilis are significant bacterial causes, and for the latter, aggressive treatment with penicillin is recommended (Bolan, 1995).

Unfortunately, an increasing number of *Haemophilus influenzae* b strains are becoming resistant to ampicillin and now to chloramphenicol so that the previously effective use of these drugs no longer guarantees a satisfactory outcome, and a third-generation cephalosporin is to be preferred – cefotaxime and ceftriaxone have been successful (Lebel *et al.*, 1989a; Schaad *et al.*, 1990). Penicillin remains the drug of choice for the treatment of meningococcal and pneumococcal meningitis but resistant meningococci are being recorded (Sutcliffe *et al.*, 1988). Penicillin-resistant pneumococci are also now becoming a problem (Weingarten *et al.*, 1990). In such circumstances, a third-generation cephalosporin is appropriate.

Gram-negative bacillary meningitis also responds to third-generation cephalosporins, and ceftazidime or a combination with an aminoglycoside is recommended for *Pseudomonas* (Norrby, 1985). Group B streptococci respond to penicillin or ampicillin if resistance is suspected. *Listeria* should be treated with ampicillin and *Staphylococcus aureus* with flucloxacillin, oxacillin or nafcillin, and vancomycin for the penicillin intolerant (Schlesinger *et al.*, 1987). For anaerobic infections we recommend the combination of penicillin, chloramphenicol and metronidazole. Treatment of infections which complicate implanted devices such as shunts almost always requires removal of the device. Vancomycin with rifampicin is usually effective. The place of the quinalones in meningitis has yet to be established. We recognize that many of these antibiotics are not available in tropical countries for various reasons, not least of which is cost. In these circumstances best use must be made of the drugs which are available and we believe that parenteral administration, usually intravenously, is necessary. Ideally, drug therapy should continue for 10 days. Any sources of infection must be eradicated.

It has been discussed before that a complex series of interactions occurs when bacteria invade the neuraxis and this is accompanied by the release of various substances, some of which contribute to the development of inflammation, the effects of which are not always advantageous to the host. Much research is currently taking place to determine which form of treatment, adjunctive to antibiotics, is beneficial. The anti-inflammatory action of corticosteroids has been studied in this context and the evidence to date is that dexamethasone given as early as possible in a dose of 0.15 mg kg^{-1} body weight for at least 4 days reduces morbidity (Lebel *et al.*, 1988, 1989b; Havens *et al.*, 1989; Odio *et al.*, 1991; Townsend and Scheld, 1993). Non-steroidal anti-inflammatory drugs, targeted monoclonal antibodies, pentoxifylline, leukocyte endothelial cell adhesion molecular antagonists, platelet-activating factor receptor antagonists and free radical scavengers are all undergoing investigation at present (Townsend and Scheld, 1993). Intracranial pressure is raised, particularly in the first 2 days and it should be possible to anticipate this and treat, if necessary by monitoring intracranial pressure (Minns *et al.*, 1989).

Chemoprophylaxis should be given to household and 'kissing' contacts of patients with meningococcal meningitis, and several drugs are available. At present, rifampicin for 2 days is recommended, but resistant strains are appearing, and ceftriaxone and ciprofloxin are alternatives (Cuevas and Hart, 1993). Prophylaxis with rifampicin should be given to infant (less than 2 years old) household contacts of *Haemophilus* meningitis cases. An alternative is to give protective chemotherapy to contacts, and results from further trials are awaited.

Prevention of bacterial meningitis is now a possibility with immunization, which is yet in its infancy and promises much for the future. Very encouraging results have been obtained against *Haemophilus* meningitis (Cartwright, 1992; Peltola *et al.*, 1992) and against meningococcal (Frasch, 1989) and pneumococcal disease (Broome and Breiman, 1991).

CONCLUSION

Bacterial meningitis remains a killer disease in tropical countries and elsewhere. Mortality from the disease continues to be high. Those who have the worst prognosis are those whose conscious level is reduced on admission, who suffer from a delay in diagnosis and do not receive antibiotics appropriate to the pathogenic bacteria. Sophisticated medical facilities are not universally available but their lack can be compensated for by clinical acumen and close attention to supportive treatment.

REFERENCES

Akpede GO and Sykes RM (1992) Convulsions with fever as a presenting feature of bacterial meningitis among preschool children in developing countries. *Developmental Medicine and Child Neurology* **34**: 524–529.

Anderson M (1984) Bacterial meningitis. In: *Recent Advances in Clinical Neurology*, vol. 4 (eds WB Matthews and GH Glaser), pp 87–121. Edinburgh: Churchill Livingstone.

Ashwal S, Tomasi L, Schneider S, Perkin R and Thompson J (1992) Bacterial meningitis in children: pathophysiology and treatment. *Neurology* **42**: 739–748.

Bolan G (1995) Management of syphilis in HIV-infected persons. In: *The Medical Management of AIDS* (eds ME Sande and PA Volberding), pp 537–554. Philadelphia: WB Saunders.

Broome CV and Breiman RF (1991) Pneumococcal vaccine – past, present and future. *New England Journal of Medicine* **325**: 1506–1508.

Bryan JP, de Silva HR, Tavares A, Roche H and Scheld WM (1990) Etiology and mortality of bacterial meningitis in northeastern Brazil. *Reviews of Infectious Diseases* **12**: 128–135.

Cabral DA, Flodmark O, Farrell K and Speert DP (1987) Prospective study of computer tomography in acute bacterial meningitis. *Journal of Pediatrics* **111**: 201–205.

Carpenter RR and Petersdorf RG (1962) The clinical spectrum of bacterial meningitis. *American Journal of Medicine* **33**: 262–275.

Cartwright KAV (1992) Vaccination against *Haemophilus influenzae* b disease. *British Medical Journal* **305**: 485–486.

Cuevas LE and Hart CA (1993) Chemoprophylaxis of bacterial meningitis. *Journal of Antimicrobial Chemotherapy* **31**: S79–91.

Darnell RB (1993) The polymerase chain reaction: application to nervous system disease. *Annals of Neurology* **34**: 513–523.

Duffy GP (1969) Lumbar puncture in the presence of raised intracranial pressure. *British Medical Journal* **1**: 407–409.

Durand ML, Calderwood SB, Weber DJ, Miller SI, Southwick FS, Caviness VS and Swartz MN (1993) Acute bacterial meningitis in adults. *New England Journal of Medicine* **328**: 21–28.

Eisenstein BI (1990) The polymerase chain reaction: a new method of using molecular genetics for medical diagnosis. *New England Journal of Medicine* **322**: 178–183.

Frasch CE (1989) Vaccines for prevention of meningococcal disease. *Clinical Microbiological Reviews* **2**: S134–138.

Friedland IR, Paris MM, Rinderknecht S and McCracken GH (1992) Cranial computed tomographic scans have little impact on management of bacterial meningitis. *American Journal of Diseases of Children* **146**: 1484–1487.

Geiseler PJ, Nelson KE, Levin S, Reddy KT and Moses VK (1980) Community acquired purulent meningitis: a review of 1316 cases during the antibiotic era, 1954–1976. *Reviews of Infectious Diseases* **2**: 725–754.

Havens PL, Wenderberger KJ, Hoffman GM, Lee MB and Chusid MJ (1989) Corticosteroids as adjunctive therapy in bacterial meningitis. A meta analysis of clinical trials. *American Journal of Diseases of Children* **143**: 1051–1055.

Horwitz SJ, Boxerbaum B and O'Bell J (1980) Cerebral herniation in bacterial meningitis in childhood. *Annals of Neurology* **7**: 524–528.

Kaplan SL and Feigin RD (1978) The syndrome of inappropriate secretion of antidiuretic hormone in children with bacterial meningitis. *Journal of Pediatrics* **92**: 758–761.

Klein JO, Feigin RD and McCracken GH (1986) Report on the task force on diagnosis and management of meningitis. *Pediatrics* **78S**: 959–982.

Klein NJ, Heyderman RS and Levin M (1992) Antibiotic choices for meningitis beyond the neonatal period. *Archives of Diseases in Childhood* **67**: 157–161.

Lebel MH, Freij BJ, Syrogiannopoulos GA, Chrane DF, Hoyt MJ, Stewart SM, Kennard BD, Olsen KD and McCracken GH (1988) Dexamethasone therapy for bacterial meningitis. *New England Journal of Medicine* **319**: 964–971.

Lebel MH, Hoyt MJ and McCracken GH (1989a) Comparative efficacy of ceftriaxone and cefuroxime for treatment of bacterial meningitis. *Journal of Pediatrics* **114**: 1049–1054.

Lebel MH, Hoyt J, Waagner DC, Rollins NK, Finitzo T and McCracken GH (1989b) Magnetic resonance imaging and dexamethasone therapy for bacterial meningitis. *American Journal of Diseases of Children* **143**: 301–306.

Lorber J and Sunderland R (1980) Lumbar puncture in children with convulsions associated with fever. *Lancet* **52**: 188–191.

Marton KI and Gean AD (1986) The spinal tap: a new look at an old test. *Annals of Internal Medicine* **104**: 840–848.

Minns RA, Engleman HM and Stirling H (1989) Cerebrospinal fluid pressure in pyogenic meningitis. *Archives of Disease in Childhood* **64**: 814–820.

Norrby SR (1985) Role of cephalosporins in the treatment of bacterial meningitis in adults. Overview with special emphasis on ceftazidime. *American Journal of Medicine* **79**: 56–61.

Odio CM, Faingezicht I, Paris M, Nassar M, Baltodano A, Rogers J, Saez-Llorens X, Olsen KD and McCracken GH (1991) The beneficial effects of early dexamethasone administration in infants and children with bacterial meningitis. *New England Journal of Medicine* **324**: 1525–1531.

Peltola H, Kilpi T and Anttila M (1992) Rapid disappearance of *Haemophilus influenzae* type b meningitis after routine childhood immunisation with conjugate vaccines. *Lancet* **340**: 592–594.

Price RW and Worley JM (1995) Management of neurologic complications of HIV-1 infection and AIDS. In: *The Medical Management of AIDS* (eds ME Sande and PA Volberding), pp 261–288. Philadelphia: WB Saunders.

Quagliarello V and Scheld WM (1992) Bacterial meningitis: pathogenesis, pathophysiology and progress. *New England Journal of Medicine* **327**: 864–872.

Rennick G, Shann F and de Campo J (1993) Cerebral herniation during bacterial meningitis in children. *British Medical Journal* **306**: 953–955.

Roos KL, Tunkel AR and Scheld WM (1991) Acute bacterial meningitis in children and adults. In: *Infections of the Central Nervous System* (eds WM Scheld, RJ Whitley and DT Durack), pp 335–409. New York: Raven Press

Rubin RH and Hooper DC (1985) Central nervous system infections in the compromised host. *Medical Clinics of North America* **69**: 281–293.

Schaad UB, Suter S and Gianelli-Borrardori A (1990) A comparison of ceftriaxone and cefuroxime for the treatment of bacterial meningitis. *New England Journal of Medicine* **322**: 141–147.

Schlesinger LS, Ross SC and Schaberg DR (1987) *Staphylococcus aureus* meningitis: a broad based epidemiological study. *Medicine (Baltimore)* **66**: 148–156.

Schwartz B, More PS and Broome CV (1989) The global epidemiology of meningococcal disease. *Clinical Microbiological Reviews* **2**: S118–124.

Simberkoff MS, Moldover NH and Ranal J (1980) Absence of detectable bacterial and opsonic activities in normal and infected human cerebrospinal fluids: a regional host defence deficiency. *Journal of Laboratory and Clinical Medicine* **95**: 362–372.

Sutcliffe EM, Jones DM, El-Sheikh S and Percival A (1988) Penicillin insensitive meningococci in the UK. *Lancet* **i**: 657–658.

Swartz MN and Dodge PR (1965) Bacterial meningitis – a review of selected aspects. *New England Journal of Medicine* **272**: 725–731, 779–787, 842–848, 898–902.

Sze G and Zimmerman RD (1988) The magnetic resonance imaging of infections and inflammatory diseases. *Radiological Clinics of North America* **26**: 839–859.

Townsend GC and Scheld WM (1993) Adjunctive therapy for bacterial meningitis: rationale for use, current status, and prospects for the future. *Clinical Infectious Diseases* **17**: S537–549.

Tunkel AR and Scheld WM (1993) Pathogenesis and pathophysiology of bacterial meningitis. *Clinical Microbiological Reviews* **6**: 118–136.

Tunkel AR, Wispelwey B and Scheld WM (1990) Bacterial meningitis: recent advances in pathophysiology and treatment. *Annals of Internal Medicine* **112**: 610–623.

Tureen JH, Dworkin RJ, Kennedy SL, Sachdeva M and Sande MA, (1990) Loss of cerebral autoregulation in experimental meningitis in rabbits. *Journals of Clinical Investigation* **85**: 577–581.

Weingarten RD, Markewicz Z and Gilbert DN (1990) Meningitis due to penicillin-resistant *Streptococcus pneumoniae* in adults. *Reviews of Infectious Diseases* **12**: 118–124.

9

Tuberculosis

Nadir E. Bharucha and Roberta H. Raven

Department of Neuroepidemiology, Medical Research Centre, Bombay Hospital Institute of Medical Sciences, Bombay, India

INTRODUCTION

Tuberculosis (TB), an ancient disease, remains a major world health problem and is widespread in developing countries with large populations where there is crowding, poverty, malnutrition and infection. These same factors operate in areas of urban deprivation in developed countries (Snider and Roper, 1992). Immunosuppression, primarily due to the HIV epidemic, renders more people susceptible to tuberculosis. Resistance to antituberculous drugs makes curative therapy much more difficult.

AETIOLOGY

There are two groups of bacteria responsible for TB. The first, known as the TB complex, are obligatory parasites; these are *Mycobacterium tuberculosis, M. bovis, M. ulcerans* and *M. africanum*. The second group are saprophytes, mycobacteria from the environment, which are called mycobacteria other than tuberculosis (MOTT). These include *M. avium* and *M. intracellulare* which together are known as the MAI complex and are important in the immunosuppressed host. The great majority of tuberculous manifestations in the nervous system are caused by *M. tuberculosis*.

IMMUNOLOGY

The important immune response to the mycobacterial organism is cellular rather than humoral. The effector cells are macrophages and sensitized by T lymphocytes. Macrophages ingest mycobacteria and destroy some of them. They present on their surfaces TB antigens together with major histocompatibility complex

(MHC) I and II molecules, so that sensitized T lymphocytes can recognize and remember them.

Macrophages also secrete cytokines which are necessary for activation of T lymphocytes. Sensitized T lymphocytes also secrete cytokines which activate macrophages, and attract peripheral blood monocytes which are then converted to macrophages. Macrophages are transformed into histiocytes which form granulomas. Delayed-type hypersensitivity demonstrated by the Mantoux test, is a manifestation of cell-mediated immunity.

PATHOGENESIS

After the organism has gained entry via the respiratory tract, at the time of primary complex formation, there is clinically silent blood spread to the brain with formation of subependymal or subarachnoid tubercles, the so-called Rich foci. Later, one or more of these tubercles ruptures allowing subarachnoid spread of viable bacilli and tuberculous antigen (Rich and McCordock, 1933). This leads to tuberculous meningitis. Neurological involvement may also manifest as spinal meningitis, intracranial tuberculoma, Pott's paraplegia or intraspinal granuloma.

PATHOLOGY

Tuberculous Meningitis (TBM)

The base of the brain is covered by an extensive gelatinous exudate, filling the chiasmatic cistern (Dastur and Lalitha, 1973) extending forwards along the olfactory nerves and undersurface of the frontal lobes, laterally along the middle cerebral arteries and temporal lobes, downwards over the front of the midbrain and pons to the basal cisterns and posteriorly around the tentorium cerebelli, thus encircling the brainstem and blocking the exit of the fourth ventricle (Figure 9.1). The exudate is serofibrinous, with areas of caseation and mononuclear cell infiltration. This is *acute inflammatory caseous meningitis*.

In the miliary form of TB, there are numerous small widely scattered tubercles consisting of epithelioid and giant cells. In the more chronic cases, there may be a localized 'tuberculoma en plaque' in the meninges (Figure 9.2). This is a central area of caseation surrounded by epithelioid and giant cells or an organized and fibrotic localized exudate called *proliferative meningitis*.

The cranial nerves and spinal nerve roots passing through the exudate are mechanically compromised and show ischaemic infarcts. In addition, the arteries are directly involved as they travel through the exudate. This prominent arteritis is caused by a combination of infection and immunological effects, and results in an invasion of the adventitia by predominantly mononuclear cells. The media

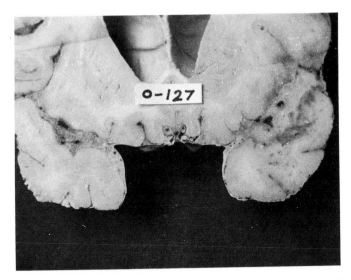

Figure 9.1 A case of tuberculosis shows exudate surrounding the optic chiasma and thick exudate in both sylvian fissures. The vessels are entrapped and show evidence of thrombosis. There is moderate hydrocephalus and a small split in septum pellucidum is evident. Courtesy of Dr S.A. Barodawalla.

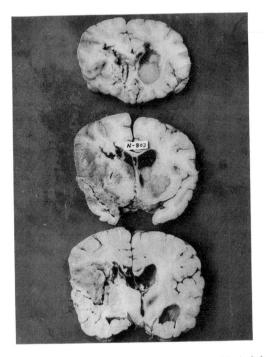

Figure 9.2 A case of multiple tuberculomas with tuberculous meningitis. Left frontotemporal region shows 'tuberculoma en plaque'. Courtesy of Dr S.A. Barodawalla.

is spared, whilst the intima shows caseation, fibrinoid degeneration and inflammatory and proliferative changes.

The Brain

Macroscopically, the brain is generally swollen and oedematous. There is often hydrocephalus, usually due to occlusion of the outlet foramina from the fourth ventricle or less commonly due to stenosis of the aqueduct or third ventricle as a result of inflammatory oedema, tuberculoma or compression of the brainstem by the surrounding exudate.

Microscopically, there is almost always an encephalitic component, and one or more of the following are present (Figure 9.3): subpial and subependymal oedema, inflammatory cell cuffs around blood vessels, and microglial proliferation. Small discrete tuberculomas and infarcts in the middle cerebral artery territory usually accompany these changes.

Tuberculous encephalopathy is unusual. In this form of TB, hypersensitivity to tuberculous protein results in generalized oedema, distension of microvasculature, perivascular demyelination and, infrequently, haemorrhages (Dastur and Udani, 1966).

Intracranial tuberculoma may be single or multiple with central necrosis surrounded by lymphocytes, plasma cells and histiocytes with many Langhans giant cells. The central lesion is surrounded by smaller satellites of epithelioid

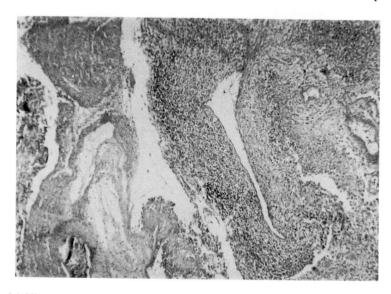

Figure 9.3 Microscopic section showing thick exudate. Vessels show granulomatous reaction and there is oedema. Courtesy of Dr S.A. Barodawalla.

cells with giant cells and incipient caseation, whereas the surrounding brain shows gliosis and oedema (Tandon and Pathak, 1973).

Spinal Cord

When there is spinal meningitis, the inflamed meninges are adherent to each other and to the cord. In addition, the underlying cord shows oedema and necrosis.

CLINICAL FEATURES

Meningitis

The earliest symptoms are non-specific. The patient has low-grade fever, headache, changes in temperament such as irritability or apathy, anorexia, abdominal pain and constipation. Typically, after 1–3 weeks, meningeal irritation develops and the headache and vomiting increase, accompanied by neck stiffness with positive Kernig's and Brudzinski's signs. The onset may be more acute or, alternatively, there may be a longer prodromal phase. In children, vomiting is the most prominent early symptom.

As the disease progresses, evidence of brain parenchymal involvement, such as seizures, drowsiness and focal neurological deficits become apparent. There may be hemiparesis and involvement of cranial nerves II, III, IV, VI, VII and VIII and, on rare occasions, involuntary movements. There may be evidence of raised intracranial pressure. Adults develop papilloedema. Young children may have a bulging fontanelle or increased head circumference.

The final stage of deep coma with abnormal extensor posturing and fixed pupils, is rarely seen nowadays when effective treatment is given.

Apart from the above, presentation of this disease may be acutely as a stroke, single or multiple seizures, cranial nerve palsies, a neuropsychiatric disorder or a slowly developing hydrocephalus. Other rare TBM manifestations include a transient, recurrent serous meningitis or a tuberculous encephalopathy, where there is predominantly a parenchymatous involvement (Kocen and Parsons, 1970).

Tuberculoma

A large tuberculoma is usually solitary. Tuberculomas present as slowly growing space-occupying lesions with seizures, focal deficits and raised intracranial pressure. They occur mainly above the tentorium in adults and below the tentorium in children, and represent a common cause of cerebral space-occupying lesions in areas where tuberculosis is prevalent.

With the introduction of CT scanning, unsuspected small tuberculomas have been found in cases of TBM. They have been known to appear and increase in size and number whilst the meningitis is coming under control with drugs. Tuberculomas have often been demonstrated to be a cause of partial seizures or secondarily generalized seizures.

Spinal Tuberculosis

There are three kinds of tuberculosis of the vertebral column, spinal cord and its coverings. The commonest kind involves tuberculous infection of bone and intervertebral disc, resulting eventually in fusion of adjacent vertebrae with deformity. This is Pott's disease. In addition, there may be compression or vascular compromise of the cord or inflammation of its coverings resulting in paraplegia.

Tuberculous spinal meningitis is the next most common form of presentation. If it is acute, it causes transverse myelitis or ascending myelitis, but when chronic, it is usually confined to one or two segments and presents like a spinal tumour, often with a combination of root and cord signs (Dastur and Wadia, 1969; Wadia and Dastur, 1969).

Spinal tuberculomas are rare and may be extradural, intradural, extramedullary or intramedullary. They usually cause compressive myelopathy and have been reviewed by Parsons and Pallis (1965).

All three forms of spinal tuberculosis may occur independently or together, with or without accompanying intracranial tuberculous infection.

DIAGNOSIS

For diagnosis of suspected TBM, examination of the cerebrospinal fluid (CSF) is mandatory. In suspected cerebral tuberculoma, neuroimaging is necessary and for suspected spinal tuberculosis, a combination of CSF examination and neuroimaging is required.

In TBM, the CSF is under pressure, usually clear but sometimes opalescent or xanthochromic. The cellular response consists of 100–500 cells mm^{-3}, usually lymphocytes. On occasion, polymorphs may predominate at the onset or later in the course of the disease. Polymorphs usually indicate a transient allergic tubercular response and subsequently the picture reverts to a lymphocytic one (Kennedy and Fallon, 1979; Ogawa *et al.*, 1987). The CSF protein is raised in TBM, generally 100–500 mg dl^{-1}, but sometimes much higher when there is a spinal block. Glucose values in the CSF are usually low (less than 50% of the blood level measured simultaneously). The CSF chloride is low, usually reflecting a low serum chloride but this is not a crucial diagnostic test. Occasionally, the initial CSF may be normal and if the diagnosis is strongly supected, lumbar puncture should be repeated in 48 hours.

Tubercle bacilli are isolated in a minority of cases of TBM. The isolation rate can be enhanced by centrifuging 10–20 ml of CSF and preparing a thick smear from the pellicle. Cultures for acid-fast bacilli take several weeks to yield results and are not helpful indicators for starting treatment.

Because of difficulties in isolating the organism, other tests have been used to obtain an accurate diagnosis. None of these is yet widely used in clinical practice. They include elevated adenosine deaminase, identification of antibody to acid-fast bacilli, identification of antigen by enzyme-linked immunosorbent assay, finding tuberculostearic acid by gas chromatography and, most recently, the polymerase chain reaction to detect mycobacterial DNA (Shankar *et al.*, 1991).

A positive tuberculin test, which only signifies exposure to tuberculosis at some time, is of value in infants and young children and in countries such as the US, where BCG vaccination is not routinely used and tuberculosis is uncommon. A negative tuberculin test is seen in about half of all patients with TBM and probably reflects anergy (Molavi and LeFrock, 1985).

An elevated erythrocyte sedimentation rate and hyponatraemia resulting from inappropriate antidiuretic hormone secretion are frequently observed in patients with TBM. Fifty to ninety per cent of patients with TBM showed evidence of pulmonary tuberculosis on chest X-ray (Molavi and LeFrock, 1985).

In meningitis, enhanced computed tomography (CT) or magnetic resonance imaging (MRI) typically reveals a combination of meningeal enhancement and hydrocephalus (Chang *et al.*, 1990) (Figure 9.4). Tuberculomas may occur with or without meningitis (Figure 9.5), but there are no features specific to tuberculomas, so they must be differentiated from other granulomas or space-occupying lesions. Other complications of meningitis, namely ischaemia, infarcts and oedema, can also be detected. Angiography is now rarely used in patients with

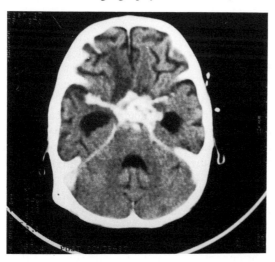

Figure 9.4 Tuberculous meningitis: contrast-enhanced computed tomography of the brain in a child. There is thick, intensely enhancing meningeal exudate within the basal cisterns, surrounding optic chiasma and pituitary stalk. The ventricles are enlarged. Courtesy of Dr Meher Ursekar.

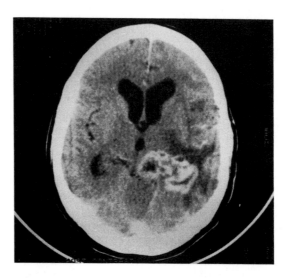

Figure 9.5 Tuberculoma: Contrast-enhanced computed tomography of the brain shows a lesion within the left temporal lobe consisting of multiple enhancing rings surrounded by vasogenic oedema. There is accompanying hydrocephalus. Courtesy of Dr Meher Ursekar.

tuberculosis of the CNS. When carried out in a patient with meningitis, it may show arterial narrowing or occlusion suggestive of arteritis.

For the diagnosis of spinal tuberculosis, either MRI or myelography in combination with CT is useful (Figure 9.6a, b). Myelography shows filling defects suggestive of arachnoiditis, or a complete block whereas CT and MRI reveal cord compression, epidural and prevertebral abscess and identify bony pathology.

Differential Diagnosis

In regions where tuberculosis is endemic, the typical clinical presentation and CSF findings of TBM do not cause diagnostic difficulty, even though bacteriological confirmation may not be obtained. It would be better to overtreat suspected cases than to delay treatment and risk additional complications. Partially treated pyogenic meningitis, fungal meningitis and viral encephalitis have to be considered in the differential diagnosis. Other rare causes of meningitis may present in a similar fashion to TBM, for example spirochaetal, listeria or parasitic disorders. Carcinomatous or lymphomatous meningitis may show similar features, and potentially treatable entities such as sarcoidosis, cerebral angiitis and Behçet's disease should not be missed. Cerebral abscess and intracranial thrombophlebitis may be difficult to differentiate clinically. Multiple therapies are sometimes necessary to cover different diagnostic options until the diagnosis is clarified (Anderson and Willoughby, 1987; Katzman and Ellner, 1990).

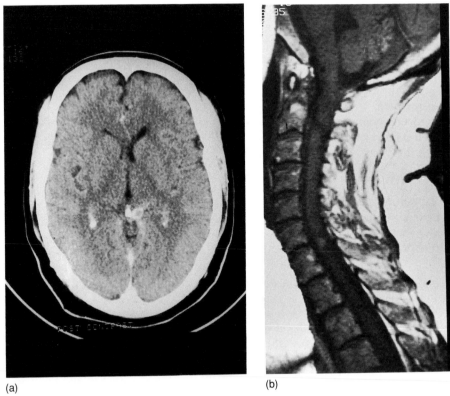

(a)   (b)

Figure 9.6 (a) Postcontrast computed tomography of brain showing a tuberculoma in basal cisterns around the midbrain on the left side. (b) Magnetic resonance image of cervical spine of same patient as in (a). T1-weighted image showing an intramedullary tuberculoma at C6 level.

Tuberculoma presents as any space-occupying lesion, but will be suspected in the appropriate clinical circumstances, for example in an Indian child with a posterior fossa mass. Biopsy may be necessary to confirm diagnosis before treatment begins, but can often be dispensed with. Spinal tuberculoma without associated vertebral disease must be differentiated from other inflammatory or compressive myelopathy which may present in an identical manner.

MANAGEMENT

Drugs currently referred to as 'first-line' antituberculous agents are streptomycin (SM), isoniazid (INH), rifampin (RMP), ethambutol (EMB) and pyrazinamide (PZA). 'Second-line' drugs, such as ethionamide, *para*-aminosalicylic acid, cycloserine, kanamycin, capreomycin and amikacin are used only if side-effects or bacterial resistance to one or more of the first-line drugs arises (Vanscoy and Willowske, 1992). Of the 'first-line' drugs, only INH, RMP and PZA are bactericidal, whilst only INH, PZA, ethionamide and cycloserine penetrate the blood–CSF barrier even when meningeal inflammation is not present. Newer second-line drugs are the fluoroquinolones, rifabutin and the macrolide antibiotics such as azithromycin. To prevent the emergence of drug-resistant bacilli (secondary drug resistance) or in case the original infection is a resistant bacillus (primary drug resistance), it is mandatory to initiate treatment with a multiple drug regimen.

A recommended regimen is to commence treatment with four drugs chosen from the following list and continue these for 18 months. These drugs are INH 10–12 mg kg^{-1}day^{-1} usually 300 mg day^{-1} for an adult, RMP 12 mg kg^{-1}day^{-1}, usually 600 mg in an adult, PZA 30 mg kg^{-1}day^{-1}, usually 1.5 g a day in an adult, EMB 15 mg kg^{-1}day^{-1} usually 800 mg day^{-1} in an adult, and SM intramuscularly 1 g day^{-1} in an adult and 20 mg kg^{-1} day^{-1} in a child.

Patients with organisms resistant to the usual therapy need specialist treatment. Those likely to have resistant organisms are patients who have relapsed during or following treatment with the standard regimen or those who have been partially treated, usually non-compliant patients. These patients should be treated with multiple drugs including second-line and new drugs (Alastair and Wood, 1993).

Nausea, vomiting and liver dysfunction are the most common toxic effects of treatment. It is important to assess liver function regularly throughout treatment. If there is symptomatic liver dysfunction or there are laboratory indications of increasing hepatotoxicity (liver enzymes raised four-fold or more), PZA, RMP and INH should be withdrawn and treatment continued with SM and EMB. As clinical and enzymatic evidence of liver dysfunction return to normal, the drugs are slowly successively reintroduced at lower doses. Dosage is gradually increased subsequently. Fortunately, development of serious hepatotoxic damage is rare. Another manifestation of drug toxicity from this regimen, is INH neuropathy due to a conditioned vitamin B$_6$ deficiency, which can be prevented by adding pyridoxine 40 mg prophylactically. Rifampicin colours body fluids orange pink. Ethambutol is known to produce optic neuritis and visual impairment. It is probably wiser not to give it to very young children who cannot complain of visual loss, and to test visual acuity and colour vision, particularly green, regularly. Streptomycin can produce hearing impairment and dizziness, particularly in the elderly.

In view of the need for prolonged costly treatment, sometimes in patients who suffer from drug toxicity and do not comply with treatment, there has been much discussion about whether a shorter course of therapy is preferable. Despite some favourable reports, short courses of treatment are not generally advocated, because of the increasing frequency of single and multiple drug-resistant strains, both primary and secondary, with the possibility of relapse. In addition, in many parts of the world there are few or no data available on drug resistance.

The use of corticosteroid therapy is controversial. It is recommended when there is evidence of rising intracranial tension, development of a focal neurological deficit suggesting an arteritis, rising CSF protein suggesting a spinal block, or clinical or neuroimaging evidence of arachnoiditis at the optic chiasma. In TBM the hypersensitivity and immune responses are closely linked and both are affected by steroids. The effect on hypersensitivity is to reduce meningeal inflammation, which is beneficial. The effect on the immune system is to suppress host defences, which may be dangerous and particularly in a patient who is already immunosuppressed, as in HIV infections. Steroids also have other widely known side-effects. Thus the question of steroid therapy has to be carefully considered for each individual case.

Blockage of CSF pathways is a common feature of TBM. In many cases this will resolve with chemotherapy, but should clinically significant hydrocephalus develop, a ventriculo–peritoneal shunt may be required.

The drug treatment of tuberculoma and of spinal TB is as described earlier. With tuberculoma, surgery is indicated only if there is inadequate response or the diagnosis is in doubt. In spinal meningitis, there appears to be little place for intrathecal hyaluronidase, and surgery has no role. Surgery, however, is useful in tuberculous spondylitis, to decompress the cord and stabilize the spine (Tandon and Pathak, 1973).

PROGNOSIS AND SEQUELAE

With modern methods of treatment, TBM is a curable disease, particularly if therapy is begun before encephalopathy or raised intracranial pressure develop (Kennedy and Fallon, 1979). If the diagnosis is delayed, sequelae are common, particularly in children. The main residual disabilities are seizures, cranial nerve palsies, deafness, blindness, hemiplegia or paraplegia. Mental retardation or behavioural and learning problems considerably restrict the child's achievement potential. Finally, in a few cases, hypothalamic damage from hydrocephalus may result in endocrine disturbances. If treatment does not start before the patient has become unconscious, or has developed signs of brainstem dysfunction, the case fatality ratio is 50%.

REFERENCES

Alastair JJ and Wood MD (1993) Treatment of multidrug resistance tuberculosis. *New England Journal of Medicine* **329**: 784–791.

Anderson NE and Willoughby EW (1987) Chronic meningitis without pre-disposing illness: a review of 83 cases. *Quarterly Journal of Medicine* **240**: 283–295.

Chang KH, Han MH, Roh JK *et al.* (1990) Gd-DTPA-enhanced MR imaging of the brain in patients with meningitis: comparison with CT. *American Journal of Roentgenology* **154(4)**: 809–816.

Dastur DK and Lalitha VS (1973) The many facets of neuro-tuberculosis – an epitome of neuropathology. In: *Progress in Neuropathology*, vol. 2 (ed. MH Zimmerman), pp 351–408. New York: Grune and Stratton.

Dastur DK and Udani PM (1966) Pathology and pathogenesis of tuberculous encephalopathy. *Acta Neuropathologica (Berlin)* **6**: 311.

Dastur DK and Wadia NH (1969) Spinal meningitides with radiculomyelopathy: Part 2. Pathology and pathogenesis *Journal of Neurological Science* **8**: 261.

Katzman M and Ellner JJ (1990) Chronic meningitis. In: *Principles and Practice of Infectious Diseases*, 3rd edn (eds GL Mandell, GR Douglas Jr, JE Bennett), pp 755–762. New York: Churchill Livingstone.

Kennedy DH and Fallon RJ (1979) Tuberculous meningitis. *Journal of the American Medical Association* **241(3)**: 264–268.

Kocen RS and Parsons M (1970) Neurological complications of tuberculosis: some unusual manifestations. *Quarterly Journal of Medicine* **39**: 17–30.

Molavi A and LeFrock JL (1985) Tuberculous meningitis. *Medical Clinics of North America* **69(2)**: 315–331.

Ogawa SK, Smith MA, Brennessel DJ and Lowy FD (1987) Tuberculous meningitis in an urban medical center. *Medicine* **66(4)**: 317–326.

Parsons M and Pallis CA (1965) Intradural spinal tuberculomas. *Neurology* **15**: 1018.

Rich AR and McCordock HA (1933) The pathogenesis of tuberculous meningitis. *Bulletin of the Johns Hopkins Hospital* **52**: 5.

Shankar P, Manjunath N, Mohan KK *et al.* (1991) Rapid diagnosis of tuberculous meningitis by polymerase chain reaction. *Lancet* **337**: 5–7.

Snider DE Jr and Roper WL (1992) The new tuberculosis. *New England Journal of Medicine* **326**: 703–705.

Tandon PN and Pathak SN (1973) Tuberculosis of the central nervous system. In: *Tropical Neurology* (ed. JD Spillane), pp 37–63. London: Oxford University Press.

Vanscoy RE and Willowske CJ (1992) Antituberculous agents. *Mayo Clinic Proceedings* **67**: 179–187.

Wadia NH and Dastur DK (1969) Spinal meningitides with radiculomyelopathy: Part 1. Clinical and radiological features. *Journal of Neurological Science* **8**: 239.

10

Leprosy

Thomas R. Swift and Thomas D. Sabin

Medical College of Georgia, 1459 Laney Walker Blvd, Augusta, GA 30912, USA

INTRODUCTION

The Bible, Indian and Chinese manuscripts reveal that leprosy was widespread and familiar in ancient times. When G. Armour Hansen reported his observations on tissues from his Norwegian patients in 1864 he became the first to link a bacterium to a human disease. Neisser laid false claim to this discovery and Hansen's difficulties were compounded when he tried to inoculate a patient's conjunctiva with leprosy bacilli without informed consent (Mange, 1992). This organism is now known as the acid-fast *Mycobacterium leprae* and has several extraordinary properties:

(1) There is a consistent invasion of nerves. Nerves are usually very resistant to other bacterial infections but the authors have never seen a definite case of leprosy without clinical evidence of nerve involvement.
(2) *M. leprae* does not reproduce at core body temperature of 37°C. The optimal growth rate occurs at 27–30°C which results in a 'superficial' disease affecting cooler tissues including skin, nerves, testes, anterior one-third of the eye and the upper respiratory tract. The viscera are spared (Brand, 1959; Shepard, 1965).
(3) Genetically susceptible armadillos, mouse foot pads and thymectomized irradiated rats can be used to grow bacilli but *M. leprae* has not yet been satisfactorily cultured on artificial media.

Since there are some 10 million affected people in the world (about 6000 in the United States), leprosy is the cause of the most common treatable neuropathy in the world. The diagnosis is still often missed, especially in sophisticated Western medical centres where an anti-myelin-associated glycoprotein associated neuropathy would easily be diagnosed. Delay in treatment is a major problem because the disease usually progresses and the resulting disability with late treatment may be severe, even though mycobacteria may be eliminated.

MODE OF TRANSMISSION

Despite the opportunity for good epidemiological studies, the exact mode of transmission is uncertain. The failure to grow *M. leprae* on artificial media precludes critical studies such as attempting to culture the organism from arthropods in the dwellings of patients. Nasal secretions and skin contact appear to be the most likely means of communicability. In most populations, over 95% of individuals are naturally immune. The disease is generally thought to be of low infectivity but the epidemiological data seem equally compatible with an actively contagious illness which is capable of infecting only a small percentage of population.

GENERAL MANIFESTATIONS

Although there is only one *M. leprae* there are differences in the natural host resistance to invasion by the organism and this immune state sculptures the clinical features of the disease (Ottenhoff, 1994). The classification of leprosy is based on the host immunity and therefore the disease exists in several clinical and pathological subtypes. The terminology of subtypes has been changed several times over the years which may make the old literature confusing. The currently used terminology groups cases of polar low-resistance type as *lepromatous*, high-resistance cases as *tuberculoid* and the range of cases between these polar forms as *borderline*. The neurology of leprosy is in close register with the other features of each of these varieties of leprosy.

Tuberculoid Leprosy

When host resistance is very high the powerful cell-mediated immune (CMI) attack on the organisms is reflected by the development of an epithelioid granuloma with rare bacilli. Patients with tuberculoid leprosy and healthy exposed individuals both have intact T-cell dependent immunity to *M. leprae*. This CMI checks bacillary proliferation and dissemination, yet is directly responsible for the skin and nerve lesions. Further understanding of the antigenic components of *M. leprae* may clarify this paradox, and even lead to a vaccine. Clinically there is one, or very few, asymmetrical, well-demarcated, often hypopigmented skin lesions which are both anaesthetic and anhydrotic with an active raised erythematous border and a tendency to undergo self-healing (Figure 10.1a). The nerve trunks neighbouring these lesions are apt to be palpably or even visibly enlarged (Figure 10.1b). The central part of the lesion may be completely cleared of bacilli so that diagnostic biopsy may often be obtained only at the active border. Lepromin skin testing is positive. These lesions are most frequent on the outer extremities, face, upper back and

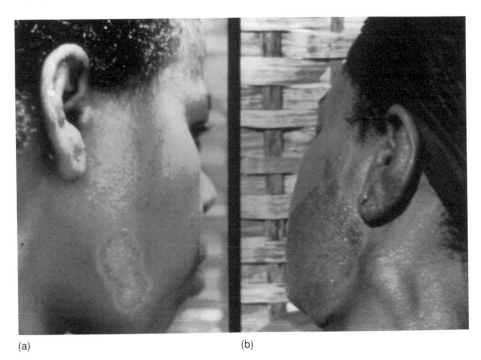

(a)   (b)

Figure 10.1 (a) A typical tuberculoid leprosy lesion with distinct raised border and hypopigmentation. Sensory loss coincides with the skin lesion. (b) Marked enlargement of the auricular nerve is evident as the nerve passes over the sternocleidomastoid muscle.

buttocks. These seem to be sites on the body where skin contact with infected material could have occurred.

Lepromatous Leprosy

At the other end of the spectrum of host resistance, leprosy bacilli are abundant with haematogenous dissemination throughout the body (Powell and Swan, 1955). Multiplication to enormous numbers occurs. The quiescent immune response is reflected in the microscopic appearance of histiocytes which contain huge numbers of 'healthy'-appearing solidly-staining bacilli with very little actual inflammatory response. An extremely specific defect in T-cell responsiveness to *M. leprae* is believed to be the cause of the heavy bacterial burden in this form of leprosy. Passive deposition of the bacilli occurs in the viscera, including the brain, but no active invasion or replication of the bacilli occurs in these 'warm' tissues. During this time of unchecked bacillary multiplication, the skin usually becomes thickened with the sheer burden of organisms. Nasal stuffiness gives way to mouth breathing. The mouth then becomes cool, as does the oral pharynx, and as they do so, they become infiltrated with organisms. Eventually, airway obstruction and suffocation did occur in the days before effective antibiotics were used, but this is seldom seen today. Infiltration of the skin is associated with a variety of lesions including macules, nodules, papules, or even a diffuse form of infiltration which causes only a subtle waxy sheen. In lepromatous leprosy, the diagnosis is easily established by biopsy of one of the skin lesions in a 'cool' area and observing the abundant organisms when properly demonstrated by the Fite modification of the acid-fast stain (Hastings *et al.*, 1968).

Borderline Leprosy

The type of cases which lie between the tuberculoid and lepromatous forms are known as borderline leprosy and represent a complex mixture of features of the two polar forms which reflect gradations in host resistance to the invasion of *M. leprae*. In borderline cases near lepromatous, bacilli are numerous but the disease tends to be more asymmetrical than pure lepromatous disease. The bacilli are present in smaller numbers and staining shows more 'beaded' forms. Large areas of the body may be affected. In borderline cases near tuberculoid there are a few lesions which are well demarcated and neurological deficits tend to overlay the skin lesions precisely. Borderline leprosy is inherently unstable, and host responsiveness tends to fluctuate, at times leading toward lepromatous disease (downgrading) or toward tuberculoid forms (reversal). Organisms tend to be numerous in borderline lepromatous and fewer in borderline tuberculoid.

LEPROUS NEURITIS

As can be seen from the foregoing, the unique characteristics of the leprosy bacillus and the variations in host response together determine the unique nature of the neuropathy in a given patient. Since the bacillus invades peripheral nerve, particularly Schwann cells, and is the only bacterial pathogen that regularly does so, it is responsible for the development of neuropathy. The bacillus multiplies optimally at 27–30°C and therefore does not cause disease of the central nervous system (CNS) or even of those parts of the peripheral nervous system where peripheral nerves are at or near core body temperature. Rather, superficial nerves and nerve networks are affected in cool areas of face, trunk and extremities resulting in a temperature-linked neuropathy (Sabin *et al.*, 1974). The extent and severity of the neuropathy are determined by the body's response to the presence of the bacillus (Ottenhoff, 1994). In tuberculoid leprosy, organisms are few, contained by a host response that is vigorous, and early and severe nerve damage occurs, but in a sharply limited area. In contrast, in lepromatous leprosy, organisms are present in very high numbers, but the tissue response is passive and nerve damage, though widespread, is less severe and occurs later. In borderline or intermediate leprosy, nerve damage occurs on a spectrum, being more limited in extent but severe on the tuberculoid end, and more diffuse but milder on the lepromatous end of the spectrum.

In neurology, the prepared clinician often must anticipate what he or she will find in order to be able to discern the pattern. To diagnose leprous neuritis, the disease must first be suspected, and the temperature-linked neuropathy specifically sought for. In finding a temperature-related pattern of nerve loss the clinician will be rewarded by the ability to diagnose leprosy specifically, and often to diagnose the type of leprosy present with a high degree of certainty, even in cases where bacilli may no longer be present and histological evidence of disease has long since disappeared or where the patient may be concealing the disease.

Lepromatous Leprosy

In lepromatous leprosy a constant bacteraemia occurs, depositing organisms throughout the body. Proliferation of organisms then occurs in cool tissues: facial promontories, the upper respiratory tract, helices of the ears and ear-lobes, the testes, extensor surfaces of upper and lower extremities, and the anterior one-third of the eyes. It is in these areas that dermal nerves and nerve networks are heavily infiltrated and where cutaneous sensory loss eventually occurs. The peripheral nerves in deeper and warmer tissues are spared, so that muscle weakness, loss of tendon jerks, and diminished vibration sensation are much less common than loss of cutaneous sensations of pinprick and temperature and later, touch. In early lepromatous leprosy there may be very little sensory loss despite the presence of many organisms in the skin and nerves demonstrated on biopsy. As the disease progresses, loss of cutaneous sensation begins to appear on ears, nose, upper lip, chin, forehead, extensor surfaces of hands, forearms, anterior legs and dorsum of feet (Sabin, 1969; Sabin and Ebner, 1969). There will be little loss of sensation on the palm of hands, arch of the feet, ventral forearms, antecubital fossae, under the scalp, in the axillae and groin, and in the gluteal cleft. The palms and soles are spared at this time owing to the increased temperature under the insulating corium. With progression, the areas of sensory loss spread and become larger, involving warmer and warmer areas, to reach a stage where a large portion of the skin surface is anaesthetized. The tip of the nose, malar areas, breasts, central abdomen and buttocks are the next to be involved. The pattern now becomes defined not so much by selective involvement of cool areas but rather by sensory sparing in warmest areas: on the scalp, the anterior neck, in the depths of the nasolabial folds, in the sternal area, axillae, groin, gluteal cleft, perineum, and even between the toes and fingers in the antecubital and popliteal fossae and centre of the back where the skin lies closest to paraspinal muscles (Figure 10.2). Corneal anaesthesia gives way to secondary infection and blindness.

The tight link of the neuropathy to temperature leads to unique findings:

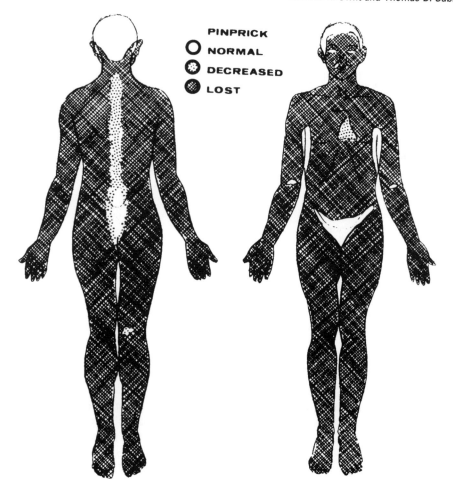

Figure 10.2 Very advanced pattern of temperature-linked sensory loss due largely to intracutaneous destruction of nerve endings. Only the warmest regions of the body surface show intact pinprick sensation. From Sabin *et al.* (1993) with permission.

preservation of sensation under habitually worn tight clothing which keeps the skin warm, such as a belt or watch band, and even the preservation of sensation in skin over vascular malformations (Sabin, 1970) (Figure 10.3). While nerve networks in the skin are being infiltrated and destroyed, so also are nerve trunks involved in areas where they are close to the body surface and therefore cool; a 15 cm segment of the ulnar nerve at and just proximal to the elbow and a small segment just proximal to the wrist, the radial nerve at the wrist, the peroneal nerve at the ankle and knee, and the great auricular nerve (Sabin *et al.*, 1974). The most superficial branches of the facial nerve are involved as they pass through the cooler tissues of the face (Monrad-Krohn, 1923). The median nerve

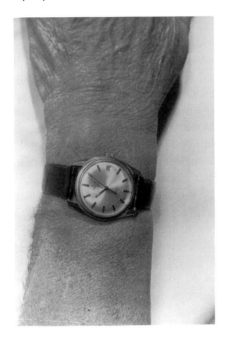 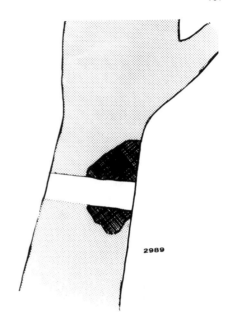

Figure 10.3 Sparing of sensation under a watch-band.

may be involved proximal to the wrist. The posterior tibial nerve is involved at the ankle. With disease progression, nerve enlargement also progresses and involves longer segments of the nerves but because of the absence of a tissue response the enlarged nerves may continue to conduct impulses for long periods of time.

Eventually, however, involvement of these named nerves reaches the point of producing motor and sensory deficits, and a pattern of temperature-linked multiple mononeuropathies is added to the temperature-linked cutaneous sensory loss. This may produce interesting combinations of neurological deficits. As an example, if a patient who already has sensory loss on the dorsum of the hand but not on the palmar surface develops an ulnar neuropathy at the elbow, he will now have sensory loss on the palmar surface and digits in the distribution of the ulnar neuropathy and develop the typical claw hand as well.

The reasons why nerve trunk enlargement leads to dysfunction in lepromatous leprosy are not clear, but in many cases nerve trunk deficits appear suddenly, during the course of erythema nodosum leprosum where immunologically mediated acute inflammatory reactions are occurring in the nerve in areas where a great deal of mycobacterial antigen is present. In addition to the ulnar neuropathy, defects commonly seen from nerve trunk involvement include peroneal neuropathy with foot drop, tibial nerve involvement with clawing of the toes, facial weakness which is patchy, usually bilateral, and less commonly weakness of wrist and finger extension from involvement of the radial nerve at the elbow. Median nerve involvement occurs where it becomes superficial just proximal to the wrist, producing weakness of thumb abduction and flexion.

The facial weakness in leprosy has unusual features that easily distinguish it from the more familiar Bell's palsy (Monrad-Krohn, 1923) (Figure 10.4a, b). The zygomatic branch of the nerve to the orbicularis oculi frequently is involved leading to lagophthalmos and ectropion of the lower eyelid. Imperfect closure of the lids occurs, allowing the cornea, already dry and usually insensitive, to become secondarily infected, eventually leading to blindness. Similarly, involvement of nerve branches to the orbicularis oris and other mouth muscles leads to weakness and ectropion of the lips. The deeper branches of the facial nerve are commonly spared. The buccinator muscle is usually intact and may produce characteristic buccinator wrinkling which replaces the nasolabial fold. If a branch of the temporal division of the nerve to the frontalis happens to run under the scalp, it may be spared, so that on attempted wrinkling of the forehead only the lateral part of the forehead and lateral eyebrow may be raised, producing a devilish appearance if bilateral. At times, the involved branches of the facial nerve which are enlarged may be directly palpated.

To summarize, in lepromatous leprosy there is a superimposition of major

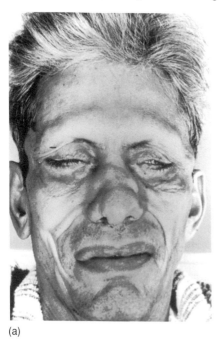 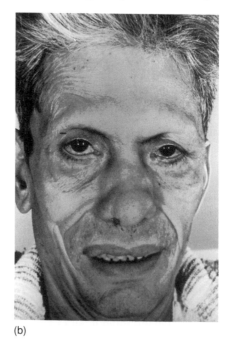

(a)   (b)

Figure 10.4 (a) The patchy nature of the facial paralysis is evident in the outpouching of the lateral upper lip and bilateral incomplete eye closure. (b) Attempting eyebrow elevation demonstrates bilateral paralysis of the medial corrugators of the forehead and right lateral corrugators. From Sabin (1971) with permission.

nerve deficits on a background of intracutaneous temperature-related loss of pinprick, temperature and touch sensation.

When reaction, in this case erythema nodosum leprosum (ENL) supervenes, as it does eventually in 40–60% of patients, there may be the development of additional nerve lesions, at times quite suddenly. Along with this neuritis there is almost always the systematic appearance of skin lesions, iritis and orchitis, which may be devastating and invariably require prompt treatment with high-dose corticosteroids or thalidomide.

Tuberculoid Leprosy

At the other end of the leprosy spectrum, tuberculoid leprosy produces early and severe nerve damage, but localized to a circumscribed area of the skin. The process destroying cutaneous and subcutaneous nerves is an epithelioid granuloma which is also responsible for the visible skin lesions (Sabin *et al.*, 1993).

Typically, there is a raised erythematous patch on the skin from few to many centimetres in size, often with a satellite lesion or two (Figure 10.5). Nerves are destroyed within the skin lesion and, on testing with a pin, an area of sensory loss is found that coincides exactly with the hypopigmented skin lesion. Since sympathetic nerves are involved, the lesion also shows no sweating and is dry. Beyond the margin of the lesion, sensation is normal. If a large nerve or branch happens to underlie the skin lesion, it too may be involved and thickened and deficits in the distribution of that nerve may occur. This suggests that organisms may travel from cutaneous nerves back to parent nerve trunks. Nerves most likely to be affected in tuberculoid leprosy are the ulnar, median, peroneal and facial. Cold abscesses may develop in such nerves (Enna and Brand, 1970), requiring surgical drainage, and nerve calcification may be visible on X-rays and nerve enlargement on computed tomographic scans (Barbancon *et al.*, 1989). Such lesions can develop in any part of the body, but spare the warmest areas.

Borderline (Intermediate) Leprosy

Between polar lepromatous and polar tuberculoid leprosy lies a spectrum of disease called borderline (Sabin *et al.*, 1993). Host response to the presence of organisms varies, being relatively low at the lepromatous end and relatively high at the tuberculoid end of the spectrum. Clinically, the pattern of cutaneous sensory loss in borderline lepromatous disease follows, in general, a temperature-linked pattern but not as perfectly as in polar lepromatous disease and skin lesions are not as numerous, confluent or symmetrical. Sensory loss may extend beyond the boundaries of the visible skin lesions. Likewise, in borderline tuberculoid disease the lesions are few, more asymmetrical, and produce earlier and more severe neural deficits which tend to be restricted to the skin lesions. In between these two varieties, in the middle of the spectrum of borderline leprosy,

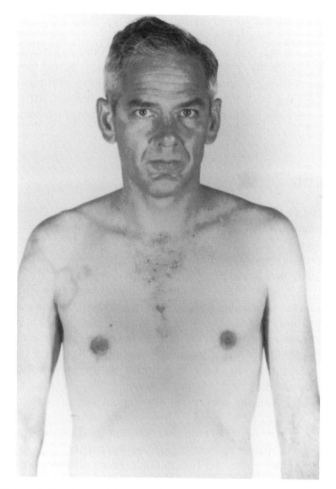

Figure 10.5 A tuberculoid lesion on right upper chest and arm with satellite lesions.

the symmetry, number of lesions, and severity vary (Figure 10.6). There is a rare variety of borderline leprosy where skin lesions are absent but nerve trunks are involved: so-called polyneuritic leprosy. These patients present with multiple trunk lesions and may cause problems in diagnosis. Nerve biopsy in polyneuritic leprosy reveals organisms.

COMPLICATIONS

If all aspects of this disease represented only a progressive bacterial infection then the disease would be a simple therapeutic problem solved by the proper selection of antibiotics to eradicate bacilli. However, physicians taking care of

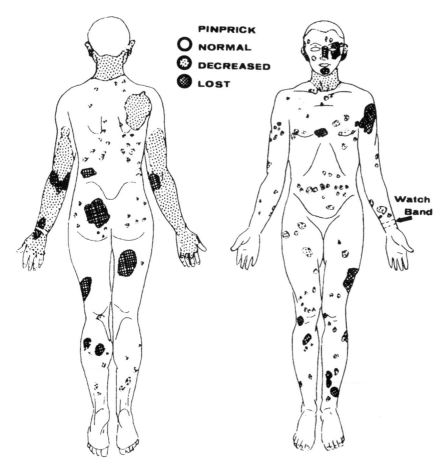

PINPRICK

O NORMAL

◉ DECREASED

● LOST

Watch
Band

Figure 10.6 Sensory loss to pinprick in a case of borderline leprosy. From Sabin *et al.* (1993) with permission.

leprosy patients find that the complications make management of the disease extremely challenging.

Leprosy Reactions

One category of complications include leprosy reactions. These consist of the development of altered immune states and vary according to the type of leprosy present (Britton, 1993). Lepromatous leprosy patients are liable to develop ENL. This consists of ENL lesions, distributed over the body in rough proportion to the density of bacilli. Biopsy reveals an arteritis with deposition of antigen–antibody complexes in the walls of small arteries where the bacterial antigen is present. The inflammatory process can cause acute painful neuritides, inflammation of the anterior chamber of the eye, fever, malaise, arthritis, orchitis as well as typical skin lesions. Occasionally, the arterial size involved is such that large skin infarcts (Lucio phenomenon) occur which heal with 'cigarette paper' scarring resembling Kohlmeir Degos disease. Various cytokines such as tumour necrosis factor alpha have been found within ENL lesions. The process appears to represent the development of circulating antibodies to mycobacterial antigen. The host's limited immunological response appears to have run amok producing a debilitating systematic disease superimposed on the leprosy.

With high-resistance forms of leprosy, reversal reactions describe a sudden increase in the tissue-mediated response resulting in acute flare-up of skin lesions along with damage to neighbouring nerves which harbour even small amounts of bacterial antigen. In borderline leprosy, a decline in tissue immunity results in slipping down the spectrum toward lepromatous disease and is termed a downgrading reaction.

Deformity Secondary to Insensitivity

Another complication of leprosy is the process of absorption of the hands and feet (Brand, 1964). Leprosy, along with hereditary sensory neuropathy, diabetic neuropathy and syringomyelia, fulfils the two conditions which permit an ongoing destruction of hands and/or feet. These two features are the loss of pain and temperature senses combined with the preserved ability to use the limb vigorously. The classic picture of a leprosy patient: blind, facially deformed, with claw hands and foot ulcers, shows the ravages of neuropathy. Without protective sensation, patients are liable to recurrent injuries of eye, hands and feet. Corneal injuries are unnoticed and untreated. Cigarette burns produce 'kissing' ulcers on adjacent fingers. The nail coming through the shoe is not removed and with every step gouges a deeper hole in the heel. Poor footwear and foot deformity together create high-pressure zones on the weight-bearing areas (metatarsal heads, calcaneus and toes) resulting in penetrating ulcers identical to those seen in any neurological condition where strength is preserved but pain sensation is lost. Penetrating ulcers are not due to 'rotting flesh', loss of 'neurotrophism', to the bacillus itself, or to vascular insufficiency. Recurrent fissures develop in skin of hands and feet made brittle by loss of sweating. Secondary infections in these fissures occur which may girdle a finger or two and result in shortening and further deformity. These fissures and other small wounds which allow common infective organisms to enter the hands and feet through ulcers, burns and cuts cause repeated bouts of osteomyelitis. Over a period of years, the fingers and feet gradually lose length and become grossly distorted. Indeed, it is the visible aspect of the disease affecting the hands, the feet and the face which probably accounts for the social stigma leprosy patients have suffered.

NEUROPATHOLOGY

Grossly enlarged nerves may be heavily infiltrated with leprosy bacilli in lepromatous disease and still function fairly well. However, ultimately the combination of progressive infiltration, enlargement of the nerve with associated liability to pressure changes and chronic trauma along with leprosy reactions conspire and nerves lose function. When reactions occur this may be a hyperacute process. The bulk of the neuropathological and electrophysiological observations point to an axonal disease but clearly Schwann cells are heavily infiltrated with bacilli. In high-resistance forms of the disease, the involvement of nerve by epithelioid granuloma and the vigorous tissue response seem to develop at the time of early infection, so that in tuberculoid leprosy a localized neurological deficit is established along with skin lesions whereas nerves in lepromatous leprosy that are involved in a widespread fashion tend to function for much longer.

TREATMENT

The mainstay of treatment since the 1940s has been the sulphones, particularly dapsone, but because of the development of bacterial resistance to dapsone in recent years recommendations have been undergoing modification. Clofazimine (Lamprene B663) is an iminophenazine which not only has antibacterial action but also ameliorates ENL. Extensive purplish discoloration of the skin and gastrointestinal upset frequently make this drug unacceptable. Crystalline deposits of this drug have been found in the conjunctiva, intestinal mucosa, liver, spleen and mesenteric lymph nodes. Current suggestions for tuberculoid or high-resistance borderline cases include a combination of dapsone and rifampicin. Dapsone is given at 100 mg daily and rifampicin 600 mg daily for a period of 6 months, but the dapsone is continued for 3 to 5 years. Lamprene is often added if dapsone resistance has been suspected or documented in mouse footpad testing. Lepromatous and borderline near lepromatous cases generally are treated with the same regimen of dapsone and rifampicin but the dapsone is continued from 10 years to life. These recommendations are undergoing frequent review and the reader is urged to contact the Gillis Long Hansen's Disease Center at Carville, Louisiana (tel. 504–642–4722) where telephone consultation is available regarding drug regimens. Expert advice regarding biopsy interpretations, patient referral and various other specific problems in management is available from the staff there.

Leprosy reactions require prompt treatment. In ENL high-dose corticosteroids should be used, particularly if there is threat to functionally important nerves. A dose of prednisolone 60–80 mg per day, or even higher, may be required. Thalidomide is the drug of choice for ENL at 300–400 mg per day. Great caution is required for women of child-bearing age but again arrangements can be made at the Gillis Long Hansen's Disease Center for the use of this drug. While its mechanism of action remains unclear, thalidomide has been shown to reduce the secretion of tumour necrosis factor alpha by monocytes and alters the radio of CD4+ to CD8+ lymphocytes. Remarkably rapid improvement in peripheral nerve function in ENL has been observed with this form of treatment. Iridocyclitis is treated with mydriatic and steroid eye drops. Reversal reactions in high-resistance leprosy also must be treated with high doses of steroids. Thalidomide only works with ENL and therefore is not indicated in the reactions associated with tuberculoid or borderline leprosy.

Leprosy rehabilitation is an extremely important aspect of treatment because for the individual patient the deformities of their face, hands and feet are more important manifestations of the disease than the bacterial counts in their biopsies. Frequent eye examinations may detect early damage in those patients with anaesthetic corneas. Surgical correction of the lagophthalmos due to facial nerve involvement is also vital in these patients. The patient must undergo intensive training to learn what environmental factors endanger insensitive but actively used hands and feet. Special footwear can be designed which is highly successful in curing and preventing plantar ulceration and the attendant cycle of soft tissue infection, osteomyelitis, bone absorption and deformity. Neurologists would do well to borrow the techniques that have been developed by leprosy workers to apply to their patients with other neuropathies.

DIFFERENTIAL DIAGNOSIS

As may be seen from the foregoing, the pattern of temperature-linked sensory, autonomic and motor deficits, once recognized, make most cases of leprosy relatively easy to diagnose, and quite distinct from the more usual polyneuropathies so much more familiar to most neurologists. The common conditions producing symmetrical glove-stocking polyneuropathies such as diabetes or alcoholic-nutritional disease result in a neuropathy in which nerve damage occurs in a length-dependent fashion affecting the longest and largest axons earliest, while affecting proximal areas of the body and head only very late in the course of disease or not at all. In these more familiar neuropathies, sensory loss begins first on the tip of the great toe and proceeds proximally as the disease becomes more severe, involving progressively more proximal areas. When the level of sensory loss approaches the knee, the fingertips begin to be involved because the length of axons to fingertips and knees is about equal and length is the determinant of dysfunction in a length-dependent neuropathy. With further progression, the anterior abdomen, and later the chest and finally the head and face may become involved. Contrast this pattern with the temperature-linked loss of sensation in leprosy which may affect the proximal forearm while sparing the palm, or affect the patellar area while sparing between the toes. Confusion may result in differentiating a stocking-glove neuropathy from leprosy if only the distal extremities are examined. The face, ears, and other cooler areas must be examined to define the temperature-linked pattern.

A second difference is in the nature of the sensory modalities lost. In the glove-stocking polyneuropathy, vibration and position senses along with touch are usually the first to become abnormal. In leprosy, these tend to be preserved. Tendon jerks are lost early in glove-stocking polyneuropathies but are retained in leprosy.

The nerve enlargement in leprosy potentially could produce confusion with other hypertrophic neuropathies such as hereditary motor and sensory neuropathy, Dejerine–Sottas disease, amyloidosis, neurofibromatosis and chronic demyelinating neuropathies. But in leprosy, nerves are segmentally enlarged only where they are cool, and associated temperature-linked patterns of sensory loss should make the diagnosis obvious.

Painful leprous neuritis occurring during ENL could be confused with other neuropathic pains such as tabes dorsalis, Fabry's disease and shingles but in the first reflexes are absent and vibration and position sense are impaired, in the second the characteristic skin and renal lesions are present, and in the third the vesicular skin lesions are diagnostic.

Leprous neuritis is sometimes confused with other conditions because of painless injuries, trophic ulcers and absorption of digits. These diseases include syringomyelia, universal insensitivity to pain, tabes dorsalis, hereditary sensory neuropathies, amyloidosis, and certain types of diabetic neuropathies. In fact, patients with these diseases often were found in leprosaria, mistakenly believed to have leprosy. But the unique nature of leprous neuritis should make differentiation from these conditions relatively easy.

REFERENCES

Barbancon O, Rath S and Alqubati Y (1989) Hansen's disease: computed tomography findings in peripheral nerve lesions. *Annals De Radiologie* **32**: 579.

Brand PW (1959) Temperature variation and leprosy deformity. *International Journal of Leprosy* **27**: 1.

Brand PW (1964) In: *Leprosy in Theory and Practice*, 2nd edn (eds RG Cochrane and TF Davey), p 447. Bristol: John Wright.

Britton WJ (1993) Immunology of leprosy. *Transactions of the Royal Society of Tropical Medicine Hygiene* **87(5)**: 508–514.

Enna CD and Brand PW (1970) Peripheral nerve abscess in leprosy. *Leprosy Review* **41**: 175.

Hastings RC, Brand PW, Mansfield RE and Ebner JD (1968) Bacterial density in the skin in lepromatous leprosy as related to temperature. *International Journal of Leprosy* **42**: 33.

Mange PF (Sept/Oct 1992) Hansen and his discovery of *Mycobacterium leprae*. *The Star*: 5–8.

Monrad-Krohn GH (1923) *The Neurological Aspect of Leprosy*. Christiana: Jacob Dybward.

Ottenhoff JHM (1994) Immunology of leprosy: Lessons from and for leprosy. *International Journal of Leprosy* **42**: 108–121.

Powell CS and Swan LL (1955) Leprosy: pathologic changes in 50 consecutive necropsies. *American Journal of Pathology* **31**: 1131.

Sabin TD (1969) Temperature-linked sensory loss: a unique pattern in leprosy. *Archives of Neurology* **20**: 257.

Sabin TD (1970) Preservation of sensation in a cutaneous vascular malformation in lepromatous leprosy. *New England Journal of Medicine* **282**: 1084.

Sabin TD (1971) Neurological features of lepromatous leprosy. *American Family Physician* **4**: 84.

Sabin TD and Ebner JD (1969) Patterns of sensory loss in lepromatous leprosy. *International Journal of Leprosy* **37**: 239.

Sabin TD, Hackett ER and Brand PW (1974) Temperatures along the course of certain nerves affected in leprosy. *International Journal of Leprosy* **42**: 33.

Sabin TD, Swift TR and Jacobson RR (1993) Leprosy. In: *Peripheral Neuropathy*, 3rd edn (eds PJ Dyck and PK Thomas), p 1354. Philadelphia: WB Saunders.

Shepard CC (1965) Temperature optimum of *Mycobacterium leprae* in mice. *Journal of Bacteriology* **90**: 1271.

11

Brucellosis

Raad A. Shakir

Department of Neurology, Middlesbrough General Hospital, Middlesbrough, Cleveland, UK

INTRODUCTION

Brucellosis still causes major morbidity in many countries world-wide. The infection is intracellular and usually causes a mild disease in man. The nervous system may be affected both in the acute and more likely in the chronic stages of the disease. The illness is most commonly acquired through ingestion of unpasteurized contaminated milk or its products or from contact with infected animals and is an occupational hazard in those who are in contact with infected animals.

HISTORY

Brucellosis was first described as a clinical entity 'Mediterranean gastric remittent fever' by J. A. Marston in 1860. David Bruce (1865–1931) described the organism as a 'micrococcus' in 1887 with the help of a Maltese microbiologist Dr Carruana-Secluna. Bruce later moved to Africa and identified *Trypanosoma brucei* as the cause of sleeping sickness.

Bang, a Danish veterinarian, identified an intracellular bacillus as the cause of abortion in cattle (Bang's bacillus). For many years no relation was thought to exist between Bruce's micrococcus and Bang's bacillus. Many others contributed to the development of our knowledge of brucellosis but two have to be specifically mentioned. The first is Mary Elizabeth Steel, the daughter of a Scottish doctor who married David Bruce; she was trained in microbiology and was instrumental in her husband's work. The second is Alice Evans a microbiologist from the United States, who was not only the first person to prove that *Micrococcus melitensis* and Bang's bacillus were different species of the same genus but also worked for many years to establish that milk was the source of the infection. It was her work that led to the pasteurization of cow's milk.

The first report on the isolation of *M. melitensis* from the brain was made in

Malta by the brilliant assistant of David Bruce, Surgeon Captain M. Louis Hughes. His classic monograph (1897) dedicated to his mentor Lord Lister is the clearest clinical description of brucellosis which he suffered from himself. Hughes was killed in the second Boer war at the age of 32 years. *Brucella melitensis* was isolated from the cerebrospinal fluid (CSF) by Lemaire in 1924 and *B. suis* was first isolated from a patient with meningoencephalitis who died of a ruptured cerebral mycotic aneurysm (Sanders, 1931). Various neurological syndromes have been reported; encephalitis, myelitis, radiculitis, neuropsychiatric manifestations, chronic meningitis, and subarachnoid haemorrhage from ruptured mycotic aneurysm (De Jong, 1936; Nichols, 1951; Spink, 1951; Fincham *et al.*, 1963).

EPIDEMIOLOGY

The number of human cases of brucellosis reported is increasing, although many countries have been declared brucellosis-free for many years. The reasons for the increased incidence is probably related to several factors; previous under-reporting, increase in animal industries with defective methods of processing, continued use of traditional methods of milk and cheese preparation and animal husbandry, in addition to the expense of implementing modern animal control programmes (Ariza *et al.*, 1993; Gilbert, 1993). It is impossible to determine clearly the incidence of brucellosis in common with many other non-fatal infections (Lopez-Merino *et al.*, 1992), there is lack of reliable statistics, and absence of reporting systems. There are additional specific reasons; many countries do not consider brucellosis as a notifiable disease, and because the disease does not present a clear clinical picture, it is often missed.

Human disease generally follows animal brucellosis. *B. melitensis* is the commonest and the most severe cause of human disease. *B. abortus*, *B. suis* and *B. canis* can all cause human disease. The other two species *B. ovis* and *B. neotome* are not known to affect man (Madkour and Gargani, 1989).

Human brucellosis is reported throughout the world and fresh cases are still seen in the Mediterranean basin, Asia, Africa, Central and South America (Animal Health Year Book, 1994). *B. melitensis* is acquired from goats, sheep and camels (Cooper, 1992); *B. abortus* is usually acquired from cattle. Other animals are also affected; for example, pigs, hares and reindeer have *B. suis* which is mainly seen in Central and South America. The disease is an occupational hazard in many other parts of the world. Farmers, veterinarians, abattoir, dairy and laboratory workers have all been reported to be at a special risk.

In endemic areas, the disease affects young adults with a male predominance. The most common method of transmission is through consumption of unpasteurized dairy products; in many endemic areas unpasteurized goat's cheese is a major source of infection. Ingestion of raw or partly cooked meat is another source of infection. In occupationally related cases, transmission through skin abrasions and cuts is probably the commonest method, aerosol transmission is another method in occupationally related cases including abattoir and laboratory workers (Ruben *et al.*, 1991).

THE ORGANISM

Genus *Brucella* has six nominal species. The first to be recognized, *B. melitensis*, is the commonest cause of human disease. *B. abortus* has a wider distribution with a lower pathogenicity but still causes human disease. *B. suis* and *B. canis* are the only others known to cause human disease. *Brucella* is a Gram-negative coccobacillus or short rod 0.5–1.5 μm in length, 0.5–0.8 μm in width. The organism is devoid of a capsule, endospores or flagella. It is rather slow to grow, many strains are carboxyphilic and require increased CO_2 tension for growth. *Brucella* is sensitive to disinfectants, resistant to drying and freezing, but sensitive to heat. Pasteurization kills the organism (Corbel, 1993). *Brucella* species are sensitive to antibiotics, including tetracyclines and rifampicin. *Brucella* is a facultative intracellular bacteria and can stay for years intracellularly, thereby requiring prolonged courses of antibiotics for eradication.

PATHOLOGY

The organism enters the bloodstream, usually through the gastrointestinal tract. The lymphatic system seems to be affected first and the organism reaches lymph nodes, spleen and bone marrow. During this initial spread, acute brucellosis can be seen as a mild febrile illness. However, the nervous system can be affected in an acute meningoencephalitic picture. The most important and disabling part of the infection is the chronic form. Various organs are affected in addition to the lymphatic system. Joints and bones seem to be the most vulnerable, but any other organ can be affected, for instance the heart, lungs, kidneys, eyes and the nervous system. The disease in its chronic stage takes the form of a non-caseating granuloma (Figure 11.1), except with *B. suis*, where it can be caseating and similar to tuberculosis. In the nervous system, it has been shown also to cause secondary demyelination. The meninges can be affected in a picture of a chronic inflammation with adhesions in the subarachnoid space. Perivascular lymphocytic infiltration, arachnoid thickening, anterior horn cell degeneration as well as degeneration of ascending and descending tracts occurs (Fincham *et al.*, 1963; Abramsky, 1977; Larbrisseau *et al.*, 1978). Cerebral blood vessels have been reported to be affected with mycotic aneurysms and subsequent subarachnoid haemorrhage. Cerebral oedema is seen, and perivascular lymphocytic infiltration with plasma cells and macrophages causing arteritis and vascular occlusions result in ischaemia and infarctions. Inflammation of the perineurium leading to cranial neuritis and radiculitis is also reported. The granuloma which affects the vertebral bodies and the intervertebral disc spaces can secondarily affect the spinal cord and the nerve roots causing neurological dysfunction. The

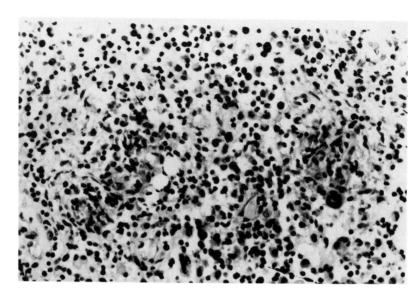

Figure 11.1 Photomicrograph showing granulomatous reaction with macrophages and multinucleated giant cells with diffuse inflammatory cell reaction.

commonest area of the vertebral column affected by *Brucella* spondylitis is the lower lumbar region; spinal root involvement at that level is not common as the granuloma affects the vertebral endplate and spreads gradually to affect the vertebral body, ligaments and dura before it reaches the nerve roots. The sacroiliac joints are commonly affected in many cases before other parts of the spinal column (Al-Deeb *et al.*, 1988).

IMMUNOLOGY

Macrophages are infected early and they are able, without sensitization, to kill *Brucella* organisms. Two weeks after infection, the number of bacteria in the liver and spleen decreases dramatically, due to the activation of the macrophages by sensitized T lymphocytes. Chronicity of *Brucella* infection is probably due to the failure of the macrophages to kill the bacteria initially or to the failure of the macrophages to be sensitized by the T cells. The exact role of the humoral response in the immunopathological mechanism of infection with brucella is not as well understood as the cellular response (Baldwin and Winter, 1994). The fact that the organism is intracellular makes it more difficult to be attacked by antibodies. IgM antibodies are the first to rise a week after the onset of the infection, reaching a peak after 4 weeks but persist for a long period extending to years. IgG antibodies appear about 4 weeks after the onset of infection, but decrease faster than IgM antibodies. IgA antibodies appear later and also persist for a long time.

CLINICAL FEATURES

The general manifestations of systemic brucellosis are beyond the remit of this chapter. There are, however, some general points worth remembering because of their influence on the nervous system. The disease may be asymptomatic, it can present with an acute or chronic febrile illness or it may present with specific organ involvement. Any organ can be affected and the disease can mimic other chronic granulomatous conditions or rheumatological diseases (Lulu *et al.*, 1988). When there is neurological involvement, other manifestations should not be overlooked. The nervous system is only affected in about 5% of general brucellosis cases (Shakir *et al.*, 1987), although higher figures have been reported on a smaller sample (Abramsky, 1977). The nervous system can be affected in a variety of ways; both acute and more chronic presentations are recognized (Shakir *et al.*, 1987; Bahemuka *et al.*, 1988; Al-Deeb *et al.*, 1989; Lubani *et al.*, 1989).

Acute Neurobrucellosis

The cause of this clinical manifestation is poorly understood. It is usually the first manifestation of *Brucella* infection and may be due to a direct toxic effect of the organism. There is a short history of hours or a few days, with a non-specific syndrome of headache, drowsiness, fever, seizures, coma with signs of meningeal irritation and increased intracranial pressure with bilateral papilloedema. Head computed tomography (CT) scans show small ventricles and features suggestive of increased pressure. Cerebrospinal fluid (CSF) examination confirms the raised pressure with a lymphocytic pleocytosis. The total protein content is raised with a low glucose in some cases. Blood and CSF cultures for *Brucella* are only positive in about a quarter of patients. Serology shows a raised blood and CSF antibody titre on standard agglutination and enzyme-linked immunosorbent assay (ELISA).

Chronic Neurobrucellosis

The manifestations of chronic neurobrucellosis are protean. The involvement can be due to a granuloma causing focal signs, meningoencephalitis with chronic inflammatory reaction, demyelination, vasculitis with perivascular chronic inflammatory infiltrate and arterial occlusion leading to areas of infarction, chronic meningitis, chronic inflammation of the perineurium with multiple cranial or peripheral nerve involvement, and large cerebral artery involvement with mycotic aneurysms and subsequent haemorrhage. Extra-axial compression results from *Brucella* spondylitis; the lumbar vertebral bodies and discs are the commonest site of affection but any part of the spinal column can be affected. The cauda equina and the spinal cord are therefore liable to extradural compression by a granuloma (Mohan *et al.*, 1990; Mousa *et al.*, 1990).

Meningoencephalitis

Any combination can be present of hemiparesis, ataxia, frontal lobe symptoms in the form of memory disturbances, speech difficulties, brainstem dysfunction with diplopia, dysphagia, dysarthria, and single or multiple cranial nerve palsies, most commonly the VIII nerve. This clinical syndrome can evolve over several weeks or a few months and symptoms can vary during its evolution suggesting a waxing and waning clinical state which may be confusing. The picture can be of a pure central nervous system disease which makes the diagnosis likely to be confused with conditions causing pure white matter or central symptomatology.

Demyelination

This has been reported for a long time as a pathological manifestation of neurobrucellosis (Fincham *et al.*, 1963). Demyelination of the corticospinal tracts has been noted on autopsy. Periventricular high signal intensity lesions suggestive of demyelination are noted on magnetic resonance images (MRI) (Figure 11.2). The demyelination can be a secondary phenomenon, and some

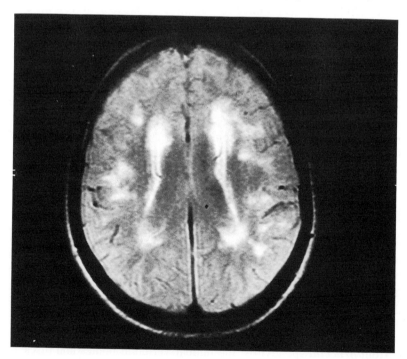

Figure 11.2 Brain MRI, T2-weighted image. Periventricular high signal lesions in a 25-year-old woman with CSF culture proven *Brucella melitensis* chronic neurobrucellosis. Courtesy of Dr S.M. Al-Deeb, Riyadh Armed Forces Hospital, Saudi Arabia.

authors have proposed a hypothesis that multiple sclerosis is a manifestation of brucellosis (Murrell and Mathews, 1990). In addition, there are reports of retrobulbar neuritis and papillitis due to brucellosis (Abd Elrazak, 1991). There are also autopsy reports of typical demyelination as seen in multiple sclerosis in cases of active brucellosis (Marconi, 1966). Oligoclonal bands in the CSF (Silva *et al.*, 1980) and abnormal evoked responses are well documented in neurobrucellosis (Khuraibut *et al.*, 1988). These findings suggest the presence of an active immunologically mediated pathological reaction in the central nervous system which may be the primary cause of the neuropathological lesions of neurobrucellosis or perhaps an epiphenomenon as a reaction to the infection.

Myeloradiculitis

Neurobrucellosis may present with a lower motor neurone picture, most commonly involving the lumbar plexus. Back pain, progressive paraparesis, areflexia, and variable sensory loss with sphincteric disturbances are the main features. Lumbar radiculitis is usually unilateral and clinically difficult to distinguish from sciatica due to lateral intervertebral disc protrusion. These signs may sometimes merge with the central type of presentation and therefore modify the clinical picture. The back pain can be chronic and continue for months or even years, and probably occurs as a result of radicular inflammation but is more likely due to associated sacroiliitis and lumbar spondylitis. These osteoarticular manifestations are perhaps best seen on isotope bone scans.

Peripheral Neuritis

This is usually a mononeuritis affecting mainly the cranial nerves due to inflammation of the perineurium. Any cranial nerve can be affected but the commonest is the VIII nerve with deafness which can be profound (Thomas and Kameswaran, 1993). Facial, trigeminal, extraocular and motor bulbar nerves are all known to be affected. Motor and rarely sensory chronic polyradiculopathy mainly affecting the lower limbs is the most common peripheral presentation and a picture similar to poliomyelitis has been reported (Debono, 1964). Clinically it is manifested by flaccid paraparesis, muscle wasting, areflexia and variably mainly large fibre sensory loss with impairment of proprioception. Demyelination of spinal roots has been noted on autopsy (Fincham *et al.*, 1963). Generally, peripheral nervous system involvement is less common, but an acute polyradiculoneuropathy is well recognized (Garcia *et al.*, 1989).

Cerebral Arteritis

This pathological manifestation either causes secondary ischaemia or mycotic aneurysms leading to subarachnoid haemorrhage (Hernandez *et al.*, 1988;

McLean *et al.*, 1992). Cardiac embolization due to *Brucella* endocarditis is an important complication which can cause major problems if not recognized and treated (Jacobs *et al.*, 1990).

DIAGNOSIS

In endemic areas a conclusive diagnosis of neurobrucellosis can only be ascertained with positive culture of the organism from blood, CSF, bone marrow or lymph nodes but this is possible only in about a quarter of clinically and serologically typical cases. Bone marrow culture should be the method utilized whenever possible (Gotuzzo *et al.*, 1986).

Serological tests vary in specificity and sensitivity and should always be interpreted according to the previous immunity and exposure. The Rose Bengal plate test is the standard screening test generally available which detects both IgM and IgG antibodies, but its value in endemic areas with a high prevalence of infection is limited. The standard agglutination test (SAT) is the most widely used and it agglutinates IgG, IgM and IgA antibodies. There is an appreciable false positive and false negative reaction and, in addition, high titres may not be indicative of disease activity in endemic areas. Titres of $\geq$ 1:100 may be diagnostic in non-endemic areas but are commonly seen in asymptomatic individuals in endemic areas (Araj *et al.*, 1986). The 2-mercaptoethanol test which extracts IgG and IgA antibodies is considered to be more indicative of disease activity (Young, 1991).

ELISA is more sensitive for the diagnosis of brucellosis generally and neurobrucellosis in particular (Ariza *et al.*, 1992). The value of ELISA in blood and CSF in neurobrucellosis has been shown to be rather specific. As shown in Table 11.1, the CSF ELISA was positive in all those with neurological symptoms and signs with CSF activity and negative in those without neurological involvement and normal CSF parameters. There were no false positives in patients with pyogenic meningitis. Blood cultures for *Brucella* were positive in 27% and CSF culture in 13% in neurobrucellosis cases (Araj *et al.*, 1988).

Cerebrospinal Fluid

The CSF examination has been reported to show an abnormality in all cases. Moderate elevation of the total protein content with lymphocytic pleocytosis is nearly universal and in a large study not a single patient with neurobrucellosis had a completely normal CSF, being higher in those with polyradiculoneuropathy than those with meningoencephalitis, whereas lymphocytosis is highest in those with acute meningoencephalitis with figures of 1200 cells l^{-1} (80–90% lymphocytes). Low CSF glucose content is noted in about a fifth of cases (Shakir *et al.*, 1987). Positive *Brucella* culture may be elusive. *B. melitensis* can be cultured in 25% of cases. Blood and bone marrow cultures should be

TABLE 11.1 Serological and culture findings in patients with neurobrucellosis, brucellosis without neurological involvement, pyogenic meningitis and controls (adapted from Araj *et al.*, 1988)

Brucella*	Percentage of positive findings in tested groups					
Test	Brucellosis with CNS infection (*n*=45)		Brucellosis without CNS infection (*n*=66)		Meningitis other than brucellosis (*n*=62)	Controls (*n*=144)
	CSF	Blood	CSF	Blood	CSF	CSF
ELISA						
IgG	100	100	0	100	0	0
IgM	20	81	0	77	0	0
IgA	85	100	0	100	0	0
MA	25	75	0	79	0	0
RB	22	73	0	72	0	0
Culture	13	27	0	23	+	0

* Titres for IgG ($\geq$ 1:200), IgM ($\geq$ 1:100), IgA ($\geq$ 1:100); MA, microagglutination($\geq$ 1:40); RB, Rose Bengal slide agglutination (undiluted).
+ Pyogenic bacteria, mycobacteria, cryptococcus, syphilis.

performed in all patients to maximize the yield. Culture results may take several weeks to come through during which time the diagnosis relies on clinical, radiological and immunological evidence (Bashir *et al.*, 1985). A raised IgG fraction and oligoclonal bands are noted in some patients (Silva *et al.*, 1980).

Neurophysiological Investigations

In acute neurobrucellosis, an EEG is important in patients with meningo-encephalitis who may have clouding of consciousness and seizures. The EEG may show epileptiform activity or a generalized encephalopathic picture. The record will also help to differentiate the condition from other causes of acute encephalitis as it only shows features of a diffuse encephalopathic process with generalized slowing without focal discharges. Electromyography (EMG) is valuable in cases of proximal polyradiculopathy. It shows denervation activity on needle EMG, with delay of F wave latencies and a mild slowing of motor, and to a lesser degree sensory conduction velocities. Evoked potentials are useful in chronic meningoencephalitis. Visual evoked potentials (VEPs) are delayed in patients with retrobulbar neuritis. Brainstem auditory evoked responses (BAERs) are reported to be delayed not only in those patients with sensorineural deafness but those with normal hearing suggesting a central brainstem delay of auditory conduction (Khuraibut *et al.*, 1988; Yaqub *et al.*, 1992).

Imaging

Radiology

Plain X-rays remain valuable in detecting bone and joint abnormalities especially sacroiliitis and lumbar spine involvement (Ariza *et al.*, 1993). Myelography may show partial or complete spinal block due to granulomatous compression (Figure 11.3). Vertebral involvement is thought to start at the superior endplate of the vertebral body, and then spread to involve the body of the vertebra causing bone softening and mechanical instability. The intervertebral disc is secondarily affected and part of it may herniate into the softened

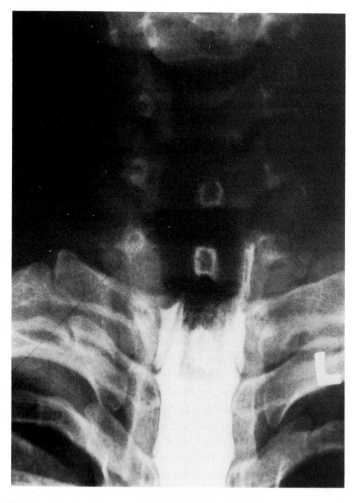

Figure 11.3 Myelography, showing complete block at the level of T1.

endplate with extension of the granulation tissue into the epidural space (Al-Deeb *et al.*, 1988).

CT Scanning

Lumbar CT may show pure spondylitis or spondylodiscitis with epidural granuloma. Head CT is mandatory in acute meningoencephalitis, when there is papilloedema or coma, especially when brain abscess is suspected (Kalelioglu *et al.*, 1990).

MRI Scanning

Brain and spinal cord MRI scans give valuable information. Periventricular white matter high signal intensity lesions on T2-weighted images are well recognized (Figure 11.2) (Sharif *et al.*, 1990). In the spinal cord, granulomatous compression is well demonstrated as well as the response to antibiotic therapy as shown in Figure 11.4a, b. This suggests that medical rather than surgical treatment is adequate in clinically and serologically confirmed cases.

Bone Scanning

This imaging technique shows the widely spread arthritis which affects 25% of all patients with chronic brucellosis (Lulu *et al.*, 1988). Unilateral sacroiliitis, lower lumbar spondylitis as well as arthritis affecting the sternoclavicular, intercostal, large and small limb joints are all known to occur (Bahar *et al.*, 1988; Madkour *et al.*, 1988).

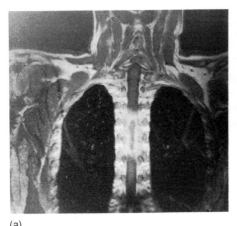 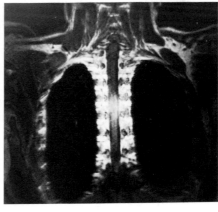

(a) (b)

Figure 11.4 MRI of a dorsal granuloma with positive *Brucella melitensis* serology before (a) and one month after (b) antibiotic therapy. There was substantial clinical improvement. Courtesy of Mr J.J. McCabe, Maudsley Hospital, London.

Other Investigations

Blood counts including white blood cells, ESR and other acute-phase reactants are non-specific and of limited value. Liver enzymes including alkaline phosphatase are not helpful.

DIFFERENTIAL DIAGNOSIS

In the acute phase all other causes of an encephalitis, including herpes encephalitis have to be considered. The CSF is non-specific and a partially treated bacterial meningitis is a possibility which should not be overlooked.

Other chronic granulomatous infections are the main conditions that may be simulated by neurobrucellosis. Tuberculosis with spondylitis and meningitis has to be excluded and this may have to await the CSF culture result. Clinical judgement has to be utilized when a decision on initiation of therapy needs to be made. In both conditions the use of polymerase chain reaction (PCR) is being investigated, but this is a demanding test with limited applicability world-wide. In spinal cord compression, tuberculosis tends to affect the dorsal rather than the lumbar vertebrae while generally the case is the reverse with brucellosis (Iqbal and Khan, 1990; Cordero and Sanchez, 1991). Other chronic infections have to be considered, including Lyme disease and syphilis.

Sarcoidosis can present with many similar features (James, 1990), and systemic lupus erythematosis and rheumatoid arthritis have to be considered as well. Two conditions worth special mention are multiple sclerosis (MS) and Behçet's syndrome. In endemic areas the clinician has to be very careful in making a diagnosis of MS without conclusively excluding brucellosis. Many features are common, the clinical presentation and the abnormal investigations can easily lead to confusion. The CSF abnormalities including high gamma-globulin and oligoclonal bands, the abnormal evoked responses and the MRI findings all make differentiation difficult at times. The waxing and waning course of brucellosis can give an impression of a remitting and relapsing condition like MS.

Behçet's disease affects the nervous system in a similar fashion (Shakir et al., 1990). The presence of orogenital ulcers and skin vasculitis should be carefully considered.

TREATMENT

This depends on the clinical presentation. In acute meningoencephalitis, recovery is the rule and this usually occurs rapidly within 2–3 days with, and sometimes without, the use of antibiotics. Initially, when the diagnosis is not clear, treating other possible entities is justified, especially herpes encephalitis.

For acute meningoencephalitis, a 2-week course of tetracycline and rifampicin is all that is required.

In the chronic forms, a 3-month combined course of rifampicin 600–900 mg daily, doxycycline 100–200 mg daily and 6 weeks of streptomycin 0.5–1 g i.m. daily is needed. Streptomycin should not be used in those with deafness. Prednisolone has been found to be useful especially in cases with diffuse central involvement, arachnoiditis or cranial nerve involvement (Al-Deeb *et al.*, 1988). Improvement is monitored clinically and radiologically. Antibodies are not a good guide in monitoring disease activity. A Jarish Herxheimer-like reaction is well recognized on initiation of therapy (Young, 1983; Shakir *et al.*, 1987).

PROGNOSIS

Acute meningoencephalitis cases make an excellent recovery. The prognosis is less good in the chronic forms. Compressive granulomas respond to therapy reasonably well, but chronic meningoencephalitis and polyradiculopathy respond less favourably and many patients remain with a neurological deficit despite complete resolution of CSF abnormalities. In such cases longer courses of rifampicin and doxycycline for 6 months are advised.

REFERENCES

Abd Elrazak M (1991). *Brucella* optic neuritis. *Archives of Internal Medicine* **151**: 776–778.

Abramsky O (1977) Neurological features as presenting manifestations of brucellosis. *European Neurology* **15**: 281–284.

Al-Deeb SM, Yaqub BA, Sharif HS and Al-Rajeh SM (1988) Neurobrucellosis. In: *Handbook of Clinical Neurology*, vol. 8(52) (eds PJ Vinken, GW Bruyn and HL Klawan), pp 581–601. Amsterdam: Elsevier Science Publishers.

Al-Deeb SM, Yaqub BA, Sharif HS and Phadke JG (1989) Neurobrucellosis: clinical characteristics, diagnosis and outcome. *Neurology* **39**: 498–501.

Animal Health Year Book (1994) Cases of animal diseases (Zoonoses) in human population. *FAO Animal Production and Health Series* no. 33, pp 131–135. Rome: FAO.

Araj GF, Lulu AR, Saadah MA, Mousa AM, Stannagard IL and Shakir Ra (1986) Rapid diagnosis of central nervous system brucellosis by ELISA. *Journal of Neuroimmunology* **12**: 173–182.

Araj GF, Lulu AR, Khateeb MI, Saadah MA and Shakir RA (1988) ELISA versus routine tests in the diagnosis of patients with systemic and neurobrucellosis. *Acta Pathologica Microbiologica Immunologica Scandinavica* **96**: 171–176.

Ariza J, Pellicer T, Pallares R, Foz A and Gudiol F (1992) Specific antibody profile in human brucellosis. *Clinical Infectious Diseases* **14**: 131–140.

Ariza J, Pujol M, Valverde J *et al.* (1973) *Brucella* sacroiliitis: findings in 63 episodes and current relevance. *Clinical Infectious Diseases* **16**: 761–765.

Bahar RH, Al-Suhaili AR, Mousa AM, Nawas MK, Kaddah N and Abdel-Dayem HM (1988) Brucellosis: appearance on skeletal imaging. *Clinical Nuclear Medicine* **13**: 102–106.

Bahemuka M, Shemena AR, Panayiotopoulos CP, Al-Aska AK, Obaied T and Daif AK (1988) Neurological syndromes of brucellosis. *Journal of Neurology, Neurosurgery and Psychiatry* **51**: 1017–1021.

Baldwin CL and Winter AJ (1994) Macrophages and *Brucella. Immunology Series* **60**: 363–380.

Bashir R, Al-Kawi MZ, Harder EJ and Jenkins J (1985) Nervous system brucellosis: diagnosis and treatment. *Neurology* **35**: 1576–1581.

Cooper CW (1992) Risk factors in transmission of brucellosis from animals to humans in Saudi Arabia. *Transactions of the Royal Society of Tropical Medicine and Hygiene* **86**: 206–209.

Corbel MJ (1993) Microbiological aspects of brucellosis. *Saudi Medical Journal* **14**: 489–502.

Cordero M and Sanchez I (1991) Brucellar and tuberculous spondylitis. A comparative study of their clinical features. *Journal of Bone and Joint Surgery-British Volume* **73**: 100–103.

Debono JE (1964) Brucellosis simulating acute anterior poliomyelitis. *Lancet* **i**: 1132–1133.

De Jong RN (1936) Central nervous system involvement in undulant fever, with the report of a case and survey of the literature. *Journal of Nervous and Mental Disease* **83**: 430–442.

Fincham RW, Sahs AL and Joynt RJ (1963) Protean manifestations of nervous system brucellosis. *Journal of the American Medical Association* **184**: 269–276.

Garcia T, Sanchez JC, Maestre JF, Guisado F, Vilches RM and Morales B (1989) Brucellosis and acute inflammatory polyradiculoneuropathy. *Neurologia* **4**: 145–157.

Gilbert GL (1993) Brucellosis: continuing risk. *Medical Journal of Australia* **159**: 147–148.

Gotuzzo E, Carrillo C, Guerra J and Llosa L (1986) An evaluation of diagnostic methods for brucellosis – the value of bone marrow culture. *Journal of Infectious Diseases* **153**: 122–125.

Hernandez MA, Anciones B, Frank A and Barriero P (1988) Neurobrucellosis and cerebral vasculitis. *Neurologia* **3**: 241–243.

Iqbal QM and Khan O (1970) Brucellosis of the spine. *Journal of the Royal College of Surgeons of Edinburgh* **35**: 395–397.

Jacobs F, Abramowicz D, Vereerstraeten P, Le Clerc JL, Zech F and Thys JP (1990) Brucella endocarditis: the role of combined medial and surgical treatment. *Reviews of Infectious Diseases* **12**: 740–744.

James DG (1990) A mimic of sarcoidosis: brucellosis. *Sarcoidosis* **7**: 87–88.

Kalelioglu M, Ceylan S, Koksal I, Kuzeyli K and Akturk F (1990) Brain abscess caused by *Brucella abortus* and *Staphylococcus aureus* in a child. *Infection* **18**: 386–387.

Khuraibut AJ, Shakir RA, Trontelj JV, Butinar D and Al-Din ASN (1988) Brainstem auditory evoked potential (BAEP) abnormalities in brucellosis. *Journal of Neurological Sciences* **87**: 307–313.

Larbrisseau A, Maravi E, Agulera F and Martinez-Lage JM (1978) The neurological complications of brucellosis. *Canadian Journal of Neurological Sciences.* **5**: 369–376.

Lemaire G (1924) Meningite a melitocoques: alterations importantes du liquide cephalo-rachidien. *Bulletin de la Société de Médecine Paris* **48**: 1636–1644.

Lopez-Merino A, Migranas-Ortiz R, Perez-Miravete A *et al.* (1992) Seroepidemiology of brucellosis in Mexico. *Salud Publica de Mexico* **34**: 230–240.

Lubani MM, Dudin KI, Araj GF, Manandhar DS and Rashid FY (1989) Neurobrucellosis in children. *Pediatric Infectious Disease Journal* **8**: 79–82.

Lulu AR, Araj GF, Khateeb MI, Mustafa MY, Yusuf AR and Fenech FF (1988) Human brucellosis: a prospective study of 400 cases. *Quarterly Journal of Medicine* **66**: 39–54.

Madkour MM and Gargani G (1989) Epidemiological aspects. In: *Brucellosis* (ed MM Madkour), pp 11–28. UK: Butterworths.

Madkour MM, Sharif HS, Abed MY and Al-Fayes MA (1988) Osteoarticular brucellosis: results of bone scintigraphy in 140 patients. *American Journal of Roentgenology* **150**: 1101–1105.

Marconi G (1966) Su un caso di sclerosi multipla acuta insorta dopo un'infezione da *Brucella abortus*. *Rivista di Patologia Nervosa e Mentale* **87**: 548–565.

McLean DR, Russell N and Khan MY (1992) Neurobrucellosis:clinical and therapeutic features. *Clinical Infectious Diseases* **15**: 582–590.

Mohan V, Gupta RP, Markland T and Sabri T (1990) Spinal brucellosis. *International Orthopeadics* **14**: 63–66.

Mousa AM, Bahar RH and Araj GF *et al.* (1990) Neurological complications of *Brucella* spondylitis. *Acta Neurologica Scandinavica* **81**: 16–23.

Murrell TG and Mathews BJ (1990) Multiple sclerosis, one manifestation of neurobrucellosis? *Medical Hypothesis* **33**: 43–48.

Nichols E (1951) Meningoencephalitis due to brucellosis with a report of a case in which *B. abortus* was recovered from the cerebrospinal fluid, and review of the literature. *Annals of Internal Medicine* **35**: 673–693.

Ruben B, Band JD, Wong P and Colville J (1991) Person to person transmission of *Brucella melitensis*. *Lancet* **337**: 14.

Sanders WE (1931) Undulant fever meningitis. *Journal of the Iowa Medical Society* **21**: 510–511.

Shakir RA, Al-Din ASN, Araj GF, Lulu AR, Mousa AR and Saadah MA (1987) Clinical categories of neurobrucellosis: a report of 19 cases. *Brain* **110**: 213–223.

Shakir RA, Sulaiman K, Kahn RA and Rudwan M (1990) Neurological presentation of neuro-Behçet's syndrome: clinical categories. *European Neurology* **30**: 249–253.

Sharif HS, Clark DC and Aabed MC *et al.* (1990) Granulomatous spinal infections: MR imaging. *Radiology* **177**: 101–107.

Silva CA, Rio ME, Maia-Goncalves A *et al.* (1980) Oligoclonal gammaglobulin of cerebrospinal fluid in neurobrucellosis. *Acta Neurologica Scandinavica* **61**: 42–48.

Spink WW (1951) What is chronic brucellosis? *Annals of Internal Medicine* **35**: 358–374.

Thomas R and Kameswaran MR (1993) Sensorineural hearing loss in neurobrucellosis. *Journal of Laryngology and Otology* **107**: 1034–1036.

Yaqub BA, Kabiraj MM, Shamena A, Al-Bunyan M, Daif A and Tahan A (1992) Diagnostic role of brain-stem auditory evoked potentials in neurobrucellosis. *Electroencephalography and Clinical Neurophysiology* **84**: 549–552.

Young EJ (1983) Human brucellosis. *Reviews of Infectious Diseases* **5**: 821–842.

Young EJ (1991) Serologic diagnosis of human brucellosis: analysis of 214 cases by agglutination tests and review of literature. *Reviews of Infectious Diseases* **13**: 359–372.

12

Tetanus

Michele Trucksis

Division of Geographic Medicine, Center for Vaccine Development, Department of Medicine, University of Maryland School of Medicine, Baltimore, MD 21201, USA

INTRODUCTION

Tetanus is caused by a neurotoxin, tetanospasmin, which is produced by the organism *Clostridium tetani*. The prevalence of the disease has decreased in the industrialized world in recent decades following the development of a safe and effective vaccine, but it is still a serious health problem in many developing countries. The history, pathogenesis, epidemiology, classification, clinical manifestations, diagnosis, treatment and prevention of this condition are described.

HISTORICAL PERSPECTIVE

One of the earliest written descriptions of clinical tetanus was detailed in *The Extant Works of Aretaeus, the Cappadocian* (Adams, 1856). Tetanus was described as 'a spasm of exceedingly painful nature, very swift to prove fatal, but neither easy to be removed'. The identification of the causal organism from soil, *C. tetani*, is attributed to Arthur Nicolaier in 1884. Kitasato and Behring first postulated that the disease state was produced by a powerful toxin rather than dissemination of the organism in the body about 1890. They also demonstrated that animals immunized with small doses of toxin acquired protective immunity and that this antitoxin serum could passively protect another animal from tetanus. Large amounts of toxin were commercially produced in horses and cows during World War I for passive immunization of the wounded. Parish (1968) estimated that these preparations may have prevented 20 000 British deaths. Tetanus toxoid was used as a safe and effective vaccine before World War II. The experience of the United States Army demonstrated its efficacy as there were only 12 cases of tetanus out of 2 734 819 hospital admissions for wounds and injuries in World War II. In contrast, there were 473 reported cases of tetanus in approximately 12 000 wounded non-immunized civilians in the battle for Manila in 1945 (Furste, 1965). Since the introduction of the tetanus vaccine, the incidence of tetanus in industrialized countries has been greatly reduced, however, cases still occur in these countries in the elderly who are not adequately immunized. In contrast, tetanus remains the most common cause of neonatal death after prematurity in developing countries where immunization programmes are inadequate.

THE PATHOGEN AND ITS TOXIN

Clostridium tetani is a motile, Gram-positive, anaerobic rod. It produces a terminal spore, which has a characteristic 'drumstick' or 'tennis racket' appearance when viewed microscopically. The spores are highly resistant to chemical disinfectants, heat and drying. They are ubiquitous, found in animal and human faeces, and can survive in dry soil for years.

Tetanus occurs when the spores of *C. tetani* are introduced into damaged or devitalized tissue. The spores are activated for vegetative growth in anaerobic conditions, allowing production of tetanospasmin, a neurotoxin. As tetanospasmin disseminates systematically, clinical tetanus develops. Simple introduction of *C. tetani* spores into tissue does not allow production of the toxin; rather, the spores must convert into vegetative forms, and then under appropriate (low) oxidation–reduction potential conditions toxin is produced.

The tetanus toxin gene (*tet*), is encoded on a 75-kb plasmid in toxigenic strains of *C. tetani* (Eisel *et al.*, 1986). The toxin is produced as a single polypeptide that is subsequently cleaved by an endogenous protease(s) to yield two subchains. The subchains, L (light, mol. wt 50 000) and H (heavy, mol. wt 100 000) are covalently linked by a disulphide bridge (Figure 12.1). A segment termed 'fragment C' has been prepared from native toxin by papain cleavage (Figure 12.1) (Helting and Zwisler, 1977); its binding specificity is similar to that of the carboxy-terminal portion of the H chain. The individual subchains are non-toxic (Matsuda and Yoneda, 1974) as is the unnicked single polypeptide chain (Bergey *et al.*, 1989). The toxin is secreted from *C. tetani* although there is no signal peptide found at the amino-terminus. The amino acid sequence of tetanus toxin reveals a close homology to available partial amino acid sequences of botulinum toxins A, B and E (Eisel *et al.*, 1986). The cysteine residues involved in the

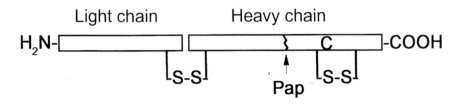

Figure 12.1 Subunit structure of tetanus neurotoxin, tetanospasmin. C, fragment C; Pap, papain.

disulphide linkage between the two subunits of tetanus toxin align with the cysteine residues in the three botulinum toxins (Eisel *et al.*, 1986). The close homology between these two toxins suggests that they are ancestrally related. These toxins are the most potent neurotoxins known to man.

PATHOGENESIS

Tetanospasmin is produced at a localized site of infection by vegetative *C. tetani* and secreted and/or released upon lysis of the organism. The toxin binds via the carboxy-terminal part of the H chain to neural ganglioside receptors such as GD_{1b} and GT_{1b} at myoneural junctions of alpha motor neurones and enters the neurone by translocation (Eisel *et al.*, 1986). Once inside the presynaptic terminal, tetanus toxin inhibits transmitter release. In addition, it is carried by retrograde axonal transport to the neuroaxis where it migrates transynaptically to other neurones, extending the process not only from the periphery into the spinal cord, but across synaptically connected neurones in the brain.

Toxin also enters the bloodstream and lymphatics, spreading to myoneural junctions throughout the body. The bloodstream dissemination of toxin accounts for initial symptoms in facial muscles and nerves with the shortest axons, as well as later symptoms in muscles of the neck, trunk and finally the extremities. The toxin can be neutralized by passively administered antitoxin before it enters the neurone; however, once it has translocated the neural membrane it is inaccessible to neutralization (Schmitt *et al.*, 1981). When the toxin gains access to the spinal cord or brainstem, it migrates synaptically into inhibitory cells. Here it prevents release of γ-aminobutyric acid (GABA) or glycine (Mellanby and Green, 1981), thus denying the alpha motor neurone its most essential inhibitory transmitters. This raises the resting firing rate of the alpha motor neurones, which results in resting muscle rigidity. In addition, the normal inhibition of other motor neurones during movements of a particular motor group, and the termination of reflexive contractions, are both dependent on the actions of these inhibitory transmitters. The motor system thus responds to an afferent stimulus with intense, sustained, simultaneous contraction of agonist and antagonist muscles that characterizes the tetanic spasm.

The sympathetic nervous system is also affected by tetanospasmin. A clinical syndrome resembling pheochromocytoma can be seen in the first or second week of clinical tetanus (Kerr *et al.*, 1968). Patients have high catecholamine levels, which cause autonomic dysfunction with labile hypertension, tachycardia, cardiac arrhythmias, pyrexia, peripheral vascular constriction and occasionally hypotension. This condition may lead to sudden death from bradycardia and/or asystole unresponsive to medications.

The nervous system effects from tetanospasmin are permanent. Recovery requires sprouting of nerve terminals and formation of new synapses.

EPIDEMIOLOGY

Tetanus occurs primarily in developing countries. Most reported tetanus cases world-wide occur in neonates, although in industrialized countries nearly all cases occur in adults. In 1991, the World Health Organization estimates neonatal tetanus claimed the lives of over 433 000 infants (Whitman *et al.*, 1992). It is second only to measles as the leading killer of children. Case fatality rates of 80–90% occur even with treatment. The incidence of neonatal tetanus is often focal and occurs in population groups where shared behaviour or the environment increase the risk of contamination of the umbilical cord stump. In some developing countries, the umbilical cord is cut with a non-sterile instrument or cow dung is applied to the umbilical stump, which increases the risk of exposure to *C. tetani* spores and the development of tetanus. Of the 433 000 infants who died of neonatal tetanus in 1991, 80% were born in South-East Asia or Africa (Whitman *et al.*, 1992).

The majority of tetanus cases follow an acute injury. In school-age children in Nigeria, injury to a lower extremity resulting in tetanus accounted for 9% of fatalities due to infectious diseases in this age group (Akang *et al.*, 1993). In adults, puncture wounds are most commonly associated with tetanus. Tetanus may also occur after non-sterile injections [intravenous drug users (Cherubin, 1968)], unskilled abortions, earpiercing, scarification rituals and female circumcision. Tetanus-prone wounds are those contaminated with soil or animal or human faeces. The lack of a known wound, however, does not exclude the diagnosis of tetanus; up to 20% of tetanus cases in some series report no acute injury (Alfery and Rauscher, 1979; Bleck 1991). Tetanus may less commonly result from chronic infection, such as chronic ear infections (DeSouza *et al.*, 1992) and decubitus ulcers (CDC, 1990; Luisto, 1993). The majority of adults with tetanus are more than 50 years old and are not fully vaccinated against tetanus (CDC, 1990; Luisto, 1993).

DEFINITION AND CLASSIFICATION

Four forms of clinical tetanus are commonly recognized. These include: local, cephalic, generalized and tetanus neonatorum (neonatal tetanus). These distinctions are useful diagnostically and reflect variations in the site of toxin action, the host, and the quantity of toxin produced.

CLINICAL FEATURES

The incubation period of tetanus in human beings is 3 to 21 days. Symptoms occur as early as 24 hours or as long as months following inoculation with the organism. The length of the incubation period is directly related to the distance from the site of production of toxin to the central nervous system, but may also be affected by the amount of toxin produced. A short incubation time is associated with severe disease. Trismus, a symptom caused by rigidity of the masseter muscles, producing inability to open the mouth (lockjaw), is the most common presenting symptom.

Generalized Tetanus

This is the most frequently recognized form of the disease. It may occur as an extension of localized or cephalic tetanus. The most common presenting symptoms are pain and stiffness of the jaw, abdomen or back, restlessness, irritability and dysphagia. Stiffness progresses to rigidity, producing risus sardonicus (rigidity of facial muscles), constriction of the chest mucles, and intense, persistent spasm of the back musculature (opisthotonos). Reflex spasms usually occur within 1–4 days of the initial symptoms. The spasms may be precipitated by minor stimuli such as light, touch or noise. They last for several seconds to a few minutes, are intensely painful (the patient remains fully conscious), and may result in respiratory compromise. Before the advent of mechanical ventilation, asphyxia from laryngeal spasm was a frequent cause of death. Intense spasms may cause vertebral or long bone fractures.

The use of intensive care medicine, neuromuscular blockade to control spasms and mechanical ventilation increases the possibility of survival in the first week of the disease. The manifestations of disease in the next period include sympathetic nervous system hyperactivity resembling a high catecholamine state such as with a pheochromocytoma. Sudden cardiac death is then the leading cause of death (Richter *et al.*, 1970; Trujillo *et al.*, 1987). Evidence of myocarditis has been reported at autopsy in fatal tetanus cases (Murphy, 1970; Mitra *et al.*, 1989).

Local Tetanus

This is the mildest form of the disease with a fatality rate of about 1% (Millard, 1954). It involves fixed rigidity of the muscles at or near the site of (injury) toxin production. Neuromuscular transmission may be affected in the muscles involved producing localized weakness of muscle groups. Localized tetanus may progress to generalized tetanus unless the condition is recognized while still localized and toxin is neutralized with antitoxin.

Cephalic Tetanus

This is a form of localized tetanus which affects the face. It is rare, occurring in less than 1% of all tetanus cases (Abde and Dekate, 1980). It is associated with head wounds and chronic otitis media (DeSouza *et al.*, 1992). Peripheral facial nerve weakness or trismus are usually the initial symptom. Other cranial nerves (III IV, IX, X and XII) may also be involved singly or in combination. The prognosis is usually poor, except in association with a chronic otitis media (DeSouza *et al.*, 1992). Cephalic tetanus may progress to generalized tetanus.

Neonatal Tetanus (Tetanus Neonatorum)

This is the most common form of tetanus world-wide. It is seen in the first 10 days of life as a result of infection of the umbilical stump. Maternal antibody will passively protect the newborn; thus, this disease is a disease of unimmunized populations. Most cases probably result from failure to use aseptic technique in umbilical cord cutting and care. The most common presentation is inability to suck, weakness and irritability in the second week of life followed by rigidity and spasms. Mortality rates of 50–90% are usual (Begue and Lindo-Soriano, 1991).

Complications

Complications encountered in patients who contract tetanus are often complications common to patients requiring intensive care treatment. Most patients require mechanical ventilation due either to the need for neuromuscular blockage to control the tetanic spasms or because tetanic spasms of the respiratory muscles (the diaphragm and intercostal muscles) or laryngeal spasm may result in apnoea. Pulmonary complications include bronchopneumonia (often a result of aspiration), atelectasis and pulmonary embolus. In addition, sepsis from intravenous catheters, urinary catheters or the primary wound occurs. Gastro-intestinal haemorrhage due to acute peptic ulcer disease may occur. Vertebral and long bone fractures may occur during tetanic spasms. Cardiac complications are often the result of sympathetic overactivity and include labile hypertension, cardiac arrhythmias and peripheral vasoconstriction.

Mortality from tetanus varies with age and type of disease. The highest mortality is seen at the extremes of age, 45–90% in neonates (Whitman *et al.*, 1992; Begue and Lindo-Soriano, 1991; El-Sherbini, 1991; Delport, 1990; Gurses and Aydin, 1993) and 50% in those over 80 years of age (Prevots *et al.*, 1992). The overall case fatality rate is 21–55% (Weinstein, 1973; CDC, 1990).

DIAGNOSIS

There is no diagnostic test available for tetanus. The diagnosis is made solely on clinical grounds. In developing countries, physicians are familiar with the clinical manifestations and the diagnosis is readily made. Tetanus is more of a diagnostic dilemma in developed countries because the diagnosis is not considered until late in the disease course. Although its late manifestations are seldom confused, its early manifestations can be mistaken for other entities, especially when a history of prior injury is not obtained.

The differential diagnosis includes tetany, strychnine poisoning, dystonic reaction, rabies, Bell's palsy, meningitis and orofacial infection.

The isolation of *C. tetani* from a wound is not helpful in the diagnosis of tetanus. The organism is difficult to isolate and isolation of the organism does not necessarily make the diagnosis. The immunization status of the patient should be established. Those individuals who are not up to date in immunization are at greater risk of developing tetanus. A serum level of 0.01 international units ml^{-1} is thought to be a protective level of antibody; however, several persons with a protective level have contracted the disease (Berger *et al.*, 1978; Passen and Andersen, 1986; Crone and Reder, 1992).

TREATMENT

Prevention of tetanus by active immunization is the first line of defence (Table 12.1). The second level of disease management is treatment of an acute wound with passive immunization (Table 12.2). Once the disease is established, most commonly in a non-immunized individual, treatment requires intensive care management.

The early recognition of tetanus is crucial, so that prompt prophylactic treatment can be initiated. Acute management includes protection of the airway with a tracheostomy and ventilation support when severe tetanospasms necessitate sedation and neuromuscular blockade. Sedation with benzodiazepines or morphine is a mainstay of treatment as is neuromuscular blockade using curare. The inciting wound should be explored and devitalized tissue debrided. Passive immunization with human tetanus immunoglobulin (250–3000 international units intramuscularly) along with antibiotics (most commonly penicillin) should be given to neutralize preformed toxin and sterilize the wound. Studies using intrathecal tetanus antitoxin therapy (primarily in neonatal tetanus) have not shown a significant improvement in survival over intramuscular antitoxin (Singh *et al.*, 1989; Abrutyn and Berlin, 1991; Begue and Lindo-Soriano, 1991). Early mortality (the first week) is usually due to respiratory failure. Once a patient's airway is protected, total curarization and mechanical ventilatory assistance prevents this complication.

The next clinical problem is the management of sympathetic system overactivity. This syndrome is associated with labile hypertension, cardiac arrhythmias and sudden cardiac death. The treatment of this syndrome is currently under debate. Successful treatment has used β-blockers including propranolol and esmolol (King and Cave, 1991), magnesium sulphate, and clonidine (Sutton *et al.*, 1990). Combination treatment with a β-blocker and alpha-blockade is successful in some cases; however, in other cases, patients have suffered fatal cardiac arrest during treatment. The fatal outcome was thought to be due to

TABLE 12.1 Immunization against tetanus

Subject/vaccine and dose	Age/interval
Children (age less than 7 years)*	
1–DPT	6–8 weeks of age
2–DPT	4–8 weeks after previous dose
3–DPT	4–8 weeks after previous dose
4–DPT	1 year after previous dose
Booster-DPT	4–6 years of age
Booster-Td	every 10 years after previous dose
Adults and children older than 7 years not previously immunized*	
1–Td	first encounter
2–Td	4–8 weeks after previous dose
3–Td	6 months – 1 year after previous dose
Booster-Td	every 10 years after previous dose
Pregnant women[+]	
Previously immunized:	
Booster-TT	during first 6 months of pregnancy (optimal) or as late as 6 weeks before delivery
Previously unimmunized:	
1–TT	first encounter during pregnancy
2–TT	4 weeks after previous dose

* American Academy of Pediatrics (Peter *et al.*, 1994);   [+] World Health Organization, Expanded Programme on Immunization (Whitman *et al.*, 1992).
Abbreviations: DPT, diphtheria and tetanus toxoids and pertussis vaccine adsorbed; Td, tetanus and reduced-dose diphtheria toxoids adsorbed; TT, tetanus toxoid.

TABLE 12.2 Guidelines for tetanus prophylaxis in wound management

Vaccination status	Clean, minor wounds		Tetanus-prone wounds*	
	Td[+]	TIG	Td[+]	TIG[‡]
Unknown or < 3 doses	Yes	No	Yes	Yes
≥ 3 doses				
Last booster < 5 years	No	No	No	No
Last booster 5–10 years	No	No	Yes	No
Last booster > 10 years	Yes	No	Yes	Yes

Recommendations of the Advisory Committee on Immunization Practices – United States (CDC, 1992)
* Wounds contaminated with dirt, faeces, soil, saliva; puncture wounds; avulsions; and wounds resulting from missiles, crushing, burns and frostbite. Wounds presenting after delay or requiring debridement due to the presence of necrotic tissue.
[+] Td: tetanus and reduced-dose diphtheria toxoids adsorbed; for children less than 7 years, DPT (diphtheria and tetanus toxoids and pertussis vaccine adsorbed) is preferred.
[‡] 250–500 units human tetanus immune globulin; given intramuscularly in another area than the Td.

myocardial depression from the use of drugs during a precipitous decrease in sympathetic activity. Local anaesthetic agents such as epidural blockage have been used in selected patients with success (Southorn and Blaise, 1986). The use of magnesium sulphate is founded in light of its known actions as a potent muscle relaxant, its ability to block neuronal and adrenal catecholamine release and its controversial ability to depress the central nervous system. This combination of properties has made it a successful agent in the treatment of tetanus (James and Manson, 1985; Lipman *et al.*, 1987). Udwadia *et al.* (1992) reported on the treatment of 32 patients with severe tetanus. They reported a mortality of only 6.3% and suggested that careful haemodynamic monitoring with judicious use of small doses (not greater than 30–40 mg i.v. per day) of diazepam for sedation to protect against marked depression of the central nervous system was less likely to lead to sudden cardiac death (Udwadia *et al.*, 1992).

PREVENTION

The safety and efficacy of the current tetanus vaccine has been proven in industrialized countries where it is routinely utilized and in many immunization programmes in developing countries. There are many success stories of a decrease in the incidence of tetanus following campaigns to immunize at-risk groups. In Egypt, an immunization campaign for vaccination of pregnant women against neonatal tetanus in 1988-1989 led to a reduction in the incidence of neonatal tetanus by 65% (El-Sherbini, 1991). In Bangladesh, a similar programme to vaccinate pregnant women against tetanus produced a reduction in the incidence of neonatal tetanus from 13.6 to 7.3 per 1000 live births (Bhatia, 1989).

Immunity is not produced by the disease itself, probably because the amount of toxin required to produce disease is much less than that required to stimulate an antibody response. Current immunization guidelines are given in Table 12.1. This protocol should prevent most cases of tetanus. In addition, acute wound care should include the use of Td and tetanus immunoglobulins as outlined in Table 12.2 (Prevots *et al.*, 1992).

CONCLUSIONS

Tetanus is a preventable disease. The tetanus toxoid vaccine is safe and effective and proven in both industrialized and developing countries. The World Health Assembly had resolved to eliminate neonatal tetanus from the globe by 1995 and several countries have made substantial progress towards this goal but pockets of disease still remain in parts of Africa and South-East Asia. In the industrialized world, including the United States, tetanus is a problem particularly of elderly adults who lack levels of protective antibody. In these countries, routine adult vaccination should be a priority.

REFERENCES

Abde VW and Dekate MP (1980) Cephalic tetanus: clinical analysis of 9 cases. *Journal of the Indian Medical Association* **74**: 111–113.

Abrutyn E and Berlin JA (1991) Intrathecal therapy in tetanus: a meta-analysis. *Journal of the American Medical Association* **266**: 2262–2267.

Adams F (1856) *The Extant Works of Aretaeus, the Cappadocian.* London: Publications of the Sydenham Society.

Akang EEU, Ekweozor C, Pindiga HU and Onyemenem TN (1993) Childhood infections in Nigeria: an autopsy study. *Journal of Tropical Medicine and Hygiene* **96**: 231–236.

Alfery DD and Rauscher LA (1979) Tetanus: a review. *Critical Care Medicine* **11**(7): 176–180.

Begue RE and Lindo-Soriano I (1991) Failure of intrathecal tetanus antitoxin in the treatment of tetanus neonatorum. *Journal of Infectious Diseases* **164**: 619–620.

Berger SA, Cherubin CE, Nelson S and Levine L (1978) Tetanus despite preexisting antitetanus antibody. *Journal of the American Medical Association* **240**: 769–770.

Bergey GK, Habig WH, Bennett JI and Lin CS (1989) Proteolytic cleavage of tetanus toxin increases activity. *Journal of Neurochemistry* **53**: 155–161.

Bhatia S (1989) Patterns and causes of neonatal and postneonatal mortality in rural Bangladesh. *Studies in Family Planning* **20**: 136–146.

Bleck TP (1991) Tetanus: pathophysiology, management, and prophylaxis. *Disease-a-Month* **37**: 551–603.

CDC (1990) Tetanus – United States, 1987 and 1988. *MMWR. Morbidity and Mortality Weekly Report* **39**: 37–41.

CDC (1992) Tetanus surveillance – United States, 1989–1990. *MMWR. Morbidity and Mortality Weekly Report* **41**: 1–9.

Cherubin CE (1968) Clinical severity of tetanus in narcotic addicts in New York City. *Archives of Internal Medicine* **121**: 156–158.

Crone NE and Reder AT (1992) Severe tetanus in immunized patients with high anti-tetanus titers. *Neurology* **42**: 761–764.

Delport SD (1990) Neonatal tetanus – an opportunity for prevention. *South African Medical Journal* **77**: 78–79.

DeSouza CE, Karnad DR and Tilve GH (1992) Clinical and bacteriological profile of the ear in otogenic tetanus: a case control study. *Journal of Laryngology and Otology* **106**: 1051–1054.

Eisel U, Jarausch W, Goretzki K *et al.* (1986) Tetanus toxin: primary structure, expression in *E. coli*, and homology with botulinum toxins. *EMBO Journal* **5**: 2495–2502.

El-Sherbini A (1991) Study of tetanus neonatorum in Tanta Fever Hospital, 1988–1989. *Journal of Tropical Pediatrics* **37**: 262–263.

Furste W (1965) Current concepts about tetanus prophylaxis. *Journal of Occupational Medicine* **7**: 5–11.

Gurses N and Aydin M (1993) Factors affecting prognosis of neonatal tetanus. *Scandinavian Journal of Infectious Diseases* **25**: 353–355.

Helting TB and Zwisler O (1977) Structure of tetanus toxin. I. Breakdown of the toxin molecule and discrimination between polypeptide fragments. *Journal of Biological Chemistry* **252**: 187–193.

James MFM and Manson EDM (1985) The use of magnesium sulphate infusions in the management of very severe tetanus. *Intensive Care Medicine* **11**: 5–12.

Kerr JH, Corbett JL, Prys-Roberts C, Smith AC and Spalding JMK (1968) Involvement of the sympathetic nervous system in tetanus. *Lancet* **2**: 236–241.

King WW and Cave DR (1991) Use of esmolol to control autonomic instability of tetanus. *American Journal of Medicine* **91**: 425–428.

Lipman J, James MFM, Erskine J *et al.* (1987) Autonomic dysfunction in severe tetanus: magnesium sulfate as an adjunct to deep sedation. *Critical Care Medicine* **15**: 987–988.

Luisto M (1989) Epidemiology of tetanus in Finland from 1969 to 1985 *Scandanavian Journal of Infectious Disease* **21**: 655–663.

Luisto M (1993) Unusual and iatrogenic sources of tetanus. *Annales Chirurgiae et Gynaecologiae* **82**: 25–29.

Matsuda M and Yoneda M (1974) Dissociation of tetanus neurotoxin into two polypeptide fragments. *Biochemical and Biophysical Research Communications* **57**: 1257–1262.

Mellanby J and Green J (1981) How does tetanus toxin act? *Neuroscience* **6**: 281–300.

Millard AH (1954) Local tetanus. *Lancet* **2**: 844–846.

Mitra RC, Das Gupta R and Sack RB (1989) Electrocardiographic changes in tetanus: a serial study. *Journal of the Indian Medical Association* **89**: 164–167.

Murphy KJ (1970) Fatal tetanus with brain-stem involvement and myocarditis in an exserviceman. *Medical Journal of Australia* **2**: 542–544.

Parish HJ (1968) *Victory with Vaccines*. Edinburgh: E. & S. Livingstone Ltd.

Passen EL and Andersen BR (1986) Clinical tetanus despite a 'protective' level of toxin-neutralizing antibody. *Journal of the American Medical Association* **255**: 1171–1173.

Peter G, Halsey NA, Marcuse EK and Pickering LK (eds) (1994) *American Academy of Pediatrics. 1994 Red Book: Report of the Committee on Infectious Diseases*. Illinois: American Academy of Pediatrics.

Prevots R, Sutter RW, Strebel PM, Cochi SL and Hadler S (1992) Tetanus surveillance – United States, 1989–1990. *MMWR CDC Surveillance Summaries* **41**: 1–9.

Richter RW, Lysons MM, Cave HG, Foster PD and Tapley HL (1970) Myocardial conduction system lesions in tetanus. *Clinical Research* **17**: 374.

Schmitt A, Dreyer F and John C (1981) At least three sequential steps are involved in the tetanus toxin-induced block of neuromuscular transmission. *Naunyn-Schmiedeberg's Archives of Pharmacology* **317**: 326–330.

Singh G, Goyal BB and Singh DP (1989) Role of intrathecal tetanus antitoxin (equine) in tetanus neonatorum. *Journal of the Indian Medical Association* **87**: 8–10.

Southorn PA and Blaise GA (1986) Treatment of tetanus-induced autonomic nervous system dysfunction with continuous epidural blockade. *Critical Care Medicine* **14**: 251–252.

Sutton DN, Tremlett MR, Woodcock TE and Nielsen MS (1990) Management of autonomic dysfunction in severe tetanus: the use of magnesium sulphate and clonidine. *Intensive Care Medicine* **16**: 75–80.

Trujillo MH, Castillo A, Espana J, Manzo A and Zerpa R (1987) Impact of intensive care management on the prognosis of tetanus: analysis of 641 cases. *Chest* **92**: 63–65.

Udwadia FE, Sunavala JD, Jain MC *et al.* (1992) Haemodynamic studies during the management of severe tetanus. *Quarterly Journal of Medicine* **83**: 449–460.

Weinstein L (1973) Current concepts: tetanus. *New England Journal of Medicine* **289**: 1293–1296.

Whitman C, Belgharbi L, Gasse F *et al.* (1992) Progress towards the global elimination of neonatal tetanus. *World Health Statistical Quarterly* **45**: 248–256.

13

Fungal Diseases

Patricia L. Hibberd

Infectious Diseases and Transplantation Units, Massachusetts General Hospital; and the Department of Medicine, Harvard Medical School, Boston, MA, USA

INTRODUCTION

While there has been a dramatic increase in the number of patients surviving for ever-increasing time periods with compromised host defences, there has been a less recognized increase in the incidence of invasive fungal infection. There are two main reasons why this patient population has been increasing world-wide. First, there has been an unprecedented epidemic of infection with the human immunodeficiency virus (HIV). The acquired immunodeficiency syndrome (AIDS) is the most advanced stage of HIV infection, characterized by profound cellular immunodeficiency resulting in opportunistic infection and malignancy. In 1993, 12 to 14 million people were estimated to be infected with HIV (American College of Physicians and Infectious Disease Society of America, 1994). These patients are not only the reservoir of future cases of AIDS, but they form the reservoir of asymptomatic carriers capable of transmitting HIV to uninfected persons. Secondly, there is a gradual but steady increase in patients who acquire host defence defects as a result of disease or treatment of disease. This second group includes patients with malignancy, especially those whose malignancy is treated with chemotherapy and/or bone marrow transplantation, patients with autoimmune disease, particularly those receiving immunosuppressive therapy, and patients with end-stage renal, liver, heart and lung disease, particularly those receiving immunosuppression after organ transplantation. The net result is an ever-increasing population at risk of invasive, and frequently life-threatening, fungal infection.

Although infection of the central nervous system (CNS) is frequently caused by bacteria, viruses or parasites, fungal meningitis is on the increase. *Cryptococcus neoformans* and *Coccidioides immitis* are the most common fungi responsible for CNS mycotic disease. These two fungi and *Histoplasmosis capsulatum* are capable of causing systemic disease in healthy people as well as immunocompromised patients. The opportunistic fungi, such as *Aspergillus*, *Candida* and the Mucoraceae, almost exclusively produce disease in immunocompromised patients. In general, invasive fungal infection results from exposure to the fungus and presence of risk factors for invasion, such as type and amount of immuno-suppression (Hibberd and Rubin, 1994). If the exposure is great enough, even patients with a normal immune system may develop fungal meningitis (as is occasionally seen with *Cryptococcus neoformans* and *Coccidioides immitis*). However, severely compromised patients with major host defence defects may develop CNS infections after minimal exposure to any of the fungi just listed, including the opportunistic ones. The three most critical host defence defects are those that depress cell-mediated immunity, those that impair neutrophil function and those that produce neutropenia. The causes of these defects range from chronic disease (e.g. diabetes, renal disease, malignancy), medications (e.g. corticosteroids, cytotoxic drugs), infection (e.g. HIV) to malnutrition and other poorly characterized conditions.

Three forms of fungal infection are recognized – primary infection, reactivation, and superinfection. Primary infection occurs after initial exposure to a fungal pathogen. Reactivation infection occurs when infection acquired many years previously may reactivate from a dormant focus due to the waning of previous immunity, e.g. due to progressive HIV infection. Reinfection occurs when previously acquired immunity wanes, such that a new exposure to the fungus results in invasive infection. The risk of developing CNS disease in a normal host is probably greatest after primary infection. In immunocompromised patients all three types of infection may result in CNS disease, frequently in conjunction with other manifestations of systemic dissemination.

CENTRAL NERVOUS SYSTEM DISEASE CAUSED BY THE SYSTEMIC MYCOSES

Cryptococcus neoformans

Cryptococcal meningitis is caused by *Cryptococcus neoformans*, a yeast-like fungus with a world-wide distribution. The fungus is found in soil, particularly soil contaminated with bird droppings. *C. neoformans* gains access to a potential host when the organism is aerosolized and inhaled. Invasion occurs in patients who have defects in cell-mediated immunity, such as AIDS patients (Powderly, 1993), those patients treated with corticosteroids, or patients with lymphoreticular malignancies (Diamond and Bennett, 1974). In HIV-infected patients, cryptococcal disease is the fourth most common cause of life-threatening infection after *Pneumocystis carinii*, cytomegalovirus and mycobacteria (Kovacs *et al.*, 1985; Eng *et al.*, 1986; Zuger *et al.*, 1986). Cryptococcal meningitis occurs in 6–10% of AIDS patients in the United States (Dismukes, 1988; Chuck and Sande, 1989; Clark *et al.*, 1990a) and 15–30% of AIDS patients in Sub-Saharan Africa (Clumeck *et al.*, 1989). It is usually diagnosed in patients whose CD4 count is less than 100 cell mm^{-3} (Crowe *et al.*, 1991; Nightingale *et al.*, 1992).

Although the portal of entry for *C. neoformans* is the lung, most pulmonary infection is asymptomatic. If haematogenous dissemination occurs in susceptible patients, the CNS is the most common site seeded, followed by skin, bone, prostate and other organs. The cryptococci produce minimal inflammation in infected tissues. In the CNS, both meninges and parenchymal brain tissue tend to be diffusely involved. Patients usually present with signs and symptoms of a subacute meningitis or meningoencephalitis, although AIDS patients may be asymptomatic (Table 13.1). The majority of patients with cryptococcal meningitis will have an abnormal chest radiograph (typically bilateral alveolar or interstitial pneumonitis), but in 15–35% of patients, this may be due to concomitant opportunistic infection, particularly *Pneumocystis carinii* (Chuck and Sande, 1989; Clark *et al.*, 1990a, b).

The differential diagnosis of cryptococcal meningitis includes the other causes of chronic meningitis/meningoencephalitis, such as tuberculosis, other fungal infections, brucellosis, syphilis, parasitic infections, HIV and other viral infections and non-infectious aetiologies. Since the differential diagnosis is broad, with a wide range of treatment options, it is important to make a specific diagnosis. In addition, diagnosis of cryptococcal meningitis (in the absence of definitive evidence of HIV infection) permits diagnosis of AIDS using the World Health Organization Clinical Case Definition of AIDS for use in Africa (WHO, 1985; Colebunders *et al.*, 1987). (See Chapter 4.)

Isolation of *C. neoformans* from any site is significant and in all patients (apparently normal hosts and immunocompromised patients) mandates a search for disseminated disease, particularly in the CNS. Therapy is indicated in all

TABLE 13.1 Clinical manifestations of fungal meningitis

	Cryptococcosis HIV infected	Cryptococcosis non-HIV infected	Coccidioidomycosis	Histoplasmosis
No symptoms	< 20%	< 10%	very rare	rare
Headache	70–90%	> 80%	70–90%	70–90%
Fever	60–90%	50–70%	50–60%	50–90%
Nausea and vomiting	40–50%	40–50%	30–40%	rare
Stiff neck	20–40%	40–60%	30–40%	40–60%
Photophobia	< 20%	30–40%	< 10%	rare
Mental status alterations	20–40%	40–60%	< 10%	10–30%
Seizures	< 10%	10–20%	< 10%	< 30%
Focal neurological defects	< 20%	< 10%	< 20%	< 50%

TABLE 13.2 Laboratory abnormalities in fungal meningitis

	Cryptococcosis HIV infected	Cryptococcosis non-HIV infected	Coccidioidomycosis	Histoplasmosis
Cerebrospinal fluid				
Glucose < 50 mg dl^{-1} (2.77 mmol l^{-1})	25–65%	60–80%	50–75%	common
Protein > 45 mg dl^{-1} (2.74 mmol l^{-1})	50–70%	> 85%	>95%	common
WBC < 20 mm^{-3}	65–80%	< 30%	< 10%	< 10%
Cryptococcal antigen ⩾ 1:8	> 90%	> 90%	not applicable	not applicable
Complement-fixing antibody	not applicable	not applicable	75–95%	not applicable
India ink	70–90%	50–60%	< 10%	< 10%
Culture positive	> 90%	> 90%	< 50%	< 50%
Opening pressure > 200 mm water	50–70%	60–80%	> 50%	variable
Serum				
Cryptococcal antigen ⩾ 1:8	> 75%	> 75%	not applicable	not applicable
Non-CNS sites				
Culture positive	40–70%	35–60%	< 20%	50–90%
CT scan				
normal	common	common	rare	common
abnormal	dilated ventricles rare focal nodules	dilated ventricles rare focal nodules	dilated ventricles obscuring of basal cisterns	basilar inflammation single or multiple brain lesions

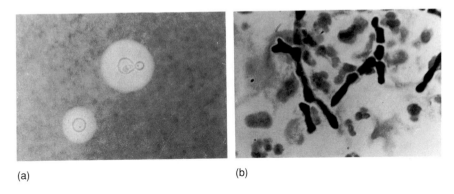

(a)   (b)

Figure 13.1   (a) *Cryptococcus neoformans* in cerebrospinal fluid; India ink preparation. (b) Gram stain of sputum showing septate hyphae with acute angle branching characteristic of *Aspergillus* species.

patients from whom *C. neoformans* is isolated except normal hosts with pulmonary cryptococcosis who may have self-limited disease.

Cerebrospinal fluid (CSF) findings and radiological findings on computed tomography (CT) are shown in Table 13.2. Preliminary diagnosis is made by detection of the characteristic polysaccharide capsule of the *Cryptococcus* on India ink stain (see Figure 13.1a), or by detection of a CSF titre of greater than 1:8 using the latex agglutination assay for cryptococcal polysaccharide antigen. Definitive identification is made by culture of CSF on Sabouraud's agar, but the organisms will grow on blood and chocolate agar incubated at 37°C for 3–10 days. Repeated attempts at isolation should be made if initial culture is negative, because small numbers of organisms may be present and missed. *C. neoformans* can frequently be cultured from urine or sputum in patients with disseminated cryptococcosis.

Prognostic factors have been most extensively studied in North American HIV-infected patients with cryptococcal meningitis, where acute mortality is 10–25% (Chuck and Sande, 1989; Clark *et al.*, 1990a; Saag *et al.*, 1992) and one-year survival is 30–50% (Chuck and Sande, 1989; Powderly *et al.*, 1992). Patients with a CSF cryptococcal antigen titre of greater than 1:1054, a CSF leukocyte count of less than 20 cells mm^{-3}, age under 35 years, isolation of *C. neoformans* from extraneural sites and hyponatraemia have been associated with a poorer prognosis (Chuck and Sande, 1989; Larsen *et al.*, 1990). Desmet *et al.* (1989) evaluated the serum cryptococcal antigen assay for screening in 450 HIV patients in Zaire: serum antigen was detected in 55 of the patients, 44 of whom had meningitis. This result contrasts with data from Hoffman *et al.* (1991) who found no cases of cryptococcal meningitis in 350 Danish HIV-infected patients screened for cryptococcal antigen. Screening for antigen will probably be most cost-effective in HIV-infected patients with fever and headache. Therapy is discussed later.

Coccidioides immitis

Unlike *Cryptococcus neoformans*, *Coccidioides immitis* is geographically restricted to the Western Hemisphere, particularly the South West states of the United States, the northern and Pacific zones of Mexico, Guatemala, Honduras and Venezuela. *C. immitis* exists in soil in the mycelial phase. Hyphal segments fragment, releasing arthroconidia which are infectious. Aerosolized arthroconidia may be inhaled; in tissue, they swell, forming large thick-walled structures (spherules). Within the spherule, repeated internal subdivisions produce large numbers of endospores which can be released and dispersed to start the cycle in other tissues when the spherule ruptures. Infections in normal patients living in endemic areas are frequent, usually asymptomatic and restricted to the lungs. About 0.5% of patients develop disseminated disease (via vascular or lymphatic spread), usually in the first few months of infection. Almost any organ in the body may be seeded, but more common sites are skin, bone and joints, meninges and genitourinary tract. Between 33 and 50% of patients with dissemination will have meningeal involvement and frequently the CNS is the only site of symptomatic disease (Bouza *et al.*, 1981). Risk factors for dissemination include extremes of age, male sex, non-Caucasian race, pregnancy and immunosuppression (Pappagianis, 1980). The risk of HIV-infected patients developing disseminated coccidiomycosis either from primary infection, reactivation or reinfection in endemic areas is greater than 10% (Gagliani and Ampell, 1990).

Histopathologically, *C. immitis* usually causes a granulomatous reaction in tissues. In the CNS, there is a predilection for the meninges, particularly at the base of the brain. Focal space-occupying lesions are rare. A granulomatous fibrosing reaction occurs as the meningitis progresses; the resulting hydrocephalus frequently requires shunting. As with cryptococcal meningitis, coccidiodal meningitis usually has a subtle and subacute onset (Vincent *et al.*, 1993). Signs and symptoms are shown in Table 13.1. CT and CSF findings are shown in Table 13.2.

The diagnosis of coccidiodal meningitis may be a difficult one to make for two reasons. Firstly, *C. immitis* is recovered from CSF in less than 50% of patients with known meningitis. Although *C. immitis* may be cultured on Sabouraud's agar, the cultures represent a severe biological hazard because they are highly infectious for the laboratory personnel who handle them. Clinicians must always alert a laboratory to this possibility, because extreme care must be taken to avoid aerosolization of the mycelial phase by using appropriate safety equipment and procedures (Johnson *et al.*, 1964). Secondly, not all patients with meningitis have other sites of involvement from which a diagnosis (either by recovery of fungus in culture or by demonstration of spherules in tissue) can be made. However, 95% of patients with coccidiodal meningitis have complement-fixing antibody in CSF obtained from lumbar or cisternal taps (Drutz and Catanzaro, 1978a, b). Demonstration of this antibody alone is sufficient to justify initiation of antifungal therapy. A presumptive diagnosis of meningitis may be made in patients with chronic meningitis, in conjunction with either evidence of systemic coccidiodomycosis or a serum complement fixation titre to *C. immitis* of 1:16 or greater. Therapy is discussed later.

Histoplasma capsulatum

Histoplasmosis is caused by *Histoplasma capsulatum*, which in its yeast form readily infects non-immune macrophages in man. Like *Coccidioides immitis*, *H. capsulatum* is geographically restricted, being found in the soil enriched with faecal material from chickens, starlings and bats in distinct areas of the tropics and temperate zones. In the United States, the endemic area is in the eastern-central part of the country, predominantly the Ohio and Mississippi river valleys. A distinct stable variant, *H. capsulatum* var. *duboisii* is found in central Africa, predominantly in the countries of West Africa. In the soil, *H. capsulatum* is in its mycelial form. Inhaled airborne spores release the infectious yeast form. In heavily endemic areas, such as the United States, the entire population is infected and probably repeatedly reinfected, because acquired cellular immunity wanes with time. These infections are usually asymptomatic and rarely of clinical consequence. Occasionally, even in a normal host, excessive inhalation of spores results in symptomatic disease. Haematogenous dissemination tends to occur in infants, the elderly, patients with malignancies (particularly lymphoma) and those with HIV infection (Johnson *et al.*, 1988). Disseminated histoplasmosis is one of the AIDS-defining diseases in the Centers for Disease Control (CDC) surveillance case definition for AIDS (CDC, 1992; Chang, 1992), and the most common AIDS-defining infection in some endemic areas. It is usually diagnosed in patients with CD4 count less than 200 cells mm^{-3}.

The burden of disease in disseminated histoplasmosis seen in North America is in organs rich in infected macrophages such as visceral lymph nodes, spleen, liver and bone marrow. In African histoplasmosis, the burden of disease is in the skin and bones. CNS involvement is uncommon in North America and as yet unknown in Africa. CNS histoplasmosis mimics tuberculosis. It causes a granulomatous reaction, particularly in the meninges at the base of the brain. Parenchymal involvement may occur as single or multiple focal granulomatous lesions. Signs and symptoms are shown in Table 13.1. CT and CSF findings are shown in Table 13.2.

Diagnosis by isolation of *H. capsulatum* from the CNS is difficult because of the paucity of viable fungi in the CSF. The fungus may take 5–45 days to grow. Cultures of bone marrow, blood, urine and sputum are more likely to be positive and may assist with diagnosis if CNS disease is present. A *Histoplasma* antigen assay is in development. Serum antibody tests are rarely useful, since serological responses rarely occur in immunocompromised patients with histoplasmosis (Kaufmann *et al.*, 1978). Therapy is discussed later.

CENTRAL NERVOUS SYSTEM DISEASE CAUSED BY OPPORTUNISTIC FUNGI

Aspergillus Species

Of the more than 350 species of *Aspergillus*, *A. fumigatus* and *A. flavus* account for almost all cases of human disease. Aspergilli are common saprophytic moulds, ubiquitous in nature. Since transmission occurs through the air, the greatest impact of *Aspergillus* infection is on the lungs. In the normal host, infection usually remains within the lungs causing a wide variety of conditions such as allergic and bronchopulmonary aspergillosis, chronic necrotizing pulmonary aspergillosis and pulmonary aspergilloma. In the immunocompromised patient, haematogenous dissemination to the CNS, eyes, bones, skin, kidneys, heart and other organs may occur following invasion of the pulmonary vasculature. Occasionally, CNS aspergillosis results from primary disease in the paranasal sinuses, with direct extension to the CNS via the draining venous sinuses or orbit. Invasive *Aspergillus* and CN aspergillosis occurs almost exclusively in severely immunocompromised patients: patients with prolonged and severe neutropenia following cytotoxic chemotherapy (particularly those with leukaemia); patients with chronic granulomatous disease; and patients receiving glucocorticoids and other immunosuppressive drugs (Rinaldi, 1983; Gerson *et al.*, 1984; Denning and Stevens, 1990). The hyphae invade blood vessels causing thrombosis with subsequent infarction and necrosis. Thus haemorrhagic necrosis and brain abscesses are the most common manifestations of CNS aspergillosis. Presentation, CT and CSF findings are shown in Table 13.3.

The differential diagnosis is broad and includes subdural empyema, epidural abscess, pyogenic meningitis or brain abscess, viral encephalitis, cryptococcal meningitis, mucormycosis, mycotic aneurysms, and non-infectious conditions such as CNS vasculitis, primary and metastatic neoplasms.

Diagnosis of CNS aspergillosis is difficult, since *Aspergillus* is rarely isolated from CSF and blood cultures. *Aspergillus* is only isolated from expectorated sputum in 10–30% of patients who have active pulmonary disease. Biopsy of the portal of entry or aspiration of the CNS abscess is frequently required to provide the prompt diagnosis needed to attempt to reverse the high mortality rate associated with CNS aspergillosis. The characteristic appearance of *Aspergillus* is shown in Figure 13.1b. The utility of serology in invasive disease is not yet established. Therapy is discussed later.

Mucoraceae

The major pathogens of the Mucoraceae include *Rhizopus*, *Mucor* and *Absidia* species. Although they are taxonomically separate from *Aspergillus* species, mucormycosis closely resembles invasive aspergillosis. These pathogens are ubiquitous saphrophytes which cause invasive disease in four types of

TABLE 13.3 Opportunistic fungi in the central nervous system – Clinical and laboratory abnormalities

	Aspergillosis	Rhinocerebral mucormycosis	Candidiasis
Clinical manifestations			
Fever	> 90%	> 50%	> 50%
Headache	75–90%	variable	variable
Stiff neck	< 10%	< 10%	< 10%
Mental status alterations	> 50%	> 90%	variable
Focal neurological deficits	> 50%	> 70%	rare
Cerebrospinal fluid			
Glucose < 50 mg dl^{-1}	rare	rare	rare
Protein > 45 mg dl^{-1}	common	common	variable
WBC < 20 mm^{-3}	rare	rare	variable
Culture positive	rare	rare	> 80%
CT scan			
Normal	rare	never	variable
Abnormal	infarction brain abscess	infarction brain abscess	rare focal lesions

patients; diabetics with ketoacidosis; severely compromised patients, particularly those with leukaemia and lymphoma; severely malnourished patients; and patients who have extensive trauma to the cutaneous and mucosal surfaces, particularly after burn injury (Lehrer *et al.*, 1980). Aerosolized spores may be inhaled or directly inoculated onto damaged skin. In susceptible hosts, blood vessels are invaded by the fungi, producing tissue infarction and a characteristic black inflammatory exudate. CNS infection occurs either after haematogenous dissemination from the portal of entry, or after contiguous spread from the palate or nasal sinuses, through adjacent sinuses and the orbit (rhinocerebral mucormycosis). Occasionally in malnourished patients, invasion may occur from the gastrointestinal tract. Presentation, CT and CSF findings are shown in Table 13.3.

The diagnosis must be suspected from clinical findings and is established by biopsy of infected areas; the Mucoraceae are rarely isolated from CSF or blood cultures. As with invasive aspergillosis, prompt diagnosis is needed to attempt to reverse the high mortality rate associated with invasive mucormycosis. Therapy is discussed later.

Candida Species

Unlike all the other fungi discussed in this chapter, *Candida* species, particularly *C. albicans*, are part of the normal oropharyngeal, gastrointestinal and vaginal flora. CNS disease due to *Candida* is rare even in patients with haematogenously disseminated disease. *Candida* frequently enters the bloodstream via intravenous catheters, particularly in patients receiving intravenous hyperalimentation (Edwards *et al.*, 1978). The patient with impaired neutrophil function is at greatest risk of developing disseminated disease, including seeding of the CNS, following fungaemia that originates from a catheter site. Disseminated disease occasionally follows bloodstream invasion from a focus in the gastro-intestinal tract (Crislip and Edwards, 1989). Occasionally *Candida* meningitis may result from infection of a ventricular shunt (Sugarman and Massanari, 1980) or a neurosurgical procedure, rather than from disseminated candidiasis.

Candida tends to cause a random distribution of intraparenchymal micro-abscesses, mainly about the middle cerebral artery. Signs, symptoms, CT and CSF findings are shown in Table 13.3. Organisms are found on Gram stain in about 40% of patients. Cultures confirm the diagnosis and allow speciation of the candidal organisms. More than 90% of cases are due to *C. albicans*. Therapy is discussed later.

TREATMENT OF FUNGAL INFECTIONS IN THE CENTRAL NERVOUS SYSTEM

Although amphotericin B is the cornerstone of therapy for fungal meningitis, it is an unsatisfactory medication for four reasons. First, entrance of amphotericin into the CSF is poor, such that intrathecal amphotericin is necessary for treatment of serious meningitis (e.g. coccidioidal meningitis). Second, toxic reactions including immediate systemic reactions (fever, chills and hypoten-sion), decreased glomerular filtration, and anaemia are common. Renal toxicity is often dose-limiting and may limit the extent and efficacy of treatment. Third, both intravenous and intrathecal amphotericin are logistically difficult to admin-ister over the prolonged periods required for treatment of meningitis or brain abscesses. Fourth, in certain immunocompromised patients, particularly those infected with HIV, lifelong therapy is necessary to prevent relapse of some fungal meningidites, e.g. cryptococcal meningitis. Intravenous medications are unsuitable for life-long maintenance therapy. For these reasons there has been much interest in the oral formulations of the new triazole antifungal agents – fluconazole and itraconazole – as alternative treatment strategies.

Other available antifungal therapies include the oral antifungal agent flucyto-sine and surgical removal of infected tissue. Flucytosine has a limited antifungal spectrum and significant haematological and gastrointestinal toxicity, but it remains in the antifungal armamentarium because, when combined with ampho-tericin, there is improved outcome in cryptococcal meningitis. In HIV-infected patients, flucytosine-induced myelosuppression is frequently prohibitive. Surgi-cal removal of infected tissue is more important than amphotericin B for treatment of mucormycosis.

Treatment of fungal meningitis remains controversial despite results from several recently published clinical studies. Table 13.4 shows the most com-monly recommended treatment regimens for the fungi discussed in this

TABLE 13.4 Treatment of fungal infections of the central nervous system

	Treatment – Amphotericin	Treatment – other agents	Maintenance	References
Cryptococcosis – HIV infected	0.7–1.0 mg kg^{-1} day^{-1} i.v. × ? 4–8 weeks (or resolution of symptoms, CSF abnormalities)	THEN Fluconazole 400 mg day^{-1} p.o. to complete 10 week ? PLUS Flucytosine 25 mg kg^{-1} p.o. every 6 hours for ? ? OR Fluconazole 400 mg day^{-1} p.o. for 10 weeks	Fluconazole 200 mg day^{-1} p.o. for life	White and Armstrong, 1994
Cryptococcosis – non-HIV infected	0.5–0.8 mg kg^{-1} day^{-1} i.v. for ? 6 weeks (longer if symptoms and CSF culture positive)	PLUS Flucytosine 37.5 mg kg^{-1} day^{-1} for ? 6 weeks	? Fluconazole 200 mg kg^{-1} day^{-1} ? duration	Larsen et al., 1990
Coccidioidomycosis	0.6 mg kg^{-1} day^{-1} i.v. for 7 days then 0.8 mg kg^{-1} every other day i.v. to total dose > 2.5 g PLUS 0.1–0.3 mg day^{-1} intrathecally for ? duration (until normal CSF, at least 1 month, ? 2 years)	OR Fluconazole 400 mg day^{-1} p.o. for 9–12 months	? Fluconazole 200–400 mg day^{-1} ? duration	Labadie and Hamilton, 1986 Wheat, 1994
Histoplasmosis	0.6 mg kg^{-1} day^{-1} i.v. for 7 days then 0.8 mg kg^{-1} every other day – total dose 10–15 mg kg^{-1}		? Itraconazole 200–400 mg kg^{-1} day^{-1} p.o. for life ? amphotericin B 50–100 mg i.v. per week	Wheat, 1994
Aspergillosis	0.8–1.0 mg kg^{-1} day^{-1} for total dose > 2 g	? PLUS Rifampin 600 mg p.o. day^{-1}	none	Denning and Stevens, 1990
Mucormycosis	0.8–1.0 mg kg^{-1} day^{-1} for total dose > 2.5 g	PLUS Primary therapy – surgical removal of infected tissue, control of underlying condition (acidosis)	none	Parfray, 1986
Candidiasis	0.8–1.0 mg kg^{-1} day^{-1} i.v. for ? duration (until no symptoms, normal CSF)	? PLUS Flucytosine 37.5 mg kg^{-1} day^{-1} for ? duration	none	Smego et al., 1984

i.v., intravenous; p.o., oral.

TABLE 13.5 Prevention and treatment of adverse effects associated with antifungal agents

	Adverse event	Prevention or treatment
Amphotericin B	Fever	Premedicate with acetaminophen, ? hydrocortisone
	Rigors	Meperidine (other narcotics)
	Renal dysfunction	If patient is sodium depleted or dehydrated premedicate with 500 ml 0.9% saline intravenously ? Repeat after amphotericin dose completed
	Thrombophlebitis	Use central catheter
	Hyperkalaemia	Slow infusion, monitor potassium
	Hypokalaemia	Potassium replacement, monitor potassium
	Arachnoiditis, etc.	associated with intrathecal administration – intrathecal corticosteroids
Flucytosine	Myelotoxicity	Keep peak serum flucytosine level $< 100\ \mu g\ ml^{-1}$ Monitor twice weekly especially in azotemia
Fluconazole and itraconazole	Drug interaction with terfenadine, astemizole ventricular arrhythmias	Avoid terfenadine and hismanal during therapy with either fluconazole or itraconazole

chapter. Approaches to treatment and prevention of toxicity of amphotericin B and flucytosine are shown in Table 13.5.

In summary, fungal meningitis tends to be a subacute or chronic process which is just as lethal as bacterial meningitis if it is untreated. Amphotericin B remains the drug of choice in most situations, although the newer triazoles have a role at least in chronic suppressive therapy. In order to prevent the anticipated continuing increase in fungal meningitis in a cost-effective way, it will probably be necessary to focus on host defence defects and/or administer prophylactic antifungal therapy to those at greatest risk (e.g. AIDS patients with very low CD4 counts). However, as use of antifungal agents increases, particularly when used for prophylaxis, there will be an attendant risk of developing drug-resistant fungi.

REFERENCES

American College of Physicians and Infectious Disease Society of America (1994) Human Immunodeficiency Virus (HIV) Infection. *Annals of Internal Medicine* **120**: 310–319.

Bouza E, Dreyer JS, Hewitt WL *et al.* (1981) Coccidioidal meningitis: An analysis of thirty-one cases and review of the literature. *Medicine* **60**: 139.

CDC (1987) Revision of the CDC surveillance case definition for acquired immunodeficiency syndrome. Council of State and Territorial Epidemiologists: AIDS Program Center for Disease Control. *MMWR. Morbidity and Mortality Weekly Reports* **36** (suppl 1): 15.

CDC (1992) 1993 revised classification system for HIV infection and expanded surveillance case definition for AIDS among adolescents and adults. *MMWR. Morbidity and Mortality Weekly Reports* **41**: 961.

Chang SW, Kate MH and Hernandez SR (1992) The new AIDS case definition – implicators for San Francisco. *Journal of the American Medical Association* **267**: 973.

Chuck SL and Sande MA (1989) Infections with *Cryptococcus neoformans* in the acquired immunodeficiency syndrome. *New England Journal of Medicine* **321**: 794–799.

Clark RA, Greer D, Atkinson W, Valainis GT and Hyslop N (1990a) Spectrum of *Cryptococcus neoformans* infection in 68 patients infected with human immunodeficiency virus. *Reviews of Infectious Diseases* **12**: 768–777.

Clark RA, Greer DL, Valainis GT and Hyslop N (1990b) *Cryptococcus neoformans* pulmonary infection in HIV-1 infected patients. *Journal of Acquired Immune Deficiency Syndrome* **3**: 480–484.

Clumeck N, Carael M and Van de Perre P (1989) The African AIDS experience in contrast with the rest of the world. In: *Opportunistic Infections in Patients with the Acquired Immunodeficiency Syndrome* (eds G Leoung and J Mills), pp 43–56. New York: Marcel Dekker.

Colebunders RL, Francis H, Izaley L *et al.* (1987) Evaluation of a clinical case definition of acquired immunodeficiency syndrome in Africa. *Lancet* **1**: 492–494.

Crislip MA and Edwards JE Jr (1989) Candidiasis. *Infectious Disease Clinics of North America* **3**: 103.

Crowe SM, Carlin JB, Stewart KI, Lucas CR and Hoy JF (1991) Predictive value of CD4 lymphocyte numbers for the development of opportunistic infections and malignancies in HIV infected persons. *Journal of Acquired Immune Deficiency Syndrome* **4**: 770–776.

Denning DW and Stevens DA (1990) Antifungal and surgical treatment of invasive aspergillosis: A review of 2,121 published cases. *Reviews of Infectious Diseases* **12**: 1147–1201.

Desmet P, Kayembe KD and De Vroey C (1989) The value of cryptococcal serum antigen screening among HIV-positive/AIDS patients in Kinghasa, Zaire. *AIDS* **3**: 77.

Diamond RD and Bennett VE (1974) Prognostic factors in cryptococcal meningitis: A study of 111 cases. *Annals of Internal Medicine* **80**: 176–181.

Dismukes WE (1988) Cryptococcal meningitis in patients with AIDS. *Journal of Infectious Diseases* **157**: 624–628.

Drutz DJ and Catanzaro A (1978a) Coccidioidomycosis (part 1). *Annual Review of Respiratory Diseases* **117**: 559.

Drutz DJ and Catanzaro A (1978b) Coccidioidomycosis (part 2). *Annual Review of Respiratory Diseases* **117**: 727.

Edwards JR Jr, Lehrer RI, Steihm ER *et al.* (1978) Severe candidal infections: clinical perspective, immune defense mechanisms and current concepts of therapy. *Annals of Internal Medicine* **89**: 91.

Eng RHK, Bishburg E, Smith SM *et al.* (1986) Cryptococcal infections in patients with acquired immunodeficiency syndrome. *American Journal of Medicine* **81**: 19–23.

Galgiani JN and Ampell NM (1990) Coccidioimycosis in human immunodeficiency virus infected patients. *Journal of Infectious Diseases* **162**: 1165–1169.

Gerson SL, Talbot GH, Hurwitz S *et al.* (1984) Prolonged granulocytopenia: the major risk factor for invasive pulmonary aspergillosis in patients with acute leukemia. *Annals of Internal Medicine* **100**: 345–351.

Hibberd PL and Rubin RH (1994) Clinical aspects of fungal infection in organ transplant recipients. *Clinical Infectious Disease* **19**: 533–540.

Hoffman S, Stenderup J and Mathieson LR (1991) Low yield of screening for crypto-coccal antigen by latex agglutination assay on serum and cerebrospinal fluid from Danish patients with AIDS or ARC. *Scandinavian Journal of Infectious Diseases* **23**: 697.

Johnson JE, Perry JE, Fekety FR *et al.* (1964) Laboratory acquired coccidioimycosis: A report of 210 cases. *Annals of Internal Medicine* **60**: 941.

Johnson PC, Khardori N, Najjar AF *et al.* (1988) Progressive disseminated histoplasmo-sis in patients with acquired immunodeficiency syndrome. *American Journal of Medicine* **85**: 152–158.

Kaufman CA, Israel KS, Smith JW *et al.* (1978) Histoplasmosis in immunocompromised patients. *American Journal of Medicine* **64**: 923–932.

Kovacs JA, Kovacs AA, Polis M *et al.* (1985) Cryptococcosis in the acquired immuno-deficiency syndrome. *Annals of Internal Medicine* **103**: 533–538.

Labadie EL and Hamilton RH (1986) Survival improvement in coccidioidal meningitis by high dose intrathecal amphotericin B. *Archives of Internal Medicine* **146**: 2013–2018.

Larsen RA, Leal MAE and Chan LS (1990) Fluconazole compared with amphotericin B plus flucytosine for cryptococcal meningitis in AIDS: a randomized trial. *Annals of Internal Medicine* **113**: 183–187.

Lehrer RI, Howard DH, Sypherd PS *et al.* (1980) Mucormycosis (part 1). *Annals of Internal Medicine* **93**: 93.

Nightingale SD, Cal SX, Peterson DM *et al.* (1992) Primary prophylaxis with fluconazole against systemic fungal infections in HIV-positive patients. *AIDS* **6**: 191–194.

Pappagianis D (1980) Epidemiology of coccidioimycosis. In: *Coccidiomycosis: A text*, (ed. DA Stevens), p 63. New York: Plenum.

Parfray NA (1986) Improved diagnosis and prognosis of mucormycosis. A clinicopatho-logic study of 33 cases. *Medicine* **65**: 113–123.

Powderly WG (1993) Cryptococcal meningitis and AIDS. *Clinical Infectious Disease* **17**: 837–842.

Powderly WG, Saag MS, Cloud GA *et al.* (1992) A controlled trial of fluconazole and amphotericin B to prevent relapse of cryptococcal meningitis in patients with the acquired immunodeficiency syndrome. *New England Journal of Medicine* **326**: 793–798.

Rinaldi MG (1983) Invasive aspergillosis. *Reviews of Infectious Diseases* **5**: 1061–1077.

Saag MS, Powderly WG, Cloud GA *et al.* (1992) Comparison of amphotericin B with fluconazole in the treatment of acute AIDS-associated cryptococcal meningitis. *New England Journal of Medicine* **326**: 83–89.

Smego RA, Perfect JR and Durack DT (1984) Combined therapy with amphotericin B and 5-fluorocytosine for candidal meningitis. *Reviews of Infectious Diseases* **6**: 781–801.

Sugarman B and Massanari M (1980) Candida meningitis in patients with CSF shunts. *Archives of Neurology* **37**: 180–181.

Vincent T, Galgiani JN, Huppert M and Salkin D (1993) The natural history of coccidioidal meningitis: VA Armed Forces cooperative study 1955–1958. *Clinical Infectious Disease* **16**: 247–254.

Wheat J (1994) Histoplasmosis and coccidiodomycosis in individuals with AIDS. A clinical review. *Infectious Disease Clinics of North America* **8**: 467–482.

White MH, Armstrong D (1994) Cryptococcosis. *Infectious Disease Clinics of North America* **8**: 383–398.

WHO (1985) Acquired Immunodeficiency Syndrome (AIDS) Workshop in AIDS in Central Africa, Banjuii, 22–25 October 1985. *Weekly Epidemiologic Reviews* **60**: 342.

Zuger A, Louie E, Holzman RS *et al.* (1986) Cryptococcal disease in patients with the acquired immunodeficiency syndrome: diagnostic features and outcome of treatment. *Annals of Internal Medicine* **104**: 234–240.

Section 3
PARASITIC CONDITIONS

14

Cerebral Malaria*

David A. Warrell

The Centre for Tropical Medicine, University of Oxford,
Nuffield Department of Clinical Medicine,
John Radcliffe Hospital, Headington, Oxford OX3 9DU, UK

INTRODUCTION

Malaria is still one of the world's major killing diseases. Two billion people, more than 40% of the world's population in more than a hundred countries, live in the malaria endemic zone. There may be as many as 300–500 million infections per year, 90% in Africa, with 1.5–3 million fatal cases most of which are African children (WHO, 1993). Although the malaria endemic area is confined to the tropics, travellers with malaria may present in any country. The total number of reported cases of malaria diagnosed in Britain has been around 2000 each year with a case fatality of about 0.2–0.4%, but there has been a striking increase in the proportion of potentially life-threatening *Plasmodium falciparum* infections from 17% in 1977 to 55% in 1993 (PHLS Malaria Reference Laboratory). Similar total numbers and mortality are reported in France, but with an even higher proportion of *P. falciparum* cases (81% in 1989). In the United States more than 1000 imported cases are reported, 39% attributable to *P. falciparum* (Center for Disease Control, 1994).

MALARIA PARASITES AND THEIR LIFE CYCLES

There are four species of human malaria parasites: *Plasmodium falciparum, P. vivax, P. malariae* and *P. ovale*. Humans are infected when sporozoites are injected, during a blood meal, by female *Anopheles* mosquitoes. They disappear rapidly into the liver where schizonts develop. After 6–16 days these schizonts rupture, releasing merozoites into the bloodstream where they invade erythrocytes. In the case of the relapsing malarias, *P. vivax* and *P. ovale*, the development of some sporozoites becomes arrested and they remain dormant as

---

*The colour plate section appears between p. 236 and p. 237

TABLE 14.1 Falciparum malaria: manifestations of severe disease

Cerebral malaria	Syndrome of respiratory distress, acidosis and anaemia (children)
Hypoglycaemia	Lactic acidosis
Renal failure	Hepatic dysfunction
Shock	Secondary bacterial infections
Pulmonary oedema	Haemostatic disturbances
'Blackwater fever'	

hypnozoites in hepatocytes capable of causing relapses months or years later. *P. falciparum* and *P. malariae* have no persisting hepatic phase but may survive in the blood, undetectable by microscopy, to give rise to recrudescence infections. Within erythrocytes, merozoites develop from rings through trophozoites to multinucleated schizonts which rupture, releasing merozoites which can infect new erythrocytes but cannot reinvade the liver. Some develop into the sexual forms, gametocytes, which, when taken up by mosquitoes, can complete a sexual cycle producing sporozoites ready for inoculation into a new human host.

Cerebral malaria is the best-known severe manifestation of falciparum malaria (Table 14.1) and is the most frequent in adults in most parts of the world. In Spitz's autopsy series of 100 cases in American servicemen, 90% were admitted to hospital in coma or with convulsions (Spitz, 1946). Among South-East Asian adults with severe falciparum malaria, 60–80% have cerebral malaria, in African children 30–70%, and in Melanesian adults in Papua New Guinea 10–15% (Lalloo *et al.*, in press).

DEFINITION OF CEREBRAL MALARIA

The term cerebral malaria implies the presence of neurological features, especially impaired consciousness. However, fever alone may produce mild disturbances of consciousness, such as irritability, confusion, obtundation, psychosis and febrile convulsions, especially in young children. To distinguish cerebral malaria, for research purposes, this diagnosis should be restricted to patients with unrousable coma (Warrell *et al.*, 1982). Unrousability is defined by the Glasgow Coma Scale (Teasdale and Jennett, 1974; Teasdale *et al.*, 1979, 1983) (Table 14.2), the patient makes a non-purposive (non-localizing) or no motor response to noxious stimuli and an inappropriate, incomprehensible or no verbal response (maximum score 7/11) (Warrell, 1989). The level of unconsciousness is chosen because the distinction between obtundation/drowsiness and unrousable coma is clear cut, whereas minor degrees of impaired consciousness are difficult or impossible to separate from effects of fever alone (Warrell *et al.*, 1982). In addition, it is essential to confirm the diagnosis of acute falciparum malaria by finding asexual forms of the parasite in a blood smear and to exclude other causes of encephalopathy, especially treatable ones such as bacterial, fungal and

TABLE 14.2 Definition of unrousable coma: modified Glasgow Coma Scale (Teasdale and Jennett, 1974; Teasdale *et al.*, 1979, 1983)

		Score
Adults		
Best verbal response:	Oriented	5
	Confused	4
	Inappropriate words	3
	Incomprehensible sounds	2
	None	1
Best motor response:	Obeys commands	6
	Localizes pain	5
	Flexion to pain: withdrawal	4
	abnormal	3
	Extension to pain	2
	None	1
	Total	2–11
	'unrousable coma'	⩽ 7
Children ('Blantyre scale') (Molyneux *et al.*, 1989)		
Eye movements:	Directed (e.g. follows mother's face)	1
	Not directed	0
Verbal response:	Appropriate cry	2
	Moan or inappropriate cry	1
	None	0
Best motor response:	Localizes painful stimulus	2
	Withdraws limb from pain	1
	Non-specific or absent response	0
	Total	0–5
	'unrousable coma'	⩽ 2

viral encephalitides. This strict research definition is necessary to allow the comparison of results of studies in different parts of the world (Warrell *et al.*, 1990). However, in clinical practice, any degree of impairment of consciousness and other signs of cerebral dysfunction demands treatment as urgent as does 'cerebral malaria' in the strict sense.

CLINICAL FEATURES

Cerebral Malaria in Adults (Warrell *et al.*, 1982, 1990; Gilles and Warrell, 1993)

In adults, the clinical features of cerebral malaria usually develop after several days of fever and other non-specific symptoms indistinguishable from those of uncomplicated malaria. Patients may sink gradually into coma (Figure 14.1) or deteriorate suddenly and persistently after a generalized seizure. For the diagnosis of cerebral malaria, coma should persist for more than 30 minutes after a generalized convulsion to make the distinction from post-ictal coma, for example following a febrile convulsion. Coma usually persists for 24–72 h. The signs of cerebral malaria in adults are summarized in Table 14.3.

Generalized convulsions are observed in about half of the adult patients: these are more common than Jacksonian-type or persistent focal seizures. Possible causes of these convulsions include the cerebral hypoxia associated with cerebral malaria (Warrell *et al.*, 1988), fever, hypoglycaemia, other metabolic disturbances such as renal failure and lactic acidosis, drugs (including some anti-

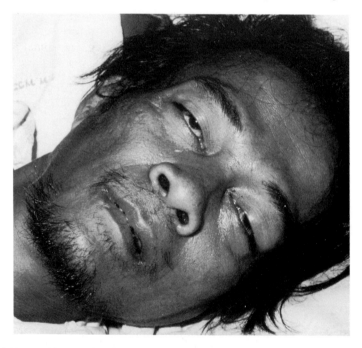

Figure 14.1 Unrousable coma in a Thai man with cerebral malaria. Copyright D.A. Warrell.

TABLE 14.3 Cerebral malaria in adults: clinical features

Impaired consciousness
Convulsions
Clenched jaw, bruxism
Symmetrical upper motor neurone lesion
Extensor posturing
Dysconjugate gaze
Retinal haemorrhages

malarials such as chloroquine and mefloquine), eclampsia in pregnant women and Reye's syndrome in children.

Mild restriction of neck movement is not uncommon and the patient's posture with neck retraction or even opisthotonos may suggest meningitis. However, neck rigidity and photophobia do not occur. In Thai adults, retinal haemorrhages (Plate 1) were seen in about 15% of cases; exudates and papilloedema were rare. Retinal haemorrhages were associated with cerebral malaria or presaged its development and carried a poor prognosis (Looareesuwan *et al.*, 1983a). Similar findings have been reported from Africa (Kayembe *et al.*, 1980) and in non-immune travellers (Dyson *et al.*, 1990).

Corneal and eyelash reflexes are intact, the pupils are equal and react normally. Dysconjugate gaze (internuclear ophthalmoplegia) is a common finding (Figure 14.2). The eyes are usually divergent with normal oculocephalic ('doll's eye') and oculovestibular (caloric) reflexes. Convergence spasm, implying an upper brainstem lesion, transient ocular bobbing, horizontal and vertical nystagmus and VIth cranial nerve palsies (Figure 14.3) have also been observed.

Forcible jaw closure (Figure 14.4) and tooth grinding (bruxism) (Figure 14.5) are common. The jaw jerk is usually brisk and a pout reflex may be elicited, indicating frontal release. A grasp reflex is rare. The gag reflex is usually preserved.

The most usual neurological pattern is of a symmetrical upper motor neurone lesion. Muscle tone and tendon reflexes are usually increased with patellar and

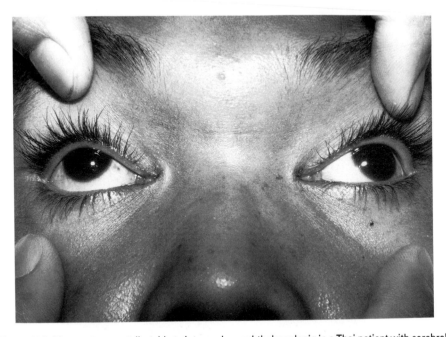

Figure 14.2 Divergent gaze attributable to internuclear ophthalmoplegia in a Thai patient with cerebral malaria. Copyright D.A. Warrell.

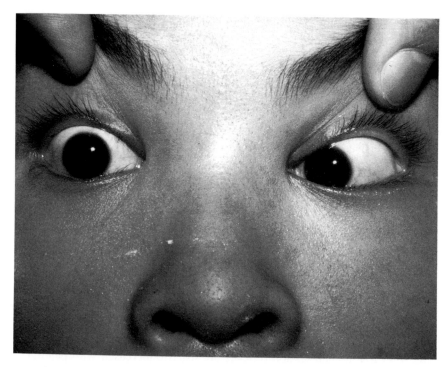

Figure 14.3 Right VIth cranial nerve lesion in a Thai girl; a sequel of cerebral malaria. Copyright D.A. Warrell.

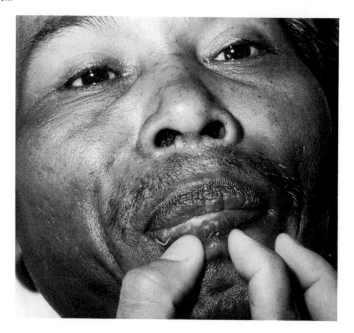

Figure 14.4 Forcible closure of the jaw and pursing of the lips in a Thai patient comatose with cerebral malaria. Copyright D.A. Warrell.

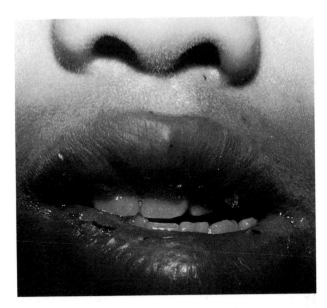

Figure 14.5 Grinding of teeth 'bruxism' in a Thai girl with cerebral malaria. Copyright D.A. Warrell.

especially ankle clonus and extensor plantar responses. Abdominal reflexes are usually absent, a useful sign for distinguishing hysterical patients with fevers of other causes in whom these reflexes are often very brisk. Some patients show a general reduction in muscle tone and tendon reflexes.

Extensor posturing, suggesting brainstem dysfunction or profound hypoglycaemia, is a common and important sign. Decerebrate (Figure 14.6a, b) and decorticate (Figure 14.7) patterns are seen, associated with sustained upward deviation of the eyes, extension of the neck, pouting and periodic sterterous breathing (Figure 14.8). Identical features are seen in patients with hypoglycaemia of other causes (Seibert, 1985), such as complicating bacillary dysentery (Bennish *et al.*, 1990) (Figure 14.9). These signs may also raise the possibility of brainstem herniation, especially in children (see below) (Plum and Posner, 1982).

Cerebral Malaria in Children (Molyneux *et al.*, 1989; Warrell *et al.*, 1990; Gilles and Warrell, 1993)

In most parts of the world where malaria is endemic, severe manifestations and complications of falciparum malaria are seen only in young children who have not yet acquired immunity as a result of frequent infections. Recent work, principally in Africa, has revealed a number of important differences in natural history, clinical features, pathophysiology and sequelae in these children compared to non-immune adults. In children, evolution and recovery of coma in

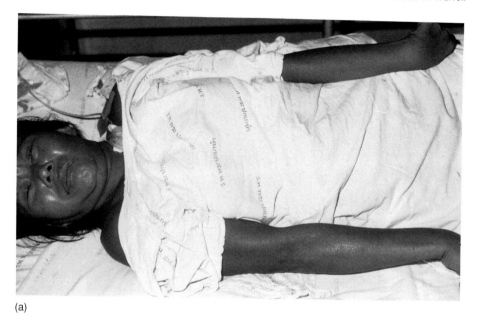

(a)

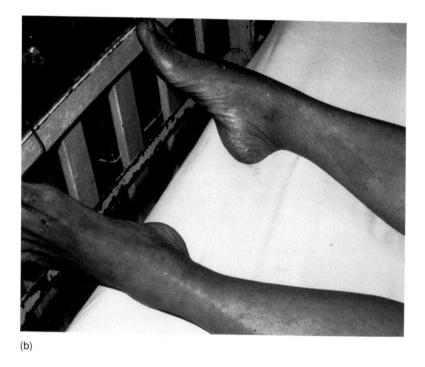

(b)

Figure 14.6 (a) Decerebrate rigidity in a Thai woman with cerebral malaria.
(b) Extension of the lower limbs in a patient with decerebrate rigidity. Copyright D.A. Warrell.

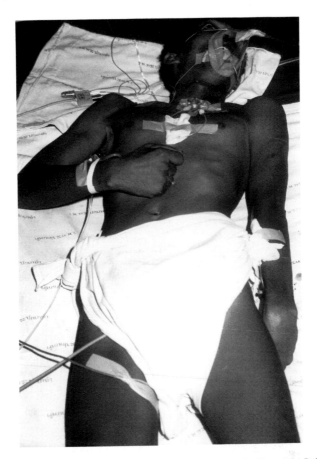

Figure 14.7 Decorticate rigidity in a Thai patient with cerebral malaria. Copyright D.A. Warrell.

cerebral malaria is more rapid than in adults. In a group of 131 children with cerebral malaria studied in Malawi the mean length of reported history was only 47 h (range 2 h to 7 days) (Molyneux *et al.*, 1989). In rural parts of the Gambia, most fatal cases of malaria had died before reaching a dispensary, clinic or hospital (Greenwood *et al.*, 1987). Half of the Malawian children had regained consciousness within 24 h of starting hospital treatment (Molyneux *et al.*, 1989). Common early symptoms include fever, anorexia, vomiting, cough (in Malawi) and convulsions. In the Malawian children, 82% had a history of convulsions, 31 out of 131 had convulsions within 3 h of admission and in 29 they occurred later in the clinical course. Convulsions were associated with delayed recovery of consciousness and an increased risk of neurological sequelae and death. For the definition of unrousable coma in young children who have not yet learnt to speak, the Glasgow Coma Scale has been modified (Table 14.2) (Molyneux *et al.*, 1989). The neurological picture of cerebral malaria in children and adults is compared in Table 14.4. The abnormalities of corneal and brainstem reflexes

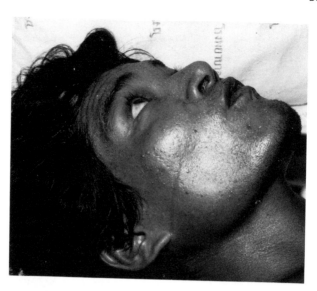

Figure 14.8 Pouting and sustained upward deviation of the eyes in a Thai patient with cerebral malaria. Copyright D.A. Warrell.

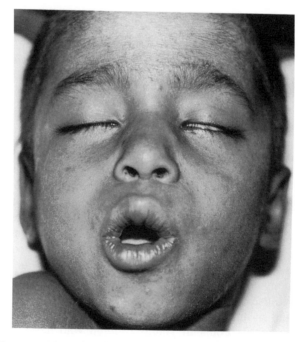

Figure 14.9 Pouting and upward deviation of the eyes in a Bangladeshi child with profound hypoglycaemia as a complication of bacillary dysentery (Bennish *et al.*, 1990). Copyright Dr R.E. Phillips.

TABLE 14.4 Manifestations of cerebral malaria in children and adults

	Children	Adults
Coma	+	+
Convulsions	> 70%	~50%
Dysconjugate gaze	+	+
Symmetrical upper motor neurone lesion	+/–	+
Hypotonia	+	+/–
Extensor posturing, opisthotonos	+	+
Absent reflexes: corneal	+	–
oculocephalic	+	–
oculovestibular	+	–
pupillary	+	–
Respiratory arrhythmias	+	+/–
Rostrocaudal deterioration	+	–
Raised lumbar CSF opening pressure	100%	20%
Permanent neurological sequelae	> 10%	< 5%

(Figure 14.10) and the evidence of rostrocaudal deterioration in some children observed in Kilifi, Kenya (Newton *et al.*, 1991a, 1994), is particularly striking. With the finding of raised intracranial pressure in all children in this group (Figures 14.11, 14.12), these neurological signs and their progression, suggest the possibility of brainstem herniation (Plum and Posner, 1982; Newton *et al.*, 1991a). Extensor posturing, which was common in Malawian and Kenyan children, although a recognized neurological manifestation of hypoglycaemia

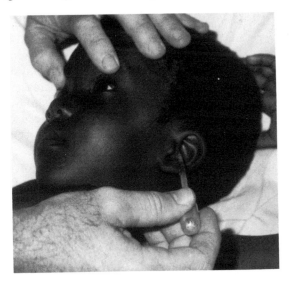

Figure 14.10 'Caloric test' of the oculovestibular reflex in a Kenyan child with cerebral malaria. Copyright D.A. Warrell.

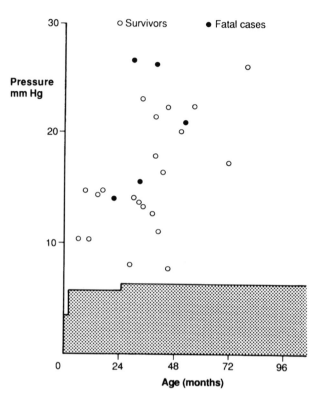

Figure 14.11 Cerebrospinal fluid opening pressures in 26 Kenyan children with cerebral malaria (Newton *et al.*, 1991).

(Seibert, 1985), was equally common in hypoglycaemic and normoglycaemic children and is also a feature of midbrain dysfunction associated with brain herniation (Plum and Posner, 1982). Children with cerebral malaria are often flaccid (Figure 14.13), whereas adults usually exhibit increased muscle tone.

Retinal haemorrhages have been found in 16% of children with cerebral malaria in Zambia (Haslett, 1991) and in 6–8% of African children in other series (Newton *et al.*, 1991b), in 35% of children with cerebral malaria in Malawi (Lewallen *et al.*, 1993). In Malawi, the abnormalities included retinal haemorrhages, cottonwool spots, intraretinal oedema, narrowed and obstructed arteries, venous distention and tortuosity and papilloedema. Papilloedema and retinal oedema outside the posterior vascular arcades carried a bad prognosis (Lewallen *et al.*, 1993).

SEQUELAE

Neurological sequelae are more common in children than in adults, affecting 10% or more patients (Molyneux *et al.*, 1989; Brewster *et al.*, 1990). Common

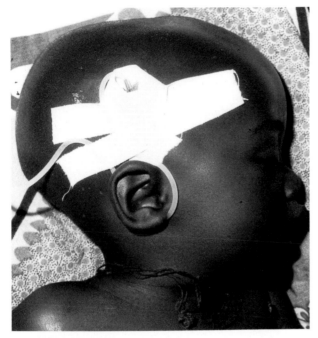

Figure 14.12 Bulging anterior fontanelle in a Kenyan child with cerebral malaria. Copyright D.A. Warrell.

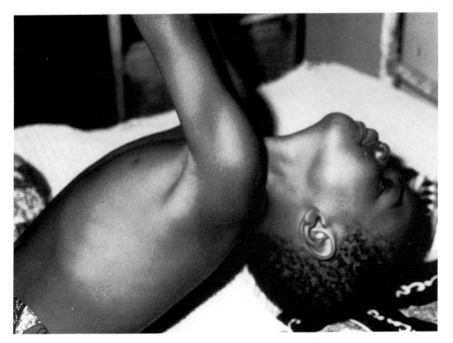

Figure 14.13 Flaccid tone in a Kenyan child with cerebral malaria. Copyright D.A. Warrell.

TABLE 14.5 Childhood cerebral malaria:
neurological sequelae (Brewster *et al.*, 1990)

Hemiplegia
Cortical blindness
Aphasia
Ataxia
Decerebration
Generalized spasticity
Psychosis, behavioural disturbance
Tremors
Mental retardation
Epilepsy

sequelae are listed in Table 14.5. In some cases of hemiplegia (Collomb *et al.*, 1967, 1968), carotid artery occlusion has been demonstrated by angiography (Collomb *et al.*, 1967; Omanga *et al.*, 1983). The frequency of intellectual impairment after cerebral malaria is being explored by prospective studies.

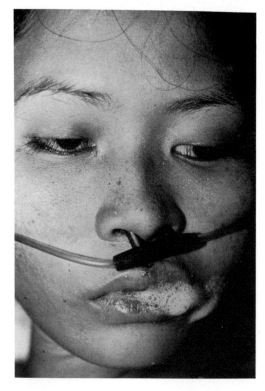

Figure 14.14 Postpartum acute pulmonary oedema in a Thai woman with cerebral malaria. Copyright Professor Sornchai Looareesuwan.

Neurological sequelae were seen in only 5% of Thai adults (Warrell *et al.*, 1982); they included transient paranoid psychosis or delirium, cranial nerve lesions (especially VIth), extrapyramidal tremor, signs of cerebellar dysfunction (see later) and prolonged coma and in other studies polyneuropathy, mononeuritis multiplex and Guillain–Barré syndrome were observed.

INVOLVEMENT OF OTHER SYSTEMS IN PATIENTS WITH CEREBRAL MALARIA

Cerebral malaria may be associated with any of the other manifestations and complications of severe falciparum malaria listed in Table 14.1, including jaundice, disseminated intravascular coagulation (Plate 2), pulmonary oedema (Figure 14.14) and 'blackwater fever' (Figure 14.15).

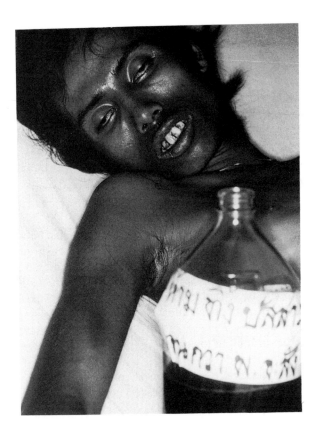

Figure 14.15 'Blackwater fever' in a Thai patient with cerebral malaria and acute renal failure. Copyright Dr R.E. Phillips.

MORTALITY OF CEREBRAL MALARIA

The mortality of strictly defined cerebral malaria is about 15–25% in adults and children even when good medical care can be provided (Warrell *et al.*, 1990) but, in well-equipped intensive care units this can be reduced to less than 5% (Salord *et al.*, 1991).

DIAGNOSIS OF CEREBRAL MALARIA

Malaria must be included in the differential diagnosis in any severely ill and febrile patient. In travellers, the infection can be acquired during 'stopovers' in malarious areas on rare occasions, even if they did not leave the aircraft. A diagnosis of malaria is more likely in those who did not take precautions against mosquito bites while in the endemic area and did not take antimalarial chemo-prophylaxis or took their drugs irregularly or stopped prematurely. Unusual routes of infection include blood and platelet transfusion, contaminated needles, marrow/tissue transplants and transplacental infection. Infection has also been reported in people living near international airports ('airport malaria').

LABORATORY DIAGNOSIS

Urgent attempts should be made to confirm the diagnosis of malaria by examining peripheral blood films every 8–12 hours. Thin and thick blood films (Plates 3 and 4) should, ideally, be made at the bedside using 'capillary blood' straight from the patient which has not been stored with anticoagulant. Slides should be examined by an experienced parasitologist as scanty parasitaemias are easily overlooked and a number of artefacts can confuse the uninitiated. Newer diagnostic methods include QBC (quantitative buffy coat) and 'Para Sight F' dipstick antigen capture assay. These can approach the sensitivity and specificity of conventional microscopy. If a patient with fever and impaired consciousness or other neurological signs could have been exposed to malaria, antimalarial chemotherapy should be started immediately even if blood smears are repeatedly negative. Severely ill patients should be treated for falciparum malaria even if only the 'benign' species, *P. vivax*, *P. ovale* or *P. malariae* are found in blood films, as it may be difficult to identify ring forms of *P. falciparum* with certainty in such infections.

The diagnosis of cerebral malaria can be confirmed at autopsy by finding the characteristic tight packing of erythrocytes containing the pigmented mature forms in cerebral venules and capillaries in sections or smears of brain tissue (Plate 5). If it is not possible to open the skull, needle necropsies may be made through the superior orbital fissure, foramen magnum, nostril and ethmoid bone or fontanelles (in infants and young children) (Warrell *et al.*, 1990).

OTHER INVESTIGATIONS

There is always evidence of a severe haemolytic anaemia. Neutrophil leukocytosis and thrombocytopenia are common. There may be evidence of coagulopathy. Total and direct plasma bilirubin concentrations are usually increased, serum albumin concentrations reduced and aminotransferases, $5'$ nucleotidase and especially lactic dehydrogenase concentrations elevated but not the levels seen in viral hepatitis. Serum creatine phosphokinase concentrations are elevated in some patients suggesting generalized rhabdomyolysis (De Silva and Goonetilleke, 1988; Miller KD *et al.*, 1989a; Miller JH *et al.* 1994). About one-third of patients with cerebral malaria have evidence of renal dysfunction (blood urea more than 13 mmol 1^{-1}; serum creatinine more than 176 µmol 1^{-1} (Phillips *et al.*, 1984; Sitprija, 1988; Trang *et al.*, 1992). Lactic acidosis is associated with hypoglycaemia and renal failure. Hypoglycaemia is a common and important abnormality in patients with cerebral malaria and may not be suspected clinically because the symptoms (anxiety, tachycardia, breathlessness, faintness, convulsions) are attributed to malaria (White *et al.*, 1983a, 1987). Common electrolyte abnormalities include hyponatraemia (Miller *et al.*, 1967; Holst *et al.*, 1994), hypocalcaemia (Warrell *et al.*, 1990) and hypophosphataemia (Warrell *et al.*, 1990). Blood cultures may yield Gram-negative rod bacteria (*E. coli*, *Pseudomonas*, *Salmonella*, etc.) (Warrell *et al.*, 1982, 1990; Mabey *et al.*, 1987).

Microscopy and culture of cerebrospinal fluid (CSF) is essential in patients with cerebral malaria to exclude other treatable CNS infections (Warrell *et al.*, 1982, 1990). If lumbar puncture must be delayed for any reason, the patient should be given empirical treatment for bacterial meningitis (Newton *et al.*, 1991). In cerebral malaria, the CSF may contain up to 15 lymphocytes per µl and increased protein concentrations, but in patients who have had repeated generalized convulsions, a pleocytosis of up to 80 cells μl^{-1} (mainly leukocytes) may occur (Wright *et al.*, 1993).

Protein, red cells, red cell casts and haemoglobin are often found in the urine which is literally black in patients with severe intravascular haemolysis – 'Blackwater fever'.

CT and MRI imaging of the brain in adults shows evidence of cerebral swelling and oedema in a minority of cases. In Thailand, cerebral oedema was an agonal phenomenon (Looareesuwan *et al.*, 1983b). Focal lesions, suggesting infarction or haemorrhage, have been demonstrated (Pham-Hung *et al.*, 1990; Millan *et al.*, 1993) and, in a patient with persistent vertical nystagmus, MRI evidence of central pontine myelinolysis was obtained 14 days after admission (Kampel *et al.*, 1993). In a patient with local epilepsy after recovering from cerebral malaria, a small lesion was demonstrated by CT which eventually resolved as did his symptoms.

In Kenyan children with cerebral malaria, brain swelling was found without evidence of acute hydrocephalus or vasogenic oedema. Evidence of extensive ischaemic damage was found in children with severe neurological sequelae (Newton *et al.*, 1994).

TABLE 14.6 Differential diagnosis of cerebral malaria

Encephalitides: viral, bacterial, fungal (e.g. cryptococcal), protozoal (e.g. trypanosomal)

Systemic infections with encephalopathy: enteric fevers ('cerebral typhoid'), septicaemia, viral haemorrhagic fevers (e.g. Korean, Argentine, Bolivian and Venezuelan haemorrhagic fevers, Rift Valley fever and Kyasanur Forest disease)

Metabolic encephalopathies: hepatic, renal, respiratory and circulatory failure, hypoglycaemia of other causes

Eclamptic toxaemia

Malignant hypertension, cerebrovascular accidents

Heat stroke (especially in unacclimatized visitors to the tropics who have taken excessive exercise)

Toxic encephalopathies (e.g. organophosphorus poisoning)

A variety of non-specific EEG abnormalities have been reported (Collomb *et al.*, 1977). In Kenyan children with cerebral malaria, subclinical seizure activity was found (C.R.J.C. Newton, personal communication).

DIFFERENTIAL DIAGNOSIS OF CEREBRAL MALARIA (Table 14.6)

The differential diagnosis of cerebral malaria includes a variety of encephalitides, systemic infections and toxic and metabolic encephalopathies including hypoglycaemia, cerebrovascular accidents and heatstroke. It is important to realize that, particularly in tropical endemic areas, the finding of falciparum parasitaemia in a patient with impaired consciousness does not prove that malaria is the cause of coma or the sole diagnosis. In holoendemic areas there may be a high prevalence of asymptomatic parasitaemia in the community.

PATHOLOGY OF CEREBRAL MALARIA

At autopsy the brain often appears oedematous and is heavy. There are no published reports of grooving of the cerebral peduncles ('Kernohan's notch'), (Kernohan and Woltman, 1929), displacement of Greenhall's line to suggest diencephalic downthrust (Esiri and Oppenheimer, 1989) or evidence of herniation of the cerebellar tonsils through the foramen magnum. The small vessels, particularly of the grey matter (Plate 6) and meninges, are congested with parasitized erythrocytes containing malaria pigment. This explains the characteristic slatey grey colour of the surface of the brain in cerebral malaria (Plate 7). In larger vessels there is margination of parasitized erythrocytes along the endothelium (Plate 8). Up to 70% of erythrocytes in the cerebral vessels are parasitized and these are more tightly packed than in other organs (MacPherson *et al.*, 1985). The degree of sequestration of parasitized erythrocytes in the cerebral microvasculature correlates with depth of coma (Riganti *et al.*, 1990). Electron-dense knob-like protuberances of the parasitized erythrocyte membrane are points of contact with the vascular endothelium whose surface is distorted by pseudopodial projections. Numerous petechial ring haemorrhages are seen in the white matter. These result from haemorrhage from end arterioles proximal to occlusive plugs of parasitized erythrocytes. Typically, the erythrocytes forming the ring haemorrhage are unparasitized. The cause of perivascular destruction of neurones, demyelination and formation of Dürck's granulomata (small collections of microglial cells) is uncertain but they may develop at sites of ring haemorrhages. MacPherson *et al.* (1985) and Turner *et al.* (1994) found no inflammatory cells, platelets or fibrin plugs in the cerebral blood vessels and no evidence of immune complex deposition. However, Maung-Maung-Oo *et al.* (1987) discovered *P. falciparum* antigens and IgG deposits in the capillary basement membrane and other authors have found margination of mononuclear cells in cerebral capillaries in the brains of patients who died with falciparum malaria (Porta *et al.*, 1993; Parnaik *et al.*, 1994).

The histopathological basis of retinal haemorrhages in cerebral malaria appears to be sequestration of parasitized erythrocytes with evidence of cytoadherence and rosetting inside ocular capillaries and venules (Dudgeon, 1921; Mahdi *et al.*, 1989; Hidayat *et al.*, 1993).

PATHOPHYSIOLOGY OF CEREBRAL MALARIA

During the past 70 years several hypotheses have been suggested to explain the pathophysiology of cerebral malaria (Table 14.7). The three most likely mechanisms will be discussed here. (Warrell, 1987; Warrell *et al.*, 1990; White and Ho, 1992).

TABLE 14.7 Pathophysiology of cerebral malaria: hypotheses

'Mechanical hypothesis': cytoadherence (Miller, 1969), rosetting (Carlson, 1993), sequestration
'Toxin/mediator hypothesis' endotoxin (Clark, 1978), cytokines (Clark *et al.*, 1981), free oxygen radicals (Clark and Hunt, 1983), nitric oxide (Clark *et al.*, 1992)
'Permeability hypothesis' (Maegraith and Fletcher, 1972)
Immune complex damage (Adam *et al.*, 1981)
Disseminated intravascular coagulation (Punyagupta *et al.*, 1974)
Post-infective demyelination – 'vasculomyelinopathy' (Toro and Roman, 1978)

The Mechanical Hypothesis

This seems the most plausible. It postulates that the flow of parasitized erythrocytes through the cerebral microcirculation is reduced, resulting in 'stagnant hypoxaemia': a reduction of the supply of oxygen and other nutrients to the brain leading to coma. Sluggish blood flow has been attributed to the sticking of parasitized erythrocytes to vascular endothelium (cytoadherence) (Miller, 1969), decreased deformability of parasitized erythrocytes (Nash *et al.*, 1989) and to rosetting – the sticking of unparasitized erythrocytes around a parasitized erythrocyte (Carlson, 1993). There is no adequate animal model for human cerebral malaria. However, some predictions of the mechanical hypothesis are testable in human patients. Tight packing or parasitized erythrocytes in small cerebral blood vessels (sequestration) has been observed since the end of the nineteenth century (Marchiafava and Bignami, 1894).

The molecular basis for cytoadherence has been studied intensively during the past few years. The adhesin expressed on the surface membrane of the parasitized erythrocyte seems likely to be the high-molecular-weight protein *P. falciparum* erythrocyte membrane protein 1 (PfEMP1) (Berendt *et al.*, 1994). Several candidate endothelial receptors have been identified, including CD36 (formerly platelet glycoprotein IV), thrombospondin (TSP), intercellular adhesion molecule-1 (ICAM-1) (Berendt *et al.*, 1989) and vascular cell adhesion molecule (VCAM) and E-selectin (Berendt *et al.*, 1994). Recent immunohistochemical studies have shown evidence of increased expression of ICAM-1 and E-selectin in the cerebral microvascular endothelium of patients who died with cerebral malaria (Turner *et al.*, 1994). Obstruction of the cerebral microvasculature envisaged by the mechanical hypothesis should result in a reduction in total cerebral blood flow and cerebral hypoxia. In Thai adults with cerebral malaria, cerebral flood flow was found to be low in relation to arterial oxygen content, one of its major determinants (Warrell *et al.*, 1988). Cerebral oxygen consumption and cerebral arteriovenous oxygen content difference were decreased and cerebral venous pO_2 was increased. Arterial lactic acid concentration and cerebral lactic acid production were significantly higher while the patients were comatose than when they had just recovered consciousness (Warrell *et al.*, 1988) (Figure 14.16). Cerebrospinal fluid lactic acid concentration was elevated in all but one of 45 patients and was significantly higher in fatal cases than in survivors (White *et al.*, 1985). These observations confirm a switch in the brain to anaerobic glycolysis.

Cytokine Hypothesis

In African children with cerebral malaria plasma tumour necrosis factor α (TNFα) and interleukin-1α concentrations have been found to correlate with severity judged by the level of parasitaemia, hypoglycaemia, case fatality and incidence of neurological sequelae. (Grau *et al.*, 1989; Kwiatkowski *et al.*,

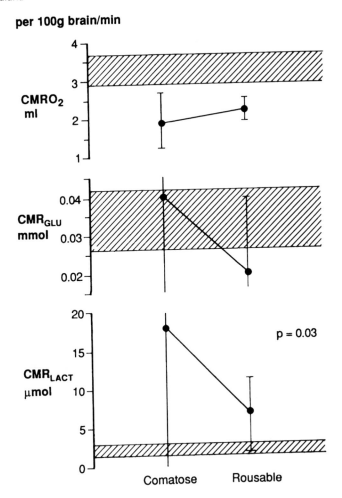

Figure 14.16 Cerebral oxygen consumption (CMR$_{O2}$), cerebral glucose consumption (CMR$_{GLU}$) and cerebral lactate production (CMR$_{LACT}$) in a group of 12 Thai adult patients with cerebral malaria. The normal ranges are shown by the hatched areas (Warrell *et al.*, 1988).

1990). The idea that cytokines, released by macrophages in response to a malarial antigen or 'toxin', might play a major role in the pathophysiology of severe falciparum malaria is an attractive one as these cytokines, and especially TNFα, exhibit a number of highly relevant properties. These include the upregulation of several candidate cerebrovascular endothelial receptors for cytoadherence, such as ICAM-1 (Berendt *et al.*, 1989), VCAM-1, E-selectin and CD36 (by interferon-γ) and induction of hypoglycaemia, coagulopathy and dyserythropoiesis. However, there are a number of inconsistencies in this hypothesis. One of the major effects of TNFα, shock, is rarely seen in cerebral malaria, plasma TNFα concentrations seem grossly inappropriate in some individuals, the biological activity of TNFα measured by immunoassay is uncertain and there is some evidence that TNFα may have a beneficial effect in killing malaria parasites. The hypothesis is being tested in African children with cerebral malaria using an anti-TNFα monoclonal antibody (D. Kwiatkowski, personal communication). In the Gambia, children homozygous for the TNF_2 allele, a variant of the TNFα gene promoter region, showed increased risk of death or severe neurological sequelae from cerebral malaria (McGuire et al., 1994).

Permeability Hypothesis

This hypothesis which was fashionable for many years (Maegraith and Fletcher, 1972) has been critically reviewed elsewhere (Warrell et al., 1986, 1990). Evidence against the permeability hypothesis, in Thai adults at least, was the finding that: (1) blood–CSF barrier permeability was not increased in comatose patients (Warrell et al., 1986); (2) cerebral oedema was seen in only a minority of comatose patients during life (Looareesuwan et al., 1983); (3) CSF opening pressures at lumbar puncture were usually normal (denying the intracranial hypertension expected if there were cerebral oedema) (Warrell et al., 1986); and (4) anti-inflammatory drugs such as dexamethasone did not prove beneficial in this condition (Warrell et al., 1982). However, this hypothesis still has its proponents (Polder, 1989; Patnoik et al., 1994).

TREATMENT

Chemotherapy (Warrell et al., 1990; WHO, 1990)

Early initiation of antimalarial chemotherapy using an appropriate drug and optimal regimen is most important. Chloroquine was the drug of choice for the treatment of severe falciparum malaria, but resistant strains now predominate throughout most parts of the endemic area and most physicians now prefer to use quinine (White et al., 1982) irrespective of the supposed geographical origin of the infection (Table 14.8). If an intravenous formulation of quinine is not immediately available, quinidine gluconate injection which is stocked by some hospitals in the United States and elsewhere for the treatment of cardiac arrhythmias, could be used to initiate treatment (Phillys et al., 1985; Miller et al., 1989). In the treatment of a disease which kills as quickly as cerebral malaria, it is essential to achieve therapeutic plasma concentrations of the drug as quickly as possible. This can be done by giving an initial loading dose (20 mg quinine dihydrochloride per kg body weight infused intravenously over 4 h) (White et al., 1983b), which need *not* be reduced in pregnant women nor in severely ill patients with renal and hepatic dysfunction (White et al., 1982). To prevent

TABLE 14.8 Cerebral malaria: chemotherapy

Quinine dihydrochloride		
Intravenous	Loading[a]	7 mg salt kg^{-1} over 30 min (infusion pump) followed immediately by 10 mg kg^{-1} over 4 h (Davis *et al.*, 1990)
	or	20 mg salt kg^{-1} over 4 h (White *et al.*, 1983b)
	Maintenance	10 mg kg^{-1} over 4 h repeated 8–12 hourly[c,d] (White *et al.*, 1983b; Davis *et al.*, 1990; Pasvol *et al.*, 1992; Winstanley *et al.*, 1993)
Intramuscular	Loading[a]	20 mg salt kg^{-1} (dilute i.v. formulation to 60 mg ml^{-1} given by deep i.m. injection divided between both anterior thighs) (Wattanagoon *et al.*, 1986; White *et al.*, 1989; Mansor *et al.*, 1990; Waller *et al.*, 1990)
	Maintenance	10 mg salt kg^{-1} 8–12 hourly[c,d] (White *et al.*, 1983b; Davis *et al.*, 1990; Pasvol *et al.*, 1992; Winstanley *et al.*, 1993)
Quinidine gluconate		
Intravenous	Loading[a]	10 mg salt kg^{-1} infused over 1–2 h (Miller *et al.*, 1989b)
	or	20 mg salt kg^{-1} infused over 4 h (Phillips *et al.*, 1985)
	Maintenance	0.02 mg salt kg^{-1} min^{-1} continuously for up to 72 h[b,c,d] (Miller *et al.*, 1989b)
	or	10 mg salt kg^{-1} infused over 4 h every 8–12 h[c,d] (Phillips *et al.*, 1985)
Artemisinin derivatives[e]		
Artesunate[f] Intravenous		
Intramuscular	Loading	3.2 mg kg^{-1}
	Maintenance	1.6 mg kg^{-1} repeated 12–24 hourly[g]
Artemether Intramuscular		

[a]Avoid loading dose if quinine, quinidine or mefloquine taken in previous 24 h
[b]Adjust rate of quinidine infusion to maintain blood level at 3–7 mg l^{-1}, and prevent prolongation of ECG QRS > 50%, QTc > 25% of pretreatment values
[c]Change to oral quinine as soon as possible and complete 7 days' treatment
[d]Add tetracycline 1 g day^{-1} in four divided doses for 7 days in non-pregnant adults in some areas
[e]Not marketed/licensed in many countries
[f]Artesunate is reconstituted with bicarbonate solution immediately before use
[g]Change to oral mefloquine (single dose 15–25 mg kg^{-1} max. 1500 mg) as soon as possible

accumulation, the maintenance dose of quinine should be reduced to half or one-third after 48 h of treatment unless the patient can swallow tablets by then. If plasma quinine/quinidine concentrations can be monitored, the maintenance dose should be reduced at any stage if these concentrations exceed 15 mg 1^{-1} (45 μmol 1^{-1}). Optimal regimens are slightly different in children because of different pharmacokinetics (Pasvol *et al.*, 1992; Winstanley *et al.*, 1993). The most important complication of quinine treatment is hypoglycaemia (White *et al.*, 1983a, 1987).

Several artemisinin derivatives have been extracted from the sweet wormwood plant (*Artemisia annua*) which has been used as treatment for febrile illnesses in China for more than a thousand years (Royal Society of Tropical Medicine and Hygiene, 1994). These have proved safe and effective in severe falciparum malaria (Hien and White, 1993). Artemether and artesunate clear parasitaemia more rapidly than quinine (Hien and White, 1993). The efficacy of artemether in comparison with quinine is being tested in large clinical trials in Vietnamese adults and African children.

Supportive Care (Warrell *et al.*, 1990, 1991)

Wherever possible, patients with cerebral malaria should be treated in an intensive care unit. Generalized seizures are common and are frequently followed by a sustained deterioration in neurological condition and complicated by aspiration pneumonia. Observed seizures should be treated immediately with a benzodiazepine such as diazepam, chlormethiazole or lorazepam. Every attempt should be made to prevent convulsions by the use of prophylactic anticonvulsants and by controlling fever (especially in children). In Thai adults a single small intramuscular dose of phenobarbital sodium (3.5 mg kg^{-1}) reduced the frequency of convulsions (White *et al.*, 1988) but higher doses (10–15 mg kg^{-1}) may be needed for prevention of fits especially in children (Winstanley *et al.*, 1992). The risk of aspiration pneumonia is reduced by aspirating stomach contents through a nasogastric tube. Deepening coma and airway obstruction are indications for elective endotracheal intubation. In adults cerebral oedema is not thought to be part of the primary pathology of cerebral malaria, but may develop terminally or during the course of prolonged intensive care if there is fluid overload or gross hypoalbuminaemia. Deterioration in the level of consciousness and appearance of neurological abnormalities (in the absence of hypoglycaemia) are indications for cranial computerized tomography to differentiate intracerebral bleeding from cerebral oedema and cerebral/medullary herniation. If intracranial hypertension is detected (e.g. by epidural transducer) or suspected, 10–20% mannitol solution can be infused over 30 minutes in a dose of 1.0–1.5 g kg^{-1}. This dose can be repeated unless the serum osmolality rises above 330 μosmol 1^{-1}. Dexamethasone in doses of 2 and 11 mg kg^{-1} were studied in two double-blind placebo controlled trials (Warrell *et al.*, 1982; Hoffman *et al.*, 1988). There was no evidence of benefit, but the duration of

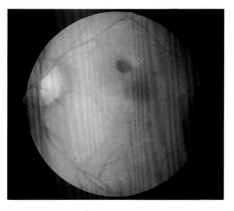

Plate 1 Retinal haemorrhages clustered round the macula in a Thai patient with cerebral malaria (Looareesuwan *et al.*, 1983). (Copyright D.A. Warrell.)

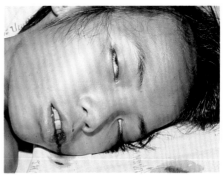

Plate 2 Profound anaemia and spontaneous bleeding from the gums in a Thai girl with disseminated intravascular coagulation complicating cerebral malaria. (Copyright D.A. Warrell.)

Plate 3 Heavy *P. falciparum* parasitaemia shown in a thin blood film from a patient suffering from cerebral malaria. (Copyright Dr M.J. Warrell.)

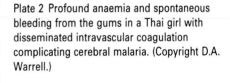

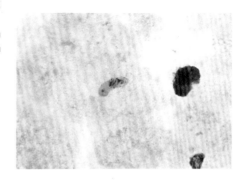

Plate 4 Thick blood film showing a female gametocyte of *P. falciparum* against a background of amorphous debris from lysed erythrocytes. (Copyright Dr M.J. Warrell.)

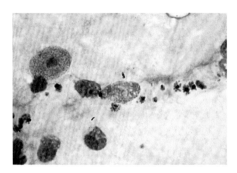

Plate 5 Postmortem needle necropsy of the brain obtained with a Vim Silverman needle through the superior orbital fissure, showing pigmented mature schizonts and trophozoites in a cerebral venule. (Copyright Dr M.J. Warrell.)

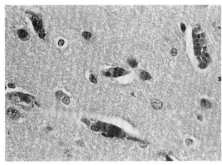

Plate 6 Human cerebral malaria: cytoadherence and sequestration of parasitized erythrocytes in small cerebral blood vessels in a brain section. (Copyright D.A. Warrell.)

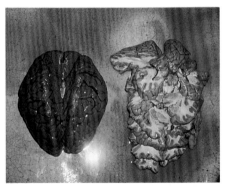

Plate 7 Brain of a patient with cerebral malaria showing typical dark plum coloration resulting from congestion of meningeal vessels with pigmented parasitized erythrocytes (left) compared with non-malarious brain (right). (Copyright Dr U. Hla Mon.)

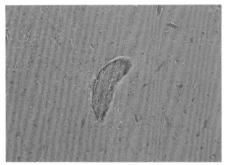

Plate 8 Human cerebral malaria: occipital cortex showing sequestration of parasitized cells in capillaries and venules. (Copyright Dr G.D.H. Turner.)

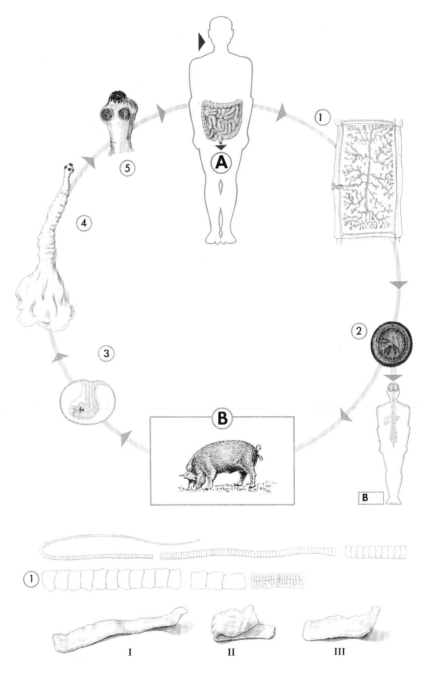

Plate 9 Life cycle of *Taenia solium*. A, Final host man only – tapeworm in small intestine: 1, mature segment of *T. solium*; 2, tapeworm egg (embryophore with six-hooked larvae). B, Intermediate host pig (exceptionally man – cysticercosis): 3, cysticercus cellulosae of *T. solium* (with crown of hooklets and four suckers) starting to evaginate; 4, evaginated cysticercus stage of *T. solium*; 5, head of pork tapeworm (with crown of hooklets. I–III, Phases of movements of freshly detached tapeworm segments.) (Courtesy of Bayer AG)

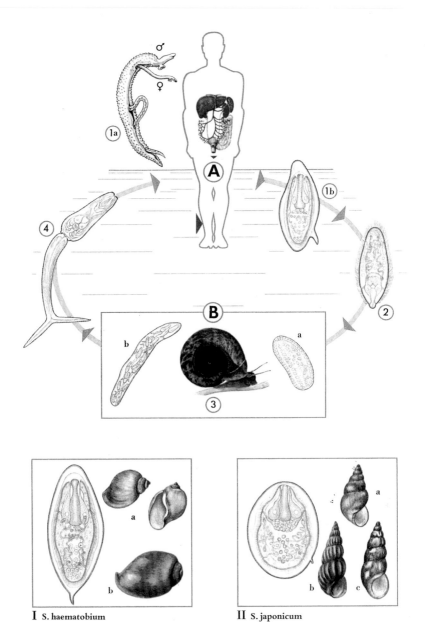

Plate 10 Life cycle of *Schistosoma* species. A, Final host – man (site of the worms, the mesenteric vessels): 1a, sexually mature pair of flukes of *S. mansoni*; b, mature egg of *S. mansoni* (lateral spine); 2, miracidium. B, Intermediate host – aquatic snails (Planorbidae, for example, *Planorbis boissyi*, *Australorbis glabratus*): 3a, sporocyst of the first order (mother sporocyst); b, sporocyst of the second order (daughter sporocyst); 4, free cercaria ('forked-tail cercaria'). I, *S. haematobium* egg with miracidium (terminal spine) – shells of the intermediate hosts of the species: a, *Bulinus truncatus* (North Africa); b, *Bulinus globosa* (West Africa). II, *S. japonicum* egg with miracidium (very small lateral spine) – shells of intermediate hosts of the genera: a, *Schistosomophora*; b, *Oncomelania*; c, *Katayama*. (Courtesy of Bayer AG.)

unconsciousness was prolonged and there was an increased incidence of infection and gastrointestinal bleeding in the dexamethasone treated group (Warrell *et al.*, 1982). A number of other agents including low-molecular-weight dextrans, heparin, prostacyclin, adrenaline, cyclosporin A and hyperbaric oxygen have been recommended at some time for the treatment of cerebral malaria, but none is of proven benefit.

The successful use of *exchange transfusion* has been reported in more than 80 cases of severe falciparum malaria, but no controlled trial has been performed (Phillips *et al.* 1985, 1990; Looareesuwan *et al.*, 1990; Warrell *et al.*, 1990; Vachon *et al.*, 1992). This technique is probably indicated in patients who have *P. falciparum* parasitaemia in excess of 10% of circulating erythrocytes, who are non-immune and who have deteriorated on conventional treatment. Exchange transfusion may reduce parasitaemia more rapidly than optimal chemotherapy alone with the added advantage of removing harmful metabolites, toxins, cytokines (but not, apparently, TNF) (Loutan *et al.*, 1992) and other mediators and restoring normal red cell mass, platelets, clotting factors, albumin and other depleted blood constituents. Potential dangers include fluid and electrolyte disturbances, cardiovascular complications, the development of ARDS (Vachon *et al.*, 1992) and infections in the transfused blood and from intravascular lines. Some of the severely ill patients treated with exchange transfusion have shown clinical improvements such as recovery of consciousness during or soon after the procedure.

Cerebral malaria is commonly associated with other manifestations and complications of falciparum malaria (Table 14.1). In particular, hypoglycaemia, severe anaemia, shock and renal failure may contribute to coma. Patients must be carefully monitored so that these abnormalities can be prevented or rapidly corrected.

OTHER NEUROLOGICAL AND NEUROPSYCHIATRIC MANIFESTATIONS OF FALCIPARUM MALARIA

Malarial Psychosis

There are many references, especially in the older literature, to a variety of psychiatric manifestations of malaria, both as the presenting feature of an acute attack of malaria and as a sequal to an episode of severe or otherwise uncomplicated malaria (Forrester, 1920; Masson, 1924; Anderson, 1927; Arbuse, 1945; Areti, 1946; Blocker *et al.*, 1968; Wintrobe, 1973). Limitations of many of these reports are failures to confirm the diagnosis of malaria and to exclude antimalarial and other drugs and other causes of the psychiatric symptoms. Thus mepacrine (quinacrine, atabrine) which was widely used for the treatment of malaria in the 1930s and 1940s, chloroquine (which was introduced in the 1950s) and more recently mefloquine, have been reported to cause mental disturbances

(Weinke *et al.*, 1991; Akhtar and Mukherjee, 1993). Chloroquine can cause insomnia, toxic confusional psychosis, personality changes, mania and suicidal impulses (Alchtar and Mukherjee, 1993). In about 4/1000 users, mefloquine has caused anxiety, restlessness, depression, amnesia, confusion, hallucinations and psychotic or paranoid reactions (F. Hoffman La Roche Ltd, Basel, Switzerland – product information). Other factors implicated in 'malarial psychosis' include alcohol, stresses associated with life or military service in tropical countries and exacerbation of pre-existing functional psychoses (Forrester, 1920; Blocker, 1968). Organic mental disturbances associated with acute malaria attacks have been identified in some cases, usually during convalescence after the fever has subsided. Features included apathy, amnesia, depression, atypical depression, acute psychosis, personality change, paranoid psychosis and delusions, such as belief that family members had been killed (Blocker, 1968; Arun Prakash and Stein, 1990). Orde Wingate, of the Allied Chindits, attempted suicide by cutting his throat while suffering from malarial psychosis (Lock, 1984), but some believed that he was suffering from atabrine poisoning. Brief reactive psychoses (Lipowski, 1980) have been observed in patients recovering from cerebral malaria (Warrell *et al.*, 1982). These symptoms rarely last for more than a few days, in contrast to those caused by functional psychoses.

Cerebellar Dysfunction

Acute cerebellar ataxia has been described as a sequel to a wide range of viral, bacterial, fungal and protozoal infections including cerebral malaria (Weiss and Guberman, 1978). There are reports in the literature of patients with falciparum malaria presenting without impairment of consciousness but with signs of cerebellar dysfunction (Anderson, 1927; Illangasekara and De Silva, 1976; Chaddha *et al.*, 1978; Chitkara *et al.*, 1984; Gupta and Dang, 1986; Arya *et al.*, 1989). Most of these cases have been reported from the Indian subcontinent. More recently, a syndrome of delayed cerebellar ataxia has been described from northern Sri Lanka (de Silva *et al.*, 1986; Senanayake, 1987). Three or four weeks after developing transient fever attributable to falciparum malaria, these patients presented with unsteadiness of gait and of the upper limbs, vertigo, dysarthria and headache. On examination there was ataxia of gait, intention tremor, dysmetria, dysdiadochokinesis, nystagmus and cerebellar dysarthria. Symptoms progressed for up to 2 weeks but completely resolved 3–16 (median 10) weeks after their onset (Senanayake, 1987). Corticosteroid treatment may have hastened recovery in one or two cases. An immunopathological mechanism for the epidemic of this syndrome in northern Sri Lanka has been suggested. It is possible that a particular strain of *Plasmodium falciparum* was responsible (de Silva, 1993). Extrapyramidal tremor has been observed as a sequel to cerebral malaria (Warrell *et al.*, 1982).

Other Neurological Manifestations of Malaria

In the past, a very wide range of neurological abnormalities were attributed to malaria. Introduction of more stringent diagnostic criteria and the discovery of other causes has dismissed malaria as the cause in some cases. For example, the polyneuropathy described in the West Indies towards the end of the nineteenth century and initially attributed to malaria (Strachan, 1897), has proved to be the result of infection by HTLV1 (tropical spastic paraparesis). Other neurological abnormalities attributed to malaria (apart from those already described as sequelae of cerebral malaria) include polyneuropathy, mononeuritis multiplex, Guillain–Barré syndrome and periodic paralysis (Vietze, 1978; Warrell *et al.*, 1990; de Silva, 1993).

REFERENCES

Adam C, Géniteau M, Gougerot-Pocidalo M *et al.* (1981) Cryoglobulins, circulating immune complexes and complement activation in cerebral malaria. *Infection and Immunity* **31**(2): 630–535.

Akhtar S and Mukherjee S (1993) Chloroquine induced mania. *International Journal of Psychiatry in Medicine* **23**(4): 349–356.

Anderson WK (1927) *Malarial Psychoses and Neuroses. Their medical, sociological and legal aspects*. London: Oxford Medical Publications.

Arbuse DI (1945) Neuropsychiatric manifestations in malaria. *US Naval Medical Bulletin* **45**: 304–309.

Arieti S (1946) Histopathologic changes in cerebral malaria and their relation to psychotic sequels. *Archives of Neurology and Psychiatry* **56**: 79–104.

Arun Prakash MV and Stein G (1990) Malaria presenting as atypical depression. *British Journal of Psychiatry* **156**: 594–595.

Arya TW, Awasthi R and Bhutani J (1989) Extrapyramidal syndrome in falciparum malaria. *Journal of the Association of Physicians, India* **37**(6): 393–394.

Bennish ML, Azad AK, Rahman O and Phillips RE (1990) Hypoglycemia during diarrhea in childhood. Prevalence, pathophysiology and outcome. *New England Journal of Medicine* **322**(19): 1357–1363.

Berendt AR, Simmons DL, Tansey J *et al.* (1989) Intercellular adhesion molecule-1 is an endothelial cell adhesion receptor for *Plasmodium falciparum. Nature* **341**: 57–59.

Berendt AR, Ferguson DJP, Gardner J *et al.* (1994) Molecular mechanisms of sequestration in malaria. *Parasitology* **108**: S19–28.

Blocker WW, Kastl AJ and Daroff RB (1968) The psychiatric manifestations of cerebral malaria. *American Journal of Psychiatry* **125**: 192–196.

Carlson J (1993) Erythrocyte rosetting in *Plasmodium falciparum* malaria–with special reference to the pathogenesis of cerebral malaria. *Scandinavian Journal of Infectious Diseases* (Supplement) **86**: 1–79.

Center for Disease Control (1994) Malaria Surveillance Summary 1991. Atlanta, GA: CDC.

Chaddha VS, Mathuri MS and Kothari RP (1978) Cerebellar syndrome in malaria. *Journal of the Association of Physicians, India* **26**: 445–446.

Chitkara AJ, Anand NK and Saini L (1984) Cerebellar syndrome in malaria. *Indian Paediatrics* **21**: 908–910.

Clark IA (1978) Does endotoxin cause both the disease and parasite death in acute malaria and babesiosis. *Lancet* **ii**: 75–77.

Clark IA and Hunt NH (1983) Evidence for reactive oxygen intermediates causing hemolysis and parasite death in malaria. *Infection and Immunity* **39**(1): 1–6.

Clark IA, Virelizier J-L, Carswell EA and Wood PR (1981) Possible importance of macrophage-derived mediators in acute malaria. *Infection and Immunity* **32**(3): 1058–1066.

Clark IA, Rockett KA and Cowden WB (1992) Possible central role of nitric oxide in conditions clinically similar to cerebral malaria. *Lancet* **340**: 894–896.

Collomb H, Rey M, Dumas S *et al.* (1967) Les hémiplégies au cours du paludisme aigu. *Bulletin de la Société Médicale Afrique Noire Langue Français* **12**(4): 791–795.

Collomb H, Dumas M, Virieu R and Konate S (1968) Accidents vasculaires cérébraux au Sénégal chez les sujets de moins de 20 ans (a propos de 47 cas). *Bulletin de la Société Médicale Afrique Noire Langue Français* **13**: 637–645.

Collomb H, Dumas M and Girard PL (1977) Parasitosis of CNS. In: *Handbook of Electroencephalography and Clinical Neurophysiology*. Vol. 15, Section V, Part A (ed. FJ Radermecker) Amsterdam: Elsevier.

Davis TME, Supanaranond W, Pukrittayakamee S *et al.* (1990) A safe and effective consecutive-infusion regimen for rapid quinine loading in severe falciparum malaria. *Journal of Infectious Diseases* **161**: 1305–1308.

De Silva HJ (1993) Cerebellar involvement in falciparum malaria: investigation of an epidemic. *Journal of the Ceylon College of Physicians.* **26**: 12–23.

De Silva HJ and Goonetilleke AKE (1988) Skeletal muscle necrosis in severe falciparum malaria *British Medical Journal* **296**: 1039.

De Silva HJ, Gamage R, Herath HKN *et al.* (1986) A delayed onset cerebellar syndrome complicating falciparum malaria. *Ceylon Medical Journal* **31**: 147–151.

Dudgeon LS (1921) *Transactions of the Ophthalmology Society, UK* **41**: 236–238.

Dupon M, Paty MC, Khune F *et al.* (1990) Paludisme et hémorragies rétiniennes. *Medecine Tropicale (Marseilles)* **50**(2): 197–199.

Esiri MM and Oppenheimer DR (1989) *Diagnostic Neuropathology. A Practical Manual.* Oxford: Blackwell.

Forrester ATW (1920) Malaria and insanity. *Lancet* **i**: 16–17.

Gilles HM and Warrell DA (eds) (1993) *Bruce-Chwatt's Essential Malariology*, 3rd edn. London: Edward Arnold.

Grau GE, Taylor TE, Molyneux ME *et al.* (1989) Tumor necrosis factor and disease severity in children with falciparum malaria. *New England Journal of Medicine* **320**: 1586–1591.

Greenwood BM, Greenwood AM, Bradley AK *et al.* (1987) Deaths in infancy and early childhood in a well-vaccinated rural, West African population. *Annals of Tropical Paediatrics* **7**(2): 91–99.

Gupta MM and Dang HS (1986) Acute cerebellar ataxia in adults (report of two cases). *Journal of Postgraduate Medicine* **32**(2): 107–109.

Haslett P (1991) Retinal haemorrhages in Zambian children with cerebral malaria (correspondence). *Journal of Tropical Pediatrics* **37**: 86–87.

Hidayat AA, Nalbandian RM, Sammons DW *et al.* (1993) The diagnostic histopathologic features of ocular malaria. *Ophthalmology* **100**: 1183–1186.

Hien TT and White NJ (1993) Qinghaosu. *Lancet* **341**: 603–608.

Hoffman SL, Rustama D, Punjabi NH *et al.* (1988) High-dose dexamethasone in quinine-treated patients with cerebral malaria: a double blind, placebo-controlled trial. *Journal of Infectious Diseases* **158**(2): 325–331.

Holst FG, Hemmer CJ, Kern P and Dietrich M (1994) Inappropriate secretion of antidiuretic hormone and hyponatremia in severe falciparum malaria. *American Journal of Tropical Medicine and Hygiene* **50**(5): 602–607.

Illangasekara VLU and De Silva S (1976) Acute cerebellar syndrome in falciparum malaria. *Ceylon Medical Journal* **22**: 130–132.

Kampel AW, Birbamer GG, Pfausler BE *et al.* (1993) Isolated pontine lesion in algid cerebral malaria: clinical features, management and magnetic resonance imaging findings. *American Journal of Tropical Medicine and Hygiene* **48**(6): 818–822.

Kayembe D, Maertens K and De Laey JJ (1980) Ocular complications of cerebral malaria. *Bulletin de la Societe Belge d'Ophtalmologie (Gent)* **190**: 53–60.

Kernohan JW and Woltman HW (1929) Incisura of the crus due to contralateral brain tumor. *Archives of Neurology and Psychiatry* **21**: 274–287.

Kwiatkowski D, Hill AVS, Sambou I *et al.* (1990) TNF concentration in fatal cerebral, non-fatal cerebral and uncomplicated *Plasmodium falciparum* malaria. *Lancet* **336**: 1201–1204.

Lalloo DG, Trevett AJ, Paul M *et al.* (in press) Severe and complicated malaria in Melanesian adults.

Lewallen S, Taylor TE, Molyneux ME *et al.* (1993) Ocular fundus findings in Malawian children with cerebral malaria. *Ophthalmology* **100**: 857–861.

Lipowski ZJ (1980) Delirium updated. *Comprehensive Psychiatry* **21**(3): 190–196.

Lock S (1984) A question of confidence. An editor's view. *British Medical Journal* **288**: 123.

Looareesuwan S, Warrell DA, White NJ *et al.* (1983a) Retinal haemorrhage, a common physical sign of prognostic significance in cerebrtal malaria. *American Journal of Tropical Medicine and Hygiene* **32**(5): 911–915.

Looareesuwan S, Warrell DA, White NJ *et al.* (1983b) Do patients with cerebral malaria have cerebral oedema? A computed tomography study. *Lancet* **i**: 434–437.

Looareesuwan S, Phillips RE, Karbwang J *et al.* (1990) *Plasmodium falciparum* hyper-parasitaemia: use of exchange transfusion in seven patients and a review of the literature. *Quarterly Journal of Medicine* **75**: 471–481.

Loutan L, Plancherel C, Soulier-Lauper M *et al.* (1992) Serum TNF in patients with severe malaria treated by exchange transfusion. *Tropical Medicine and Parasitology* **43**: 285–286.

Mabey DCW, Brown A and Greenwood BM (1987) *Plasmodium falciparum* malaria and *Salmonella* infections in Gambian children. *Journal of Infectious Diseases* **155**: 1319–1321.

MacPherson GG, Warrell MJ, White NJ *et al.* (1985) Human cerebral malaria: a quantitative ultrastructural analysis of parasitised erythrocyte sequestration. *American Journal of Pathology* **119**: 385–401.

Maegraith B and Fletcher A (1972) The pathogenesis of mammalian malaria. *Advances in Parasitology* **10**: 49–75.

Mahdi AA, Hasan M, Khan HM *et al.* (1989) Eye involvement in cerebral malaria. *Journal of Infectious Diseases* **60**(6): 1092–1093.

Mansor SM, Taylor TE, McGrath CS *et al.* (1990) The safety and kinetics of intra-muscular quinine in Malawian children with moderately severe falciparum malaria. *Transactions of the Royal Society of Tropical Medicine and Hygiene* **84**: 482–487.

Marchiafava E and Bignami A (1894) On Summer, Autumn malarial fevers. Translated from the 1st Italian edition by JH Thompson, pp 112–117. London: The New Sydenham Society.

Masson CB (1924) Effect of malaria on the nervous system with special reference to the malarial psychosis. *American Journal of Medical Sciences* **168**: 334–371.

Maung-Maung-Oo, Aikawa M, Than-Than *et al.* (1987) Human cerebral malaria: a pathological study. *Journal of Neuropathology and Experimental Neurology* **46**: 223–231.

McGuire W, Hill AVS, Allsopp CEM, Greenwood BM and Kwiatkowski D (1994) Variation in the TNF-α promoter region associated with susceptibility to cerebral malaria. *Nature* **371**: 508–511.

Millan JM, Millan JMS, Muñoz M *et al.* (1993) CNS complications in acute malaria: MR findings. *American Journal of Neuroradiology* **14**: 493–494.

Miller JH, Byers M, Whiteoak R and Warrell DA (1994) Imported falciparum malaria in British troops returning from Kenya. *Journal of the Royal Army Medical Corps* **140**: 119–123.

Miller KD, White NJ, Lott JA *et al.* (1989a) Biochemical evidence of muscle injury in African children with severe malaria. *Journal of Infectious Diseases* **159**(1): 139–142.

Miller KD, Greenberg AE and Campbell CC (1989b) Treatment of severe malaria in the United States with continuous infusions of quinidine gluconate and exchange transfusion. *New England Journal of Medicine* **321**: 65–70.

Miller LH (1969) Distribution of mature trophozoites and schizonts of *Plasmodium falciparum* in the organs of *Aotus trivergatus*, the night monkey. *American Journal of Tropical Medicine and Hygiene* **18**: 860–865.

Miller LH, Makaranond P, Sitprija V *et al* (1967) Hyponatraemia in malaria. *Annals of Tropical Medicine and Parasitology* **61**: 265–279.

Molyneux ME, Taylor TE, Wirima JJ and Borgstein A (1989) Clinical features and prognostic indicators in paediatric cerebral malaria: a study of 131 comatose Malawian children. *Quarterly Journal of Medicine* **71**: 441–459.

Nash G, O'Brien E, Gordon-Smith EC and Dormandy JA (1989) Abnormalities in the mechanical properties of red blood cells caused by *Plasmodium falciparum*. *Blood* **74**: 855–861.

Newton CRJC, Kirkham FJ, Winstanley PA *et al.* (1991a) Intracranial pressure in African children with cerebral malaria. *Lancet* **337**: 573–576.

Newton CRJC, Winstanley PA and Marsh K (1991b) Retinal haemorrhages in falciparum malaria. *Archives of Diseases in Childhood* **66**: 753.

Newton CRJC, Peshu N, Kendall B *et al.* (1994) Brain swelling and ischaemia in Kenyans with cerebral malaria. *Archives of Diseases in Childhood* **70**: 281–287.

Omanga, U, Ntihinyurwa M, Shako D and Mashako M (1983) Les hémiplégies au cours de l'accès perniceux a *Plasmodium falciparum* de l'enfant. *Annodes de Pédiatrie (Paris)* **30**: 294–296.

Pasvol G, Newton CRJC, Winstanley PA *et al.* (1992) Quinine treatment of severe falciparum malaria in African children: a randomized comparison of three regimens. *American Journal of Tropical Medicine and Hygiene* **45**: 702–713.

Patnaik JK, Das BS, Mishra SK *et al.* (1994) Vascular clogging, mononuclear cell margination and enhanced vascular permeability in the pathogenesis of human cerebral malaria. *American Journal of Tropical Medicine and Hygiene* **51**(5): 642–647.

Pham-Hung G, Truffert A, Delvallée G *et al.* (1990) Infarctus cérébral au cours d'un accès pernicieux palustre. Intérêt t diagnostique de la tomodensitométrie. *Annotes Francaises d'Anesthesie et de Reanimation* **9**: 185–187,

Phillips RE, White NJ, Looareesuwan S *et al.* (1984) Acute renal failure in falciparum malaria in eastern Thailand: successful use of peritoneal dialysis. XI International Congress for Tropical Medicine and Malaria. Calgary. Canada, September 6–11.

Phillips RE, Warrell DA, White NJ *et al.* (1985) Intravenous quinidine for the treatment of severe falciparum malaria. Clinical and pharmacokinetic studies. *New England Journal of Medicine* **312**(20): 1273–1278.

Phillips P, Nantel S and Benny WB (1990) Exchange transfusion as an adjunct to the treatment of severe falciparum malaria: case report and review. *Reviews of Infectious Diseases* **12**(6): 1100–1108.

Plum F and Posner JB (1982) *The Diagnosis of Stupor and Coma*, 3rd edn. Philadelphia: FA Davis Co.

Polder TW (1989) Morphology of cerebral malaria. Clinical and experimental study. Doctor Thesis, University of Amsterdam. Dordrecht: ICG Printing BV.

Porta J, Carota A, Pizzolato GP *et al.* (1993) Immunopathological changes in human cerebral malaria. *Clinical Neuropathology* **12**(3): 142–146.

Punyagupta S, Srichaikul T, Nitiyanant P and Petchclai B (1974) Acute pulmonary insufficiency in falciparum malaria: summary of 72 cases with evidence of disseminated intravascular coagulation. *American Journal of Tropical Medicine and Hygiene* **23**(4): 551–559.

Riganti M, Pongponratn E, Tegoshi T *et al.* (1990) Human cerebral malaria in Thailand: a clinicopathological correlation. *Immunology Letters* **25**: 199–206.

Royal Society of Tropical Medicine and Hygiene (1994) Artemisinin. Proceedings of a meeting convened by the Wellcome Trust on 25–27 April 1993. *Transactions of the Royal Society of Tropical Medicine and Hygiene* **88** (Supplement 1).

Salord F, Alloughiche B, Gaussorgues P *et al.* (1991) Severe falciparum malaria (21 cases). *Intensive Care Medicine* **17**: 449–454.

Seibert DG (1985) Reversible decerebrate posturing secondary to hypoglycaemia. *American Journal of Medicine* **78**: 1036–1037.

Senanayake N (1987) Delayed cerebellar ataxia: a new complication of falciparum malaria? *British Medical Journal* **294**: 1253–1254.

Sitprija V (1988) Nephropathy in falciparum malaria. *Kidney International* **34**: 867–877.

Spitz S (1946) The pathology of acute falciparum malaria *Military Surgeon* **99**: 555–572.

Strachan H (1897) On a form of multiple neuritis prevalent in the West Indies. *Practitioner* **59**: 477–484.

Teasdale G and Jennett B (1974) Assessment of coma and impaired consciousness. A practical scale. *Lancet* **ii**: 81–84.

Teasdale G, Murray G, Parker L and Jennett B (1979) Adding up the Glasgow Coma Scale. *Acta Neurochirurgica* **28** (Supplement): 13–16.

Teasdale G, Jennett B, Murray L and Murray G (1983) Glasgow Coma Scale: to sum or not to sum? *Lancet* **ii**: 678.

Toro G and Roman G (1978) Cerebral malaria. A disseminated vasculomyelinopathy. *Archives of Neurology* **35**: 271–275.

Trang TT, Phu NH, Vinh H *et al.* (1992) Acute renal failure in patients with severe falciparum malaria. *Clinical Infectious Diseases* **15**: 974–980.

Turner GDH, Morrison H, Jones M *et al.* (1994) An immune histochemical study of the pathology of fatal malaria. Evidence for widespread endothelial activation and a potential role for intercellular adhesion molecule-1 in cerebral sequestration. *American Journal of Pathology* **145**(5): 1057–1069.

Vachon F, Wolff M and Lebras J (1992) Exchange transfusion as an adjunct to the treatment of severe falciparum malaria. *Clin Infect Dis* **14**: 1269.

Vietze G (1978) Malaria and other protozoal diseases. *Handbook of Clinical Neurology*, vol. 35, Ch. 6, pp 143–160. Amsterdam: Elsevier.

Waller D, Krishna S, Craddock C *et al.* (1990) The pharmacokinetic properties of intramuscular quinine in Gambian children with severe falciparum malaria. *Transactions of the Royal Society of Tropical Medicine and Hygiene* **84**: 488–491.

Warrell DA (1987) Pathophysiology of severe falciparum malaria in man. *Parasitology* **94**: S53–S76.

Warrell DA (1989) Editorial. Cerebral malaria. *Quarterly Journal of Medicine* **71**(265): 369–371.

Warrell DA, Looareesuwan S, Warrell MJ *et al.* (1982) Dexamethasone proves deleterious in cerebral malaria. A double-blind trial in 100 comatose patients *New England Journal of Medicine* **306**(6): 313–319.

Warrell DA, Looareesuwan S, Phillips RE *et al.* (1986) Function of the blood–cerebrospinal fluid barrier in human cerebral malaria: rejection of the permeability hypothesis. *American Journal of Tropical Medicine and Hygiene* **35**(5): 882–889.

Warrell DA, White NJ, Veall N *et al.* (1988) Cerebral anaerobic glycolysis and reduced cerebral oxygen transport in human cerebral malaria. *Lancet* **ii**: 534–538.

Warrell DA, Molyneux ME and Beales PF (eds) (1990) Severe and complicated malaria, 2nd edn. World Health Organization Malaria Action Programme. *Transactions of the Royal Society of Tropical Medicine and Hygiene* **84** (Supplement).

Warrell DA, Phillips RE and Garrard CS (1991) Intensive care unit management of severe malaria. *Clinical Intensive Care* **2**(2): 86–96.

Wattanagoon Y, Phillips RE, Warrell DA *et al* (1986) Intramuscular quinine loading dose for falciparum malaria: pharmacokinetics and toxicity. *British Medical Journal* **293**: 11–13.

Weinke T, Trautmann M, Held T *et al.* (1991) Neuropsychiatric side effects after the use of mefloquine. *American Journal of Tropical Medicine and Hygiene* **45**(1): 86–91.

Weiss S and Guberman A (1978) Acute cerebellar ataxia in infectious disease. In: *Handbook of Clinical Neurology* (eds PJ Vinken and GW Bruyn), pp 619–639. *Infections of the Nervous System*, Part II. Amsterdam: North-Holland Publishing Co.

White NJ and Ho M (1992). The pathophysiology of malaria. *Advances in Parasitology* **31**: 83–173.

White NJ, Looareesuwan S, Warrell DA *et al.* (1982) Quinine pharmacokinetics and toxicity in cerebral and uncomplicated falciparum malaria. *American Journal of Medicine* **73**: 564–572.

White NJ, Looareesuwan S, Warrell DA *et al.* (1983b) Quinine loading dose in cerebral malaria. *American Journal of Tropical Medicine and Hygiene* **32**: 1–5.

White NJ, Warrell DA, Chanthavanich P *et al.* (1983a) Severe hypoglycemia and hyperinsulinemia in falciparum malaria. *New England Journal of Medicine* **309**(2): 61–66.

White NJ, Warrell DA, Looareesuwan S *et al.* (1985) Pathophysiological and prognostic significance of cerebrospinal fluid lactate in cerebral malaria. *Lancet* **i**: 776–778.

White NJ, Miller KD, Marsh K *et al.* (1987) Hypoglycaemia in African children with severe malaria. *Lancet* **i**: 708–711.

White NJ, Looareesuwan S, Phillips RE *et al.* (1988) Single dose phenobarbitone prevents convulsions in cerebral malaria. *Lancet* **ii**: 64–66.

White NJ, Krishna S, Waller D *et al.* (1989) An open comparison of intramuscular chloroquine and quinine in children with severe chloroquine-sensitive falciparum malaria. *Lancet* **ii**: 1313–1317.

WHO (1990) Practical chemotherapy of malaria. *Technical Report Series*, 805. Geneva: WHO.

WHO (1993) World malaria situation in 1991. *Weekly Epidemiology Records* **34**: 245–252; **35**: 253–258.

Winstanley PA, Newton CRJC, Pasvol G *et al.* (1992) Prophylactic phenobarbitone in young children with severe falciparum malaria: pharmacokinetics and clinical effects. *British Journal of Clinical Pharmacology* **33**: 149–154.

Winstanley PA, Newton CRJC, Watkins WM *et al.* (1993) Towards optimal regimens of parenteral quinine for young African children with cerebral malaria: importance of unbound quinine concentration. *Transactions of the Royal Society of Tropical Medicine and Hygiene* **87**: 201–206.

Wintrob RM (1973) Malaria and the acute psychotic episode. *Journal of Mental Diseases* **150**: 306–315.

Wright PW, Avery WG, Ardill WD and McLarty JW (1993) Initial clinical assessment of the comatose patients: cerebral malaria vs meningitis. *Pediatric Infectious Disease* **12**: 37–41.

15

Neurocysticercosis*

Noshir H. Wadia

*Director of Neurology, Jaslok Hospital & Research Centre, Consultant Neurologist for Life,
Grant Medical College & J.J. Hospital, Bombay, India*

INTRODUCTION

It is generally acknowledged that along with resurgent malaria, cysticercosis is the most common parasitic infection of the central nervous system and an important cause of death and epilepsy in developing and tropical countries. The disease in humans is caused by the larval form of the embryo of the tapeworm, *Taenia solium*, which is found in the intestine of man. The disease was once found globally, except perhaps in Australia, New Zealand, Japan and the Islamic countries, but today it affects thousands, mostly in the tropical and developing countries and some countries of Eastern Europe and Russia (Andrapov, personal communication, 1991). There is, however, a minor upsurge in the south-western United States, through migrants from endemic areas (McCormick *et al.*, 1982; Earnest *et al.*, 1987).

According to Trelles and Trelles (1978) in their excellent review, this disease was known in antiquity and some evidence of its existence goes back to the fifth century BC when Aristophanes made mention of it in one of his Comedies. It was finally Van Beneden who linked the intestinal tapeworm with the migrating cestodes in humans in 1853. Since then clinicopathological descriptions have been reported from many parts of the world, though most from South America where the disease is still heavily endemic. Trelles and Trelles (1978) have documented most of the early literature up to 1966 but mention here must be made of a series of landmark papers by medical officers of the British Army in India not fully acknowledged by them. Although reports of servicemen with cysticercosis in the British Army in undivided India have been published earlier, it was MacArthur (1934) who aroused widespread interest and showed the high incidence of epilepsy due to cysticercosis in the British Army. Morrison mentioned in that report a variety of cystic cerebral calcifications fancifully described as 'carrot', 'dunce's cap', 'tiger', 'beetle', etc. seen on radiographs,

---

*The colour plate appears between p. 236 and p. 237

and stressed their diagnostic importance. Dixon and Hargreaves (1944) and Dixon and Lipscomb (1961) further studied all the available British cases from 1892 to 1957, more clearly defining the clinical features, natural history and prognosis.

With the introduction of new laboratory tests, computed tomography (CT), magnetic resonance imaging (MRI) and new approaches in medical and surgical therapy, the diagnosis, prognosis and management of patients has improved.

LIFE CYCLE

The parasitic cycle takes place between man and pig, with man acting as the definitive host harbouring the tapeworm (Plate 9). Its scolex or head is attached to the intestinal wall by a four-cup-shaped sucker and a double row of hooklets. The body is made of several hundred segments (proglottids) which are shed in the faeces. Each proglottid contains a vast number of viable eggs or ova and these are released when it disintegrates. The *Taenia* by itself gives a few symptoms and can discharge eggs over decades. The natural intermediate host is the free-range pig which swallows the ova along with excreta. The ova converted into oncospheres lodge in the muscles and other organs in the larval form (cysticercus cellulosae) via the bloodstream. The life cycle is then continued by man who eats raw or undercooked infected (measley) pork, the larva reaching his gut to unfold into an adult worm.

Serious problems arise when man also becomes the accidental intermediate host by ingesting the ova. This can be by cross- or auto-infection. Cross-infection is either through faecal contamination of water or soil where vegetables are grown and eaten improperly washed. Another source is human night soil when used as manure. It can also happen through unclean hands of food handlers harbouring the *Taenia*. Autoinfection is through unclean hands or more rarely when the proglottids or ova regurgitate into the stomach by reverse peristalsis. It is less likely as only 4–21% of patients with cysticercosis harbour the *Taenia* (Dixon and Lipscomb, 1961; McCormick *et al.*, 1982). Thus amongst many Indians who are vegetarians or eat no pork, cross-infection is the only mode as they do not harbour a *Taenia*. The Chinese experience has been somewhat different as 53.8% of the patients of Yingkun *et al.* (1979) had 'passed long segmented worms'.

As in pig, the ova converted into oncospheres (the immature larvae) penetrate the gut, enter the capillaries and travel via the bloodstream to lodge in various tissues after burrowing through the wall of small vessels. Here it is converted into the mature larva (cysticercus cellulosae) within a few weeks leading to 'a dead end' of the cycle in humans. The commonest target organ is the central nervous system, where the cerebral grey matter, the meninges and the ventricles are favoured, but the spinal cord is largely spared. Next are the muscles followed by the subcuticular tissues, eyes and more rarely in massive infection the heart, lungs, kidneys and liver. Sotelo (1988) stated that 'for unknown reasons, the coincidence of brain and muscle cysticercosis is rare in the same patient', a fact not mentioned by others.

PATHOLOGY

The morphology of the viable cysticercus and the pathological changes and pathogenesis of the disease are discussed in detail by MacArthur (1934), Trelles and Trelles (1978), Escobar (1983), Del Brutto and Sotelo (1988) and Davis and Kornfeld (1991). Concern here is only with the evolutionary changes in the larva and the reaction of the host tissue, especially the brain and meninges.

The mature larva is cystic and has a protoscolex and a transparent fluid-filled bladder (Escobar, 1983). There is negligible local inflammatory response, permitting the parasite to survive from 2 to 6 years and even a decade (MacArthur, 1934). How it escapes the host immune defences is still an enigma (Davis and Kornfeld, 1991). When the cysticercus begins to die, the fluid within becomes turbid or 'jelly-like', and the cyst wall breaks down. This can result in the expansion of the cyst even up to several centimetres in diameter due to osmotic dysregulation (Davis and Kornfeld, 1991). More commonly breakdown of the cyst wall results in the release of parasitic antigens which cause an intense inflammatory reaction with lymphocytes, plasma cells and eosinophils and a local production of antibodies which can be detected in the cerebrospinal fluid (CSF) (Estanol *et al.*, 1989). A capsule of fibroblasts is then thrown around the cysticercus and pericystic oedema develops. Ultimately the cyst wall collapses and degenerates and the process of calcification begins which may take years to complete. The resultant pathology depends on the location, number, type, size and stage of the cysticerci in the brain parenchyma. Thus a single, large, space-occupying parenchymatous or ventricular cyst (Figure 15.1a, b) with or without hydrocephalus, or a single or multiple small parenchymatous viable cyst(s) (Figure 15.2), granuloma(s) with pericystic oedema, calcified nodule(s), or a combination thereof can be seen on pathological examination.

If the oncosphere lodges in the meninges or choroid plexus it can enter the subarachnoid spaces or ventricles and may take a different larval form, the racemose variety, in which the cyst without a protoscolex resembles a bunch of grapes: should cysticercal antigen leakage occur, a chronic inflammatory meningitis or ependymitis follows, or the cyst encased by a fibrous arachnoiditis becomes a mass obstructing CSF flow to cause hydrocephalus. More rarely a secondary inflammatory occlusion of the basal arteries may cause cerebral infarction (Del Brutto, 1992). When the cyst dies usually no calcification is seen.

Spinal cysticerci can be located in the meninges or within the spinal cord. The morphological features are no different from the brain, but the inflammation is more severe (Del Brutto and Sotelo, 1988). MacArthur (1934) maintained that the oncosphere in the muscles goes through similar but more rapid morphological changes so that the parasite may be alive in the brain and calcified dead in the muscles. The inflammatory response is usually more mute. The oncosphere lodged usually in the retina or more rarely in the anterior chamber of the eye sets up an acute inflammatory reaction leading to loss of vision. The mature larva can burst into the vitreous, become encapsulated and remain alive for years (MacArthur, 1950).

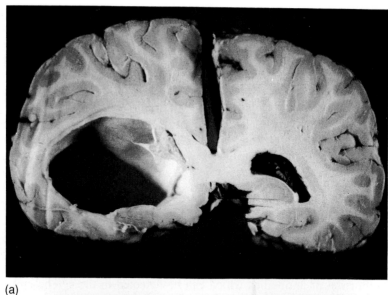

(a)

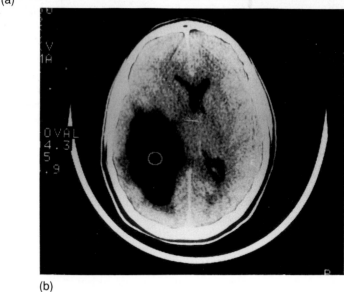

(b)

Figure 15.1 (a) Coronal section of brain with a large cysticercus in a dilated left lateral ventricle. (b) CT scan of the same patient.

EPIDEMIOLOGY

No hard epidemiological data have been generated anywhere. Nevertheless, the enormity of the parasitic infection can be gauged from the following data, despite statistical short-falls and consequent underestimates.

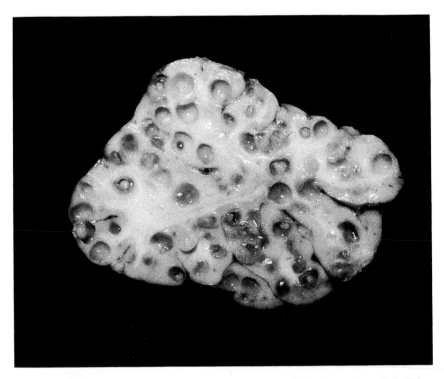

Figure 15.2 Coronal section of the occipital lobe of the brain studded with small, multiple, living cysticerci. Note that many of them have fallen out of the brain after section as there was no inflammatory reaction.

Hospital-Based Data

Trelles and Trelles (1978) extrapolating from hospital-based clinical and autopsy records estimated the incidence of cysticercosis in the general population of Peru to be 450 per 100 000 inhabitants and mentioned the likelihood of 200 000 individuals being afflicted in Latin America in 1973. Approximate prevalence rates in hospital populations range from 0.02% in Honduras to 2.4% in Brazil (Earnest *et al.*, 1987), and 3% of the patients in the neurology/neurosurgery services of Mexico City had cysticercosis (Flisser *et al.*, 1983). Vazquez and Sotelo (1992) mentioned that 50% of cases of late onset epilepsy were due to cysticercosis. In India, cysticercosis was the cause of epilepsy in 2–5% of patients studied (Mani *et al.*, 1974; Wani *et al.*, 1981; Mahajan *et al.*, 1982). In China, Yingkun *et al.* (1979) were able to study 158 cases in the neurological service of a hospital in Beijing from 1956 to 1974 and Zhi-biao *et al.* (1985) 200 cases in another hospital in 2 years. They further maintained that cysticercosis was commonly seen in other parts of China. Recently, McCormick (1985) reported that 2% of admissions to the neurology/neurosurgery services in a

Los Angeles hospital were for cysticercosis, and Scharf (1988) saw 283 such patients between 1981 and 1986 at another centre.

Autopsy Data

Trelles and Trelles (1978) mentioned that 1.82% of 11 532 autopsies carried out in the hospitals of Lima, Peru, showed cysticercosis and said that similar data had emerged from other hospitals in Latin America. In Mexico City, it was 3% (Estanol *et al.*, 1986), in Chandigarh, India it was 1.3% of 6347 consecutive autopsies (Tandon, 1983) and in Zimbabwe 0.45% (Gelfand, 1948).

Stool Examination

Stool examinations in hospital laboratories and communities have given some measure of taeniasis. Stools of 250 000 hospital patients in North India (1964–1981) revealed taeniasis in 0.5–2%. This figure rose to 12–15% in labour colonies and slums in which pigs were raised obviously unattended (Mahajan, 1982). Similarly, *Taenia solium* ova were found in 1.13% of 157 085 specimens of stools in Guatemala (Acha and Aguilar, 1964), 1.02% in the Loja region of Ecuador, 0.48% in a hospital in Rhodesia, and in 7% of the population of Timor, Indonesia (Mahajan, 1982).

Serological Studies

Mahajan (1982) reported that 2–3% of the general population in and around Chandigarh had antibody titres positive for cysticercosis and the seropositivity was greater in the rural areas and amongst the socioeconomically deprived with unhygienic habits. Similarly Flisser *et al.* (1983) found in an epidemiological survey in Mexico a seropositivity of 1% and Trelles and Trelles (1978) have mentioned that cysticercosis was confirmed in 168 out of 12 200 patients in a psychiatric hospital in Mexico by complement fixation tests.

Swine Cysticercosis

This gives an indirect indication of the prevalence of the local human form. In certain rural areas of Peru, the incidence of cysticercosis in pigs was as high as 1.66–3.83%, figures comparable to those found in Mexico, Brazil and Chile (Trelles and Trelles, 1978), while 8–10% of slaughtered pigs in areas around Chandigarh with high prevalence of taeniasis were infected with cysticerci and even protected Government farms were not entirely free (Mahajan, 1982). Mahajan reported somewhat similar figures in other developing countries (5.7% Loja, Ecuador, 0.1–8.1% Zaire, 2.13% in six Central American countries and 2.2% in Timor and Bali, Indonesia).

Asymptomatic Cases

These would be missed even in an epidemiological survey. The dimension of this can be gauged by the fact that 20% of 73 Mexican American cases in Los Angeles were detected incidentally (Gardner *et al.*, 1984) and in a necropsy series in Mexico City 80% of patients whose autopsies revealed cysticercosis had no symptoms of the disease during life (Estanol *et al.*, 1986).

CLINICAL FEATURES

The disease is said to occur equally in males and females (Sotelo, 1988) but Trelles and Trelles (1978) found it more amongst females. The highest incidence is in young adults and children are relatively spared.

The clinical features are protean and variable, and like the pathology depend on the size, number, type, location and stage of evolution of the cysticercus. Usually there are no general symptoms, but some adults and especially children do complain of headache, vomiting, fever and myalgia with or without seizures during the initial parasitaemia and invasion of the brain by the oncospheres (MacArthur, 1934; Lopez-Hernandez and Garaizer, 1982). Seizures, symptoms of increased intracranial pressure, mental disorder, focal neurological signs and those related to chronic meningitis or more rarely ocular blindness, spinal cord compression, muscular pseudohypertrophy, or a combination of these form the main clinical picture. Understandably the frequency of these vary in different reported series (Table 15.1).

Epilepsy

Recurrent seizures occur at any stage of disease. The frequency can be as high as 91.8% (Dixon and Lipscomb, 1961). The seizures may be generalized or focal, and the focus identified by visual, olfactory, hallucinatory, amnesic or other variety of aura. Often, more than one type of seizure is seen in the same person. Recurrent seizures may be the only symptom (31.1% Dixon and Lipscomb, 1961; 36.2% McCormick *et al.*, 1982) mimicking idiopathic epilepsy as increasingly revealed by CT or MRI. They may be at times hard to control with medication and death from status epilepticus is known.

Raised Intracranial Pressure

Headache, vomiting and papilloedema with or without focal neurological signs were infrequently seen by Dixon and Lipscomb (1961), but Tandon (1983) in a neurosurgical series mentioned 95% and Earnest *et al.* (1987), 38%. Headache

TABLE 15.1 Main clinical presentation of patients with cysticercosis (comparative)

Study	Dixon and Lipscomb (1961)	Canelas (1963)	Tandon (1982)	Sotelo et al. (1985a)	Earnest et al. (1987)	Venkataraman (1989)	Davis and Kornfeld (1991)*
No. of cases	450	276	42	753	200 US literature	Unspecified Indian literature	1200 world literature and personal (unspecified)
Presentation in %							
Epilepsy	91.8	53.6	45	52.4	51.9	54–94	60
Raised intracranial pressure	6.4	48.9	95	33.3	38	12–95	25
Focal CNS manifestations	2.9	26.8	62	–	28	1.2–2.5	10
Mental disorder	8.7	22.8	0	20	12	8–9	15
Chronic meningitis	–	–	–	–	–	–	25

* 10% of cases were asymptomatic and accidentally discovered.
– Not mentioned.

and vomiting with or without fever and meningismus are also symptoms of chronic basal meningitis.

Mental Disorders

Progressive loss of intellect and memory, change in behaviour, confusion, disorientation and other symptoms amounting to dementia are not uncommon, but Dixon and Lipscomb (1961) have drawn attention to manic depression, psychoneurosis and psychopathic behaviour which can lead to misdiagnosis.

Focal Signs

These vary considerably depending on the site of lesions. As the cerebral hemispheres are more involved than the hind-brain, hemiparesis, dysphasia, visual disturbance and cognitive impairment are more frequently detected than, for example, ataxia, dysarthria or diplopia. Less commonly, when the basal meninges are involved various cranial nerve palsies including optic atrophy, hypothalamic and pituitary disorder and an acute neurological deficit such as hemiplegia from cerebral infarction are seen. When the spinal cord is diseased, paraplegia and other signs of extra- or intra-medullary compression are found.

Signs Outside the CNS

MacArthur (1934) mentioned that the most helpful sign in diagnosis is the presence of a palpable subcuticular cyst, a fact as true today as it was then. Yingkun *et al.* (1979) mentioned the incidence of such nodules in Chinese patients as 41–91% and Dixon and Lipscomb (1961) found them in 54% of their cases. They rightly mentioned the need for a high index of suspicion and a thorough examination of the whole body to avoid missing even one. Appropriately questioning the patient may be rewarding. A nodule in the tongue is often noticed by the patient and requires careful palpation. The nodules may appear before, or after the nervous manifestations with an interval up to 27 years (Dixon and Lipscomb, 1961).

Ocular cysticercosis leads to sudden blindness, when the floating unfolded living larva may be visualized ophthalmoscopically. The invasion of the parasites into the muscles is usually silent, but a massive pseudohypertrophy of muscles simulating myopathy has been reported (Priest, 1926; Wadia *et al.*, 1988). Still more rarely, the heart may be invaded causing arrhythmias, cardiac failure and a heart block requiring a pacemaker (Katrak, personal communication, 1992). Whereas the clinical features just described often interlace to give a pleomorphic picture of neurocysticercosis, some patterns do emerge.

Parenchymatous Form

In the parenchymatous form when there are many viable or dying cysticerci or a large cyst, uncontrolled seizures, increasing focal deficits, intellectual deterioration with or without signs of raised intracranial pressure dominate the picture. Here the differential diagnosis from a tumour or dementia from other causes may not be easy. Similarly, a more malignant form described especially amongst children and young women may be indistinguishable from encephalitis (Earnest *et al.*, 1987; Del Brutto and Sotelo, 1988). Conversely, attention has been drawn to a more 'benign' parenchymatous form from India. In the last decade several hundred patients have been seen all over the country presenting solely with a single or multiple, focal or generalized seizure(s) in whom CT scans have shown a small, single, subcortical 'ring' or 'disc' enhancing lesion, which disappears often spontaneously after an interval (Sethi *et al.*, 1985; Ahuja *et al.*, 1989; Bansal *et al.*, 1989; Chandy *et al.*, 1991). Whereas much debate has been generated as to the cause (Wadia *et al.*, 1987; Rajshekhar *et al.*, 1993) biopsy has revealed a cysticercus in a good number (Bhatia and Tandon, 1988; Chandy *et al.*, 1989, 1991; Rajshekhar *et al.*, 1993). In fact three of the authors' patients had wrongly received antituberculous medication till their soft tissue X-rays showed calcified cysticerci. In the pre-CT era these would have been diagnosed as suffering from 'idiopathic' epilepsy. Rajshekhar *et al.* (1993) have confidently laid down clinical and CT criteria to differentiate a solitary cysticercus from a tuberculoma and considerably rested the Indian controversy. Similarly, cysticerci long dead and calcified can present with seizures alone. It appears that the parenchymatous form is the commonest one seen in India (Tandon, 1983).

Subarachnoidal Form

The subarachnoidal form presents more rapidly with symptoms and signs of low-grade meningitis with or without cranial nerve palsies which can be clinically difficult to distinguish from tuberculous, fungal or other parasitic meningitis, so common in developing tropical countries. Misdiagnosis as 'polyneuritis cranialis' can also be made. It may also declare itself with signs of raised intracranial pressure, or a space-occupying lesion, especially in the posterior fossa. Less usually the patient can present with a 'stroke' due to occlusive basal arteritis and Del Brutto (1992) has described patients with lacunar or large infarcts, transient ischaemic attacks and a progressive mid-brain syndrome.

Intraventricular Form

The intraventricular form appears with progressive or intermittent symptoms and signs of raised intracranial pressure, sometimes acute enough to demand urgent surgery. Some patients come with 'drop attacks' on movements of the head such as seen with a colloid cyst of the third ventricle or an acute obstruction of the fourth.

Disseminated Form

The disseminated form though rare has been long well known (Priest, 1926). Wadia *et al.* (1988) have pointed out that the triad of uncontrolled fits, dementia and remarkable muscular pseudohypertrophy results from the space-occupying effect of thousands of living cysticerci in the brain and muscles without much inflammatory reaction and the term 'pseudohypertrophic myopathy' was a misnomer. There is often no obvious evidence of raised intracranial pressure. There is no differential diagnosis as the combination of massively enlarged muscles and epilepsy is seen in no other human disease. McRobert (1944) vividly described his patient as a man who in a matter of 6 months had come to resemble 'a professional wrestler to the amusement of his friends and dismay of his household'.

Spinal Form

The spinal form is relatively rare and manifests with root pains, paraplegia and other signs of spinal cord compression which makes a preoperative aetiological diagnosis difficult. The compression can be extra- or intra-medullary at one level, or a cluster of racemose cysts can extend over many levels mimicking a spinal tuberculous or fungal meningitis or even an arteriovenous malformation. Extramedullary compression of the cervical cord is the commonest (Trelles and Trelles, 1978).

Having said all this, it is stressed that many patients especially those with the parenchymatous disease may remain neurologically asymptomatic. Here the disease is diagnosed on routine X-rays of the body or biopsy of a subcuticular nodule or now more increasingly with the CT or MRI. Davis and Kornfeld (1991) found 10% of such cases from 1200 in the world literature and Gardner *et al.* (1984), 20% amongst 73 Mexican Americans in Los Angeles.

INVESTIGATIONS

The arrival of newer diagnostic methods should not devalue the time-honoured ones as only these are available away from the cities of the developing world where cysticercosis most prevails.

Plain X-rays of the Muscles and Skull

MacArthur (1934) was amongst the first to draw attention to the usefulness of the X-rays of skeletal muscles to detect calcified cysticerci. X-rays revealed calcification in 391 out of 450 cases of Dixon and Lipscomb (1961). The yield is much smaller on radiographs of the skull and the differential diagnosis may not be easy from other calcifying lesions, especially toxoplasmosis.

Subcuticular Nodule or Lesion Biopsy

Histological examination of a subcutaneous nodule can clinch the diagnosis when even newer methods have failed especially when a single parenchymatous lesion is present. When available a CT-guided biopsy of the lesion is still more specific (Chandy *et al.*, 1989, 1991).

Stool Examination

Stool examination for *Taenia solium* ova should be done repeatedly. The yield is small but the presence of *Taenia* is a good indicator of cysticercosis.

Cerebrospinal Fluid Analysis

The CSF must be examined when raised intracranial pressure is excluded clinically or by CT. It reflects the activity of the disease and helps in the management of the patient. It is abnormal in 50% of patients (Davis and Kornfeld, 1991) and more if there is basal meningitis. It will show lymphocytic pleocytosis, raised protein and at times reduced glucose. Eosinophils were found in the sediment of 50% of patients with arachnoiditis (Del Brutto and Sotelo, 1988).

Immunological Tests

Several immunological tests in the serum and CSF have been devised over the years. The complement fixation (CF) test in the CSF was described by Nieto (1956) and is still being used in Mexico (Del Brutto and Sotelo, 1988), though it was replaced in most of the laboratories elsewhere by the indirect haemagglutination (IHA) test (Earnest *et al.*, 1987). The enzyme-linked immunoabsorbent assay (ELISA), the radioimmunoassay (RIA), the immunoelectrophoretic (IEP) techniques, and most recently the immunoblot test have followed with increasing specificity and sensitivity (Rosas *et al.*, 1986; Tsang *et al.*, 1989; Zini *et al.*, 1990).

Whilst Del Brutto and Sotelo (1988) found the tests in the serum to be unreliable with unacceptable false positives, Earnest *et al.* (1987) have still recommended them, but it is generally agreed that these tests have greater positivity in the CSF than serum, and this also depends on the form of cysticercosis. Zini *et al.* (1990) carried out the ELISA test using cyst fluid as antigen and found low antibody levels in the serum and absence in the CSF in the 'benign' form but high levels in both serum and CSF in the 'malignant' form. The former patients presented with easily controlled fits. Their CNS and CSF examinations were normal and the CT brain showed cysts in the brain parenchyma and the convexity leptomeninges. The 'malignant' group had recurrent seizures, abnormal CNS signs, raised intracranial pressure, an abnormal CSF and multiple cysts at the base of the brain or in the cisterns or ventricles. Antibody levels could not be correlated with the type of cysts seen on CT but were dependent on their location, being lower when the cysts were restricted to the cerebral cortex. Corona *et al.* (1986) had somewhat different results. They found on ELISA testing an overall sensitivity and specificity in the blood of 87 and 90% respectively and in the CSF of 87 and 100%. Further, the serum sensitivity of their 'benign' group was 75% compared to 93% of the malignant group and in the CSF it was 80 and 93% respectively. Rosas *et al.* (1986) have mentioned that ELISA was overall positive in only 50% of the patients when the serum alone was tested but 87% when the CSF was also examined.

The new immunoblot test had claimed much higher sensitivity (97%) and specificity (100%) even in the serum (Tsang *et al.*, 1989), though once again subsequent experience has shown that this depends on the form of the disease because in patients with only a single active parenchymatous lesion the seropositivity fell to 71 and 36% in the serum and CSF respectively (Rajshekhar *et al.*, 1991). These low results were also reflected amongst Indian patients, as only four out of seven patients with multiple parenchymatous lesions and one out of 18 with a single small enhancing lesion presumed to be a cysticercus (biopsy in only two) tested positive in the serum (Rajshekhar *et al.*, 1991).

Thus immunological tests, though useful, do have their limitations.

CT and MRI

CT and more recently MRI have become invaluable tools in the diagnosis, prognosis and treatment of cysticercosis, showing how much was missed before their advent.

CT Brain Parenchymatous Form

It has been shown that CT can image various evolutionary stages of the cysticercus from its first entry into the brain until its death (Suss *et al.*, 1986; Kramer *et al.*, 1989). When the oncosphere invades the brain parenchyma a small hypodense lesion not enhancing after contrast administration appears. With growth some enhancement is seen. This is the invasive phase. The next stage of the mature cystic larva is seen as a CSF-equivalent density round or oval lesion within which a hyperdense scolex may be identified (Figure 15.3a, b). There is no surrounding oedema or contrast enhancement representing the host response. As the larva begins to die the cyst and scolex may no longer be

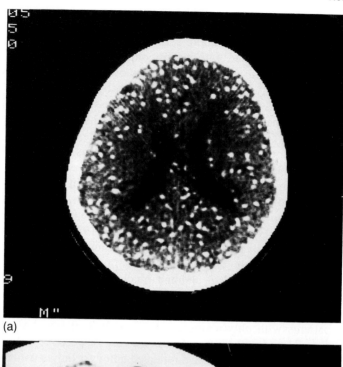

(a)

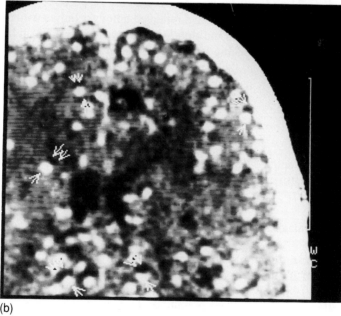

(b)

Figure 15.3 Living cysticerci. (a) Enhanced CT scan of the brain of the same patient as in Figure 15.2 imaging the vast number of living cysticerci (disseminated cysticercosis). Here the hyperdense scolices stand out more prominently producing a 'starry night' effect because the cysts are tightly squeezed. Singly the low attenuation density value cyst wall would stand out equally prominently as illustrated in the magnified view of the same scan shown in (b). Single arrows show the scolices and double arrows the cysts. Contrast produced no enhancement of cyst walls.

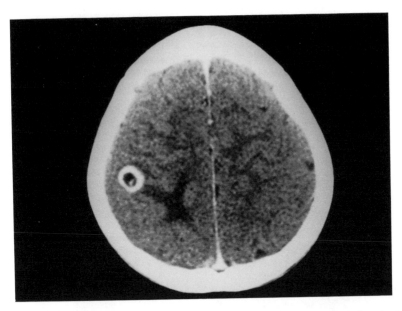

Figure 15.4 Dying cysticercus. Axial contrast – enhanced CT scan showing a ring-enhancing lesion with perifocal oedema. Here the scolex can still be identified, as at an early stage.

differentiated, but its presence is revealed by a low attenuation value area representing reactive oedema. Contrast administration reveals a ring or disc enhancing lesion within that area (Figure 15.4). Finally, in its place with larval death a high attenuation area indicating calcium appears, which increases with time. There may be one or many such lesions (Figure 15.3a, b) or a single large cyst, and larvae at different stages of evolution may be seen in the same scan. The grey white matter region is favoured, but cysts can be found anywhere.

Other Forms

Cysts in the basal meninges (subarachnoidal form) or ventricles may not be easily identified as they appear isodense with CSF and do not enhance on contrast (McCormick, 1982). Often, the cyst is not separately imaged from the ballooned ventricle (Figure 15.1b) though intraventricular contrast administration may reveal it. Diagnosis is made indirectly by the presence of the complicating hydrocephalus or distortion or disproportionate enlargement of the third or fourth ventricles. A racemose cysticercus can be identified as a cluster of cysts in the subarachnoidal cisterns or sylvian fissure (Figure 15.5) but can be missed if isodense with CSF and also be mistaken for a cystic tumour or other intracranial cyst (Suss *et al.*, 1986). In disseminated cysticercosis a 'starry night' effect is seen (Wadia *et al.*, 1988). This is produced by the hyperdense scolices of living cysticerci of the same generation standing out against the lower attenuation density value of the brain, the tightly packed cysts themselves

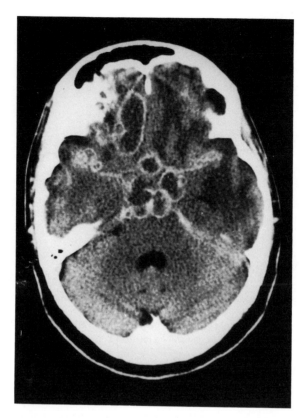

Figure 15.5 Post-contrast axial CT scan showing multiple thin-walled racemose cysts in the suprasellar and sylvian cisterns. No scolex is seen.

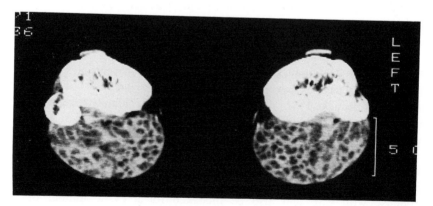

Figure 15.6 Post-contrast CT scan of the calf muscles of the same patient as in Figures 15.2 and 15.3 showing a large number of living cysticerci. Note the 'honeycomb' effect produced by the hypodense cysts against the muscle mass of higher intensity. The scolices though visualized are not as prominent (hyperdense) as in the brain. No contrast enhancement is seen.

contributing little to the image (Figure 15.3a, b). These can be mistaken for calcified dead cysticerci.

CT Muscle

CT scan of the muscles was not used in the diagnosis of cysticercosis until Wadia *et al.* (1988) pointed out the 'honeycomb' effect of a large number of living cysticerci in pseudohypertrophic muscles (Figure 15.6). The effect was produced by the low attenuation density cysts standing out against the muscle mass of higher density value. The scolices though visualized were not as prominent as in the brain. These authors have also recommended the use of CT to demonstrate cysts or calcification not revealed by soft tissues X-rays.

MRI Brain and Muscle

MR images a living parenchymatous cyst as a 5–20 mm diameter round lesion of CSF equivalent intensity on both T1- and T2-weighted images (Suss *et al.*, 1986; Tietelbaum *et al.*, 1989; Desai *et al.*, 1991a). An isodense to hyperintense scolex can be identified within most cysts producing a 'pea in the pod' appearance. (Figure 15.7a, b). In the dying cysticercus the difference between the scolex and cyst becomes unclear. The cyst fluid shows greater and increasing signal intensity than the CSF in the T1- and T2-weighted images and the pathogno-monic pericystic oedema and gliosis are also evidenced by increased signal intensity in the T2-weighted images. In between the two the wall of the cysticercus stands out distinctly being isointense to the grey matter (Figure 15.8a, b). (Desai, personal communication, 1994). The MRI with its greater sensitivity is known to reveal many cysticerci that the CT has missed, especially over the convexity, but calcification is better identified on CT. Suss *et al.* (1986) mention that it is the sensitivity to the difference between fluid and tissue water which causes the entire volume of the nodule to be imaged clearly making it larger and more conspicuous than CT. Desai *et al.* (1991b) claim that MRI can differentiate a cysticercus from a tuberculoma which the CT often cannot.

It is not always easy to identify the intraventricular cyst from the ventricle except by identifying the relatively hyperintense cyst wall separating the CSF from the cyst fluid on T1W1 images and a relatively isointense cyst wall on T2W1 images. This may be further brought out by gadolinium–DPTA enhance-ment (Desai, personal communication, 1994). The racemose cysticercus is seen as a bunch of multiple CSF signal intensity cystic lesions with well-identified walls within the CSF spaces, both on T1- and T2-weighted images. No scolices are seen.

TREATMENT

In a pleomorphic disease like neurocysticercosis, treatment has to be tailored for each patient from the available therapeutic options. With the advent of specific

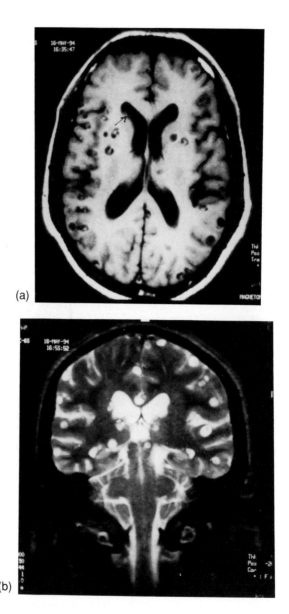

(a)

(b)

Figure 15.7 (a) Live cysticerci. T1 W1 axial brain MRI showing multiple CSF signal intensity lesions with hyperintense scolices (pea-in-the-pod appearance). (b) Same patient T2 W1 coronal MRI with multiple hyperintense live cysts. No oedema or mass effect.

drugs like praziquantel (PZQ) and albendazole (ALB) to eliminate living cysticerci, the first option is medical and the aim of therapy should be to identify through CT/MRI patients who harbour them. Comparatively, the number of these will be small because symptoms and signs mostly arise due to the

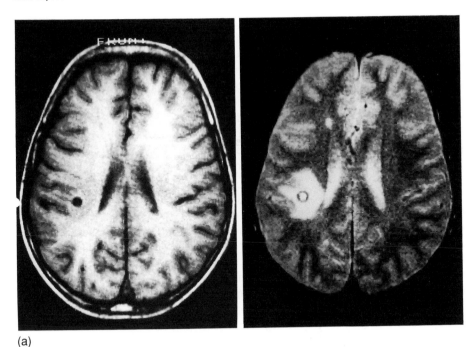

(a)

Figure 15.8 Dying cysticercus. (a) T1 W1 MRI showing a well-defined cyst with surrounding hypointense oedema. (b) T2 W1 MRI same cyst with isointense wall and surrounding hyperintense oedema.

inflammatory response as the cysticercus begins to die (Alarcon *et al.*, 1990) when specific drugs will be useless. Surgery has a smaller but still important role to play. Towards this end Sotelo *et al.* (1985a) and Del Brutto and Sotelo (1988) have suggested a new therapeutically orientated classification of 'active' and 'inactive' forms and recommended a management protocol. All forms were considered active except the calcified cysticerci and hydrocephalus due to basal fibrosis.

Medical – Specific Drugs

Praziquantel (PZQ), an isoquinoline, is a well-tolerated cysticidal drug introduced in 1980 for cysticercosis (Groll, 1982). Controlled studies by Sotelo *et al.* (1984, 1985b) confirmed its effectiveness. The usual recommended oral dose is 10–20 mg kg^{-1} three times a day for 15–21 days, but other dosage schedules have been suggested. Bittencourt *et al.* (1992) maintained that this dose is often ineffective due to the fast elimination of PZQ from the CNS. Based on monitoring of PZQ levels in body fluids, they recommended a dose of 25 mg kg^{-1} three times a day and even up to 50 mg kg^{-1} when the patient is concurrently taking strong liver enzyme inducers like phenytoin and carbamazepine as these decrease the bioavailability of PZQ significantly. They advised monitoring serum levels to prevent drug failure which they believe has caused PZQ to lose its initial therapeutic appeal. Similarly, Vazquez et al. (1987) have recommended against concurrent administration of dexamethasone as the plasma level of PZQ drops by 50%. Vasconcelos and colleagues (1987) have suggested extension of the course to 30 days, and giving a second course for 15 days if the CT scan shows no regression in cyst size. Zhi-Biao et al. (1985) have prescribed 120–180 mg kg^{-1} in divided doses over 2–4 days in Chinese patients. They maintained that 'the higher the single dose the better the result will be in spite of the same total dose'.

Albendazole (ALB) is an imidazole whose cysticidal efficacy was also recently demonstrated by Escobedo et al. (1987) and Sotelo et al. (1988). A dose of 15 mg kg^{-1} per day for one month was initially recommended but a shorter course of the same daily dose for one week (Sotelo et al., 1988) and even for 3 days (Alarcon et al., 1989) seems to be equally efficacious. Simultaneous use of dexamethasone does not appear to reduce its effectiveness as with PZQ (Takayanagui and Jardim, 1992). A comparative trial between PZQ and ALB by Sotelo and colleagues (1988) showed that both were equally good, but Takayanagui and Jardim (1992) found ALB to be clearly superior with a great reduction in the number of cysts in the CT scan after therapy (88% vs 50%). It appears that the less expensive ALB, especially if it is shown by larger trials to be effective in a 3-day course, would be the drug of choice. Del Brutto and Sotelo (1988) have now recommended initial treatment with ALB followed by assessment after 3 months by CT and another course with PZQ if there is insufficient reduction in the number of cysts.

It was generally agreed (Groll, 1982; Sotelo et al., 1984, 1988; Estanol et al., 1986; Vasconcelos et al., 1987; Del Brutto and Sotelo 1988; Alarcon et al., 1989) that these drugs were best used to destroy large or small, single or multiple viable parenchymatous cyst(s). This was based on clinical improvement and reduction in the size and number of cysts seen on CT scans after therapy as against non-treated controls. However, Kramer et al. (1990) expressed doubts about the validity of earlier trial designs and the small number of cases in each group. They maintained that the natural history of regression in neurocysticercosis indicated that there was little gain with specific drug therapy, a position which can be somewhat supported by the good number of asymptomatic and mildly symptomatic cases unearthed by CT and at autopsy mentioned earlier. Sotelo (1990) and Alarcon et al. (1990) vigorously disputed this point of view. Further Vazquez and Sotelo (1992) carried out another recent statistically analysed trial administering PZQ/ALB or both to patients compared to non-treated controls. They mentioned that patients treated for lesions without inflammation on imaging (presumably viable cysts) (group 1) had 94% fewer seizures per year than similar untreated controls (group 2), 78% fewer than patients with presumably spontaneously resolving 'inflamed' cysts (group 3) and 65% fewer than in those whose cysts were surgically removed (group 4).

Other comparative clinical and CT data are also given to prove superiority of cysticidals, although their statement that 'at the end of the study more patients in group 3 were free of cysticerci on CT scanning than group 1' raises some doubts about their claim despite the explanation that group 1 had an initial heavier parasitic burden (5 to 2.5 cysts per patient).

Not enough data are available regarding cysticidals in the treatment of the other forms. However, Del Brutto and Sotelo (1988, 1990) have recommended a trial course of these drugs in the acute encephalitic form, the subarachnoidal variety with chronic meningitis (arachnoiditis), for clumps of cysts not producing a mass effect, and even for leptomeningeal spinal cysticercosis, admitting at once that the benefits have not always been impressive.

Both PZQ and ALB are generally well tolerated, but transient gastrointestinal symptoms, dizziness and lethargy have been reported with PZQ. However, headaches, increased frequency of seizures, painful enlargement of pseudohypertrophic muscles, rise in intracranial pressure, cerebral infarction, hyperthermia, hiccups, severe itching, generalized and urticarial rash, large cutaneous bullae, rise in blood pressure, hypotension and arrhythmias and even death have been reported after administration of PZQ/ALB (Wadia *et al.*, 1988; Takayanagui and Jardim, 1992; Del Brutto, 1992; and other published and personal communications). Many of these adverse effects are believed to be due to the acceleration of the usual inflammatory reaction following release of antigen from simultaneous rapid destruction of living cysticerci. This is reflected in increased CSF pleocytosis, the severity depending on the numbers initially present. Wadia *et al.* (1988) also thought that the dermal symptoms and sudden hypotension and cardiorespiratory arrest after only three doses of PZQ could be due to an anaphylactoid reaction. Whereas it is generally believed (Del Brutto and Sotelo, 1988) that these manifestations are transient and mild requiring little or no symptomatic treatment or drug withdrawal, Wadia *et al.* (1988) and Takayanagui and Jardim (1992) have warned of the risks of this therapy.

Symptomatic Drugs

Anticonvulsants

Most patients, especially those with only seizures and one or few cysticerci and especially if the cysticerci are dying or dead, require only standard anticonvulsants. Control of fits is usually satisfactory, though Dixon and Lipscomb (1961) mentioned that it was less satisfactory than in idiopathic epilepsy. Anticonvulsants would also be required in all others with seizures whether treated with PZQ/ALB or requiring surgery, or when seizures are anticipated. Vazquez and Sotelo (1992) stated that the antiepileptic therapy could be withdrawn or dose-reduced in 44% of their patients treated with PZQ/ALB and more than half were free of seizures after 3 years, results which could not be matched by untreated or surgically operated patients.

Corticosteroids

Before the advent of PZQ/ALB dexamethasone and prednisolone were routinely prescribed to control the natural inflammatory reaction which was responsible for many of the CNS symptoms and signs. Intravenous dexamethasone, mannitol and frusemide are recommended when the more severe natural or drug-induced manifestations appear, but many prescribe prednisolone (40–60 mg day^{-1}) or dexamethasone (12–24 mg day) concurrently with PZQ/ALB for those in whom such reaction is anticipated. Wadia *et al.* (1988) have advised that patients with disseminated cysticercosis or a large parasitic load should be primed well in advance with oral dexamethasone which should be continued throughout the period of drug administration.

Surgery

Today surgery is reserved for those who cannot be treated with cysticidals. Mobile intraventricular, and accessible racemose cysts and cysts compressing the spinal cord are best excised. Ventriculoperitoneal shunting is required in patients with hydrocephalus resulting from inoperable racemose or intraventricular cysts and basal meningitis or fibrosis. It is the most common surgical procedure in this disease and has been combined at times with cysticidal therapy. Parenchymatous cysts even when occupying space are now rarely excised, especially if the diagnosis is certain. At most a CT-guided puncture to relieve the pressure is performed before cysticidals are given (Del Brutto and Sotelo, 1988). Racemose cysts can also be similarly treated though results are not so good. Rarely decompressive craniectomy is performed for cerebral oedema not subsiding with intensive medical treatment.

In summary, therapy has to be geared to get the best result, recognizing the natural history of the disease and the therapeutic options available for the various forms. The gains of active therapy with PZQ/ALB must be weighed against the risk of flaring up the disease especially when there is a very large viable parasitic load and very few symptoms or only well-controlled seizures. Often the best option is the old adage of 'wait and watch' and treat when one must. Some treatment options are suggested (Table 15.2).

PREVENTION

The only way to eradicate this scourge is by socioeconomic upliftment. In the meantime, strict market inspection of pork and education of the public about the hazards of the disease and its prevention by personal and environmental hygiene needs to be driven home. As a family source of infection is known, repeated stool examinations of all family members and food servers of the patient must be carried out and the source eradicated. The myth amongst vegetarians and those

TABLE 15.2 Some therapeutic options

Form of cysticercosis	PZQ/ALB	Steroids	Anticonvulsants	Excision	VP Shunt
Parenchymatous					
Living (cysts)					
Single large or clumps	++	+/−	+	+	−
Single small	+/−	−	+	−	−
Many or disseminated*	++	++	++	−	−
Encephalitic	++	++	++	−	−
Dying (granuloma)					
Single	−	+/−	++	+ CT guided	−
Many	−	++	++	−	−
Dead (calcified)					
With seizures	−	−	++	−	−
No seizures	−	−	−	−	−
Mixed (if many viable)	++	++	++	−	−
Subarachnoidal/ Racemose	+	+	+/−	++	++
Intraventricular	−	−	−	++	++
Spinal	+/−	−	−	++	−

++, preferred treatment; +, next option; +/−, uncertain; −, not required.
* If viable parasitic load is heavy hospital monitoring.
PZQ, praziquantel; ALB, albendazole; VP, ventriculoperitoneal.

who do not eat pork that they are not vulnerable to the disease should be dispelled.

PROGNOSIS

As mentioned earlier, the overall prognosis regarding mortality, morbidity and control of seizures is good and has improved after the advent of PZQ/ALB. However, it is variable amongst different forms. Estanol *et al.* (1986) reported that patients with parenchymal cysts or calcification without hydrocephalus presenting with seizures never require surgical treatment, respond well to cysticidals and have a good prognosis – 'benign form'. By contrast those who present with hydrocephalus, large cysts, multiple granulomas with oedema, chronic meningitis and vasculitis are more acutely ill, often require surgery and do not respond to PZQ/ALB. Fatal outcome or severe sequelae are seen in this 'malignant' form. The results of CSF shunting have not been satisfactory. Leblanc *et al.* (1986) have mentioned that intraventricular cysts do not stop growing in size after shunting and produce compression, demanding removal later. Similarly, shunting in patients with multiple racemose cysts in the basal cisterns is often unsatisfactory due to blockage of the shunt by the inflammatory debris. Del Brutto and Sotelo (1988) have mentioned a mortality of 50% and severe disability in more than 20% of survivors amongst them. Similarly spinal leptomeningitis is equally disabling. Results of excision of a large single well-defined, accessible cyst in the brain and spinal cord are most gratifying.

ACKNOWLEDGEMENTS

I wish to acknowledge with thanks, the permission given by Drs V. Shah and S.B. Desai of the Breach Candy Hospital and Research Centre, Bombay, to print some of the CT/MR scans. Figure 15.1 is printed through the kind courtesy of Dr A.P. Desai of the K.E.M. Hospital, Bombay.

REFERENCES

Acha PN and Aguilar FJ (1964) Studies on cysticercosis in Central America and Panama. *American Journal of Tropical Medicine and Hygiene* **13**: 48–53.

Ahuja GK, Behari M, Prasad K *et al.* (1989) Disappearing CT lesions in epilepsy: is tuberculosis or cysticercosis the cause? *Journal of Neurology, Neurosurgery and Psychiatry* **52**: 915–916.

Alarcon F, Escalante F, Duenas G, Montalvo M and Roman M (1989) Neurocysticercosis – short course of treatment with albendazole. *Archives of Neurology* **46**: 1231–1236.

Alarcon F, Moncayo J and Vinan I (1990) Antihelminic therapy for neurocysticercosis. *Archives of Neurology* **47**: 1060.

Bansal BC, Dua A, Gupta R *et al.* (1989) Appearing and disappearing CT scan abnormalities in India – an enigma. *Journal of Neurology, Neurosurgery and Psychiatry* **52**: 1185–1187.

Bhatia S and Tandon PN (1988) Solitary microlesions in CT: a clinical study and follow-up. *Neurology (India)* **36**: 139–150.

Bittencourt PRM, Gracia CM, Martins R *et al.* (1992) Phenytoin and carbamazepine decrease oral bioavailability of praziquantel. *Neurology* **42**: 492–496.

Canelas HM (1963) Neurocysticercosis its incidence, diagnosis and clinical forms. In: *Tropical Neurology* (eds L Van Bogaert, JP Kafer and GF Poch), p 149. Buenos Aires: Lopez Libreros.

Chandy MJ, Rajshekher V, Prakash S *et al.* (1989) Cysticercosis causing single small CT lesions in Indian patients with seizures. *Lancet* **1**: 390–391.

Chandy MJ, Rajshekher V, Ghosh S *et al.* (1991) Single, small enhancing CT lesions in Indian patients with epilepsy: Clinical, radiological and pathological consideration. *Journal of Neurology, Neurosurgery and Psychiatry* **54**: 702–705.

Corona T, Pascoe D, Gonzales-Barranco D *et al.* (1986) Anticysticercus antibodies in serum and cerebrospinal fluid in patients with cerebral cysticercosis. *Journal of Neurology, Neurosurgery and Psychiatry* **49**: 1044–1049.

Davis LE and Kornfeld M (1991) Neurocysticercosis: neurologic, pathogenic, diagnostic and therapeutic aspects. *European Neurology* **31**: 229–240.

Del Brutto OH (1992) Cysticercosis and cerebrovascular disease: a review. *Journal of Neurology, Neurosurgery and Psychiatry* **55**: 252–254.

Del Brutto OH and Sotelo J (1988) Neurocysticercosis: an update. *Reviews of Infectious Diseases* **10**: 1075–1087.

Del Brutto OH and Sotelo J (1990) Albendazole therapy for subarachnoid and ventricular cysticercosis – case report. *Journal of Neurosurgery* **72**: 816–818.

Desai SB, Shah VC, Javri DJ and Rao P (1991a) Neurocysticercosis: comparison of CT scan and MRI study of 35 cases. *Neuroradiology* **33** (supplement): 578–579.

Desai SB, Shah VC, Tavri OJ and Rao P (1991b) MRI: more specific than CT in cranial tuberculomas. *Neuroradiology* **33** (supplement): 216–218.

Dixon HBF and Hargreaves WH (1944) Cysticercosis (*Taenia solium*): a further ten year's clinical study, covering 284 cases. *Quarterly Journal of Medicine* **52**: 107–121.

Dixon HBF and Lipscomb FM (1961) Cysticercosis: an analysis and follow-up of 450 cases. *Medical Research Council special report series*, No. 299, London: 1–58.

Earnest MP, Barth Reller L, Filley CM and Grek AJ (1987) Neurocysticercosis in the United States: 35 cases and a review. *Reviews of Infectious Diseases* **9**: 961–979.

Escobar A (1983) The pathology of neurocysticercosis. In: *Cysticercosis of the Central Nervous System* (eds E Palacios, J Rodrigues-Carbajal, JM Taveras), pp 27–59. Springfield: Charles Thomas.

Escobedo F, Penagos P, Rodrigues J and Sotelo J (1987) Albendazole therapy for neurocysticercosis. *Archives of Internal Medicine* **147**: 738–741.

Estanol B, Corona T and Abad P (1986) A prognostic classification of cerebral cysticercosis: therapeutic implications. *Journal of Neurology, Neurosurgery and Psychiatry* **49**: 1131–1134.

Estanol B, Juarez H, Irigoyen MDC et al. (1989) Humoral immune response in patients with cerebral parenchymal cysticercosis treated with praziquantel. *Journal of Neurology, Neurosurgery and Psychiatry* **52**: 254–257.

Flisser A, Wodehouse E and Larralde C (1983) The epidemiology of human cysticercosis in Mexico. In: *Cysticercosis of the Central Nervous System* (eds E Palacios, J Rodriguez-Carbajal, JM Taveras), pp 7–17. Springfield: Charles Thomas.

Gardner B, Goldberg M and Heiner D (1984) The natural history of parenchymal central nervous system cysticercosis. *Neurology* **34** (supplement 1): 90.

Gelfand M (1948) Cysticercosis of brain in Africans of Rhodesia. *East African Medical Journal* **25**: 110–117.

Groll EW (1982) Chemotherapy of human cysticercosis with praziquantel. In: *Cysticercosis Present State of Knowledge and Perspectives* (eds A Flisser, K Willms, JP Laclette, C Larralde, C Ridaura and F Beltran), pp 207–218. New York: Academic Press.

Kramer LD (1990) Antihelminthic therapy for neurocysticercosis. *Archives of Neurology* **47**: 1059.

Kramer LD, Locke GE, Byrd SE and Daryabagi J (1989) Cerebral cysticercosis: documentation of natural history with CT. *Radiology* **171**: 459–462.

Leblanc R, Knowles K, Melanson D et al. (1986) Neurocysticercosis: surgical and medical management of praziquantel. *Neurosurgery* **18**: 419–427.

Lopez-Hernandez A and Garaizar C (1982) Childhood cerebral cysticercosis: clinical features and computed tomographic findings in 89 Mexican children. *Canadian Journal of Neurological Sciences* **9**: 401–407.

MacArthur WP (1934) Cysticercosis as seen in the British Army with special reference to the production of epilepsy. *Transactions of the Royal Society of Tropical Medicine and Hygiene* **27**: 343–363.

MacArthur W (1950) Cysticercosis. In: *British Encyclopaedia of Medical Practice*, vol. 4, 2nd edn (ed. Lord Horder), pp 111–225. London: Butterworths.

McCormick GF (1985) Cysticercosis: review of 230 patients. *Bulletin of Clinical Neuro Sciences* **50**: 76–101.

McCormick GF, Zee CS and Heiden J (1982) Cysticercosis cerebri: review of 127 cases. *Archives of Neurology* **39**: 534–539.

McRobert GR (1944) Somatic taeniasis (solium cysticercosis). *Indian Medical Gazette* **79**: 399–400.

Mahajan RC (1982) Geographical distribution of human cysticercosis. In: *Cysticercosis: Present State of Knowledge and Perspectives* (eds A Flisser, K Willms, TP Laclette, C Larralde, C Ridaura and F Beltram), pp 39–46. New York: Academic Press.

Mani AJ, Ramesh CK, Ahuja GK and Mani KS (1974) Cerebral cysticercosis presenting as epilepsy. *Neurology (India)* **22**: 30–34.

Nieto D (1956) Cysticercosis of the nervous system, diagnosis by means of the spinal fluid complement fixation test. *Neurology* **6**: 725–737.

Priest R (1926) A case of extensive somatic dissemination of cysticercosis cellulose in man. *British Medical Journal* **2**: 471–472.

Rajshekher V, Wilson M and Schantz PM (1991) Cysticercus immunoblot assay in Indian patients with single, small enhancing CT lesions. *Journal of Neurology, Neurosurgery and Psychiatry* **54**: 561.

Rajshekher V, Haran RP, Shankar Prakash G and Chandy MJ (1993) Differentiating solitary small cysticercus granulomas and tuberculomas in patients with epilepsy. *Journal of Neurosurgery* **78**: 402–407.

Rosas N, Sotelo J and Nieto D (1986) ELISA in the diagnosis of neurocysticercosis. *Archives of Neurology* **43**: 353–356.

Scharf D (1988) Neurocysticercosis. *Archives of Neurology* **45**: 777–780.

Sethi PK, Kumar BR, Madan VS *et al.* (1985) Appearing and disappearing CT scan abnormalities and seizures. *Journal of Neurology, Neurosurgery and Psychiatry* **48**: 866–869.

Sotelo J (1988) Cysticercosis. In: *Handbook of Clinical Neurology*, 8 (52) (eds PJ Vinken and GW Bruyn), pp 529–534. Amsterdam: Elsevier Science Publishers.

Sotelo J (1990) Antihelminthic therapy for neurocysticercosis. *Archives of Neurology* **47**: 1059–1060.

Sotelo J, Escobedo F, Rodriguez-Carbajal J, Torres B and Rubio-Donnadieu F (1984) Therapy of parenchymal brain cysticercosis with praziquantel. *New England Journal of Medicine* **310**: 1001–1007.

Sotelo J, Gurrero V and Rubio F (1985a) Neurocysticercosis. New classification based on active and inactive forms. A study of 753 cases. *Archives of Internal Medicine* **145**: 442–445.

Sotelo J, Torres B, Rubio-Donnadieu F, Escobedo F and Rodriguez-Carbajal R (1985b) Praziquantel in the treatment of neurocysticercosis: long term follow-up. *Neurology* **35**: 752–755.

Sotelo J, Penagos P, Escobedo F and Del Brutto OH (1988) Short course of albendazole therapy for neurocysticercosis. *Archives of Neurology* **45**: 1130–1133.

Suss RA, Maravilla KR and Thomson J (1986) MR Imaging of intracranial cysticercosis.

Comparison with CT and anatomopathologic features. *American Journal of Neuroradiology* **7**: 235–242.

Takayanagui OM and Jardim E (1992) Therapy of neurocysticercosis. Comparison between albendazole and praziquantel. *Archives of Neurology* **49**: 290–294.

Tandon PN (1983) Cerebral cysticercosis. *Neurology Review* **6**: 119–127.

Teitelbaum GP, Otto RJ, Lin M *et al.* (1989) MR imaging of neurocysticercosis. *American Journal of Neuroradiology* **10**: 709–718.

Trelles JO and Trelles L (1978) Cysticercosis of the nervous system. In: *Handbook of Clinical Neurology*, 35 (eds PJ Vinken and GW Bruyn), pp 291–320. Amsterdam: North-Holland Publishers.

Tsang VCW, Brand JA and Boyer AE (1989) An enzyme-linked immunoelectrotransfer blot assay and glycoprotein antigens for diagnosing human cysticercosis (*Taenia solium*). *Journal of Infectious Diseases* **159**: 50–59.

Vasconcelos D, Cruz-Segura H, Mateos-Gomez H and Alanis GZ (1987) Selective indications for the use of praziquantel in the treatment of brain cysticercosis. *Journal of Neurology, Neurosurgery and Psychiatry* **50**: 383–388.

Vazquez ML, Jung H and Sotelo J (1987) Plasma levels of praziquantel decrease when dexamethasone given simultaneously. *Neurology* **37**: 1561–1562.

Vazquez V and Sotelo J (1992) The course of seizures after treatment for cerebral cysticercosis. *New England Journal of Medicine* **327**: 696–701.

Venkataraman S (1989) Neurocysticercosis scene in India. In: *Progress in Clinical Neurosciences*, 5 (eds KK Sinha and P Chandra), pp 297–314. Ranchi: Catholic Press.

Wadia RS, Makhale CN, Kelkar AV and Grant KB (1987) Focal epilepsy in India with special reference to lesions showing ring or disc-like enhancement on contrast computed tomography. *Journal of Neurology, Neurosurgery and Psychiatry* **50**: 1298–1301.

Wadia NH, Desai SB and Bhatt M (1988) Disseminated cysticercosis – new observations including CT scan findings and experience with treatment by praziquantel. *Brain* **111**: 597–614.

Wani MA, Banerji AK, Tandon PN and Bhargava S (1981) Neurocysticercosis – some uncommon presentations. *Neurology (India)* **29**: 58–63.

Yingkun F, Shan O, Xiuzhen Z and Shulian Y (1979) Clinicoelectroencephelographic studies of cerebral cysticercosis – 158 cases. *Chinese Medical Journal* **92** (11): 770–786.

Zhi-biao Xu, Wen-Kai C, Hui-lan Z, Man-ling F and Wei-ji C (1985) Praziquantel in treatment of cysticercosis cellulosae report of 200 cases. *Chinese Medical Journal* **98** (7): 489–494.

Zini D, Farrell VJR and Wadee AA (1990) The relationship of antibody levels to the clinical spectrum of human neurocysticercosis. *Journal of Neurology, Neurosurgery and Psychiatry* **53**: 656–661.

16

African Trypanosomiasis

Michel Dumas

Institute of Neurological Epidemiology and Tropical Neurology,
Faculty of Medicine, 87025 Limoges Cedex, France

INTRODUCTION

Human African trypanosomiasis or sleeping sickness is caused by infestation with a flagellate protozoan, the trypanosome, which is inoculated by the bite of the tsetse fly *Glossina*. The particular ecological conditions of the parasites are such that sleeping sickness is only found in the intertropical regions of Africa, between the latitudes 15° North and 15° South.

HISTORY AND EPIDEMIOLOGY

The disease was recognized at the turn of the century in Liverpool by identification of *Trypanosoma gambiense* in the blood of a British officer sent home from service in Gambia. The disease was known, but not identified in the Gulf of Benin during the slave trade. Some years later, *T. rhodesiense* was isolated in Rhodesia. There was a particularly serious propagation of the disease in the first quarter of the century principally in Cameroon where it decimated populations over a wide area until Dr Jamot, a French Army doctor, set up a comprehensive programme of diagnosis and treatment. The systematic search for patients in villages and their treatment effectively eliminated this appalling disease throughout West Africa. By 1960, the disease had virtually been eradicated. Unfortunately, the relaxation of detection and treatment programmes, the degradation of sanitation and the political instability of many countries has led to a resurgence of the disease which is now found in the outskirts of large towns, where it is propagated by a rural population attracted to urban centres. Sleeping sickness is fast becoming a major public health problem in a number of countries in the intertropical zones of Africa. It is estimated that 50 million people are exposed to the disease, and the number is increasing each year, with, in affected regions, a current prevalence between 50 and 70 per 10 000.

The increasing prevalence is not helped by the absence of totally safe and effective drugs or vaccines. It is also unfortunate that the high cost of research compared with the low incomes of the populations at risk from this disease does not provide a sufficient incentive for drug development.

BIOLOGY

The vector of the trypanosome is a fly of mean length 10 mm called the tsetse fly or *Glossina*. The two wings of the fly are folded one on top of the other covering the back. Males and females live in forest or savanna where the females lay eggs in shaded, soft ground. Strictly haematophagic, they tend to bite man or animals in the heat of the day. The flies may thus become contaminated with the trypanosome which multiplies in the salivary glands of the insect. The fly remains infectious over the 3–4 months of its lifespan. Fortunately the *Glossina* is a poor vector, and only 10% of flies feeding on a host harbouring trypanosomes become infected. Moreover, the female only lays around six eggs during her lifetime.

The African trypanosome is a flagellate extracellular protozoan, morphologically different from *T. cruzi* the parasite responsible for American trypanosomiasis. This difference is still not definitely established as the trypanosome may assume an amastigotic form, especially in the cells of the choroid plexus and ependyma (Ormerod and Venkatesan, 1971; Mattern *et al.*, 1972), a point disputed by other workers. It is important to clarify this issue since it has significance not only in understanding the pathophysiology of the disease, but also on the effects of treatment.

Although there are many species of trypanosome, only two, belonging to the subgroup *T. brucei* are likely to lead to human disease: *T. brucei gambiense* found in West Africa, transmitted by *Glossina palpalis or G. trichinoides* and *T. brucei rhodesiense* found in East Africa, transmitted by *G. morsitans* or *G. swynnertoni*. They are quite similar morphologically, but have different pathogenicity. *T. brucei rhodesiense* leads to a more virulent and acute condition, although for each species of trypanosome there are strains of different virulence, which account, at least in part, for the interindividual variability in the clinical course.

After penetration into the organism, the trypanosome multiplies locally at the point of inoculation, and then propagates through the lymphatics and bloodstream where the trypanosomes continue to multiply. The parasite thus invades the whole organism, rapidly entering the central nervous system. These different stages can explain the chronology of the appearance of the clinical, biological and neurological signs.

The trypanosomes invade rapidly the central nervous system, probably within days of inoculation and possibly even within the first few hours. It is important to bear this in mind when deciding on treatment since many drugs which are active against the trypanosome do not cross the blood–brain barrier. This may account for numerous therapeutic failures. The trypanosome may remain latent in the central nervous system for long periods of time, while retaining the ability to reinvade the general circulation (Jennings *et al.*, 1979). The parasites can thus hide in the central nervous system (Evans and Brightman, 1980) where they may turn into an intracellular form, especially within cells of the choroid plexus.

Moreover, the trypanosome has the ability to alter its antigenic determinants on recognition by the host's immune system. It thus effectively transforms itself into a new trypanosome giving rise to a new crop of antibodies in the host. In this way it can evade the host's immune defences, which accounts for the hyper-gammaglobulinaemia and the pathogenesis of many tissue lesions.

A generalized immune response involving the hepatosplenolymphatic system follows infestation. The marked tropism for the central nervous system is particularly evident in mesodiencephalic structures, giving rise to perivascular inflammatory lesions with proliferation of histiocytic and plasmocytic lymphocytes. The plasmocytic lymphocytes are characteristically hypertrophied and filled with vacuoles and are referred to as Mott cells. Although the exact role of immune complexes is unclear, they are undoubtedly responsible for the generalized vasculitis predominating in heart and brain and extending to small vessels. This possibly accounts for the presence of antiheart antibodies. The renal lesions causing renal insufficiency are due to deposits of immune complexes in renal glomeruli.

The same autoimmune reactions contribute to the onset of encephalitis. Deposits of immune complexes favour liberation of plasma kinins which enhance vascular permeability leading to a breakdown of the blood–brain barrier, a critical point in the course of the disease. At this time, nerve tissue and especially myelin becomes exposed to the general circulation and immunocompetent cells. Damaged myelin can thus become a further antigen responsible for the neurological symptoms and the mesenchymatous inflammation. The disease evolves towards a demyelinating condition with lymphoplasmocytes infiltrating from the sites of perivenous leukoencephalic reactions. The antimyelin antibodies binding intact myelin lead to a self-propagating autoimmune reaction, which accounts for the marked demyelination found in the late stages of the disease.

Apart from human trypanosomiasis, there are numerous animal trypanosomiases caused by similar trypanosomes, but which are not thought to affect man. However, some animals appear to act as a reservoir for the human parasites, antelopes for *T. rhodesiense*, and probably domestic animals such as the pig and chicken for *T. gambiense*. This will clearly tend to enhance dissemination of the disease since the *Glossina* feeds equally on the blood of animals or humans. Animal trypanosomiasis kills much livestock, and thus reduces the protein supply to the population at risk, with significant public health and economic consequences.

NEUROPATHOLOGY

The main kinds of lesion commonly found are those reflecting meningoencephalitis, and consisting of infiltrates of Mott cells involving all meninges and perivascular spaces from the pericapillary and perivenous spaces diffusing into the parenchyma. Early on in the disease, electronmicroscopic examination may show the presence of trypanosomes in the choroid plexus and extravascular spaces (Van Marck *et al.*, 1981; Poltera, 1985). Obstructive vasculitis may occur in various locations, but affects predominantly white matter in the cerebral hemispheres and cerebellum. In order of frequency, the most severely involved structures are: thalamus, mesencephalon, frontal lobes, temporal lobes, cerebellum, occipital lobes and olfactory bulb. These lesions are present, but slight, during the lymphaticohaematological phase. They become major during the phase of invasion of nerve tissue, but are unrelated to the duration of the condition.

A diffuse gliosis is noted, especially in the white matter of the cerebral hemispheres and cerebellum. The myelin appears as diffuse, poorly defined pale patches, while the cerebral grey matter is always involved along with the periventricular, hypophyseal and hypothalamic formations.

CLINICAL FEATURES

The dominant clinical manifestations which portray the neurological tropism of the parasite appear after a silent period of incubation of variable duration and a lymphaticohaematological phase in which general signs predominate.

Incubation

The incubation period varies from between 2 to 3 weeks and several years, and follows an initial reaction at the site of the insect bite. This is an indurated, painful, erythematous lesion resembling a furuncle which does not, however, suppurate, and which disappears spontaneously within 3 weeks. It is accompanied by enlargement of surrounding lymph nodes, slight fever and a feeling of general malaise.

General or Lymphaticohaematological Phase

The general signs reflect the reaction of the host's immune system to the spread of the trypanosomes throughout the organism. General signs, lymphadenopathy, hepatosplenomegaly, myocarditis and skin lesions appear gradually, and may last for months or years. There are variable periods of latency and remission. These may be a function of the virulence of the strain of parasite, but are largely related to individual differences in the immune response.

Fever is a consistent sign, with a temperature fluctuating around 38°C. It is resistant to treatment, and accompanies the alteration in general state. It has no particular circadian rhythm. Lymphadenopathies are mainly localized in the cervical and subclavicular chains, especially at the trapezoids, giving rise to Winterbottom's sign. There is no surrounding inflammation, and they are small, hard, mobile and painless. They do not suppurate, but trypanosomes can be isolated at this stage from puncture aspirates.

The moderate hepatosplenomegaly is not a cardinal sign of the disease, although the hepatomegaly may be painful (15% of cases). The cardiovascular system is always involved, but in contrast to American trypanosomiasis, cardiac signs are not an essential feature of the disease. A reduced pulse pressure often in the presence of a small heart, is paradoxically accompanied by a rather characteristic concentric muscular hypertrophy. The cardiac symptomatology is probably a result of the strong immune response. An endocrine syndrome is particularly common during the progression of this phase to the neurological phase. The main features are amenorrhoea and impotence often associated with hypogonadism, although circulating levels of hypophyseal gonadotrophic hormones are not altered (Noireau *et al.*, 1988). Weight loss, hypothermia and asthenia are common. Circulating levels of hypophyseal hormones are not altered, and the disorder is either of supra- or extra-hypophyseal origin (Hublart *et al.*, 1988).

Cutaneous signs, although characteristic, are only observed in 15% of cases. The polycyclic lesions or trypanids are not easily detected on black skin. They usually appear on the trunk and limb roots, and they tend to come and go in no particular pattern. Oedema is common, especially in the lower limbs and face. Varying degrees of pruritis occur in about 50% of cases (Boa *et al.*, 1988).

Renal involvement is indicated by proteinuria. Pulmonary disorders, although common, are probably a result of secondary intercurrent infections in immunocompromised individuals.

Neurological disorders at this phase reflect the rapid invasion of meninges and brain. Three out of four patients suffer from diffuse, frequent headaches of moderate intensity. Diffuse pain (root pain, paraesthesia in the extremeties, joint pain, cramps) is particularly characteristic when associated with deep hyperaesthesia and myalgia. At this stage, there are only slight electroencephalographic disturbances indicated by a desynchronization and lability of rhythm, and the appearance of theta waves.

Phase of Cerebral Involvement

This phase with an insidious onset over a period of months or years, follows on from the phase described previously. The generalized symptomatology which predominates initially gradually gives way to more specific neuropsychiatric signs. There is usually a marked asthenia with hypothermia throughout this phase. Secondary infections should be investigated in all cases with hypothermia.

Pyramidal involvement is observed as a diffuse hyperactivity of tendon reflexes with bilateral Babinski sign, Hoffmann's sign and sometimes knee and ankle clonus. Primitive reflexes (peri-oral and cheiro-oral reflexes) appear in around 70% of cases. The intensity of these signs increases during the course of the condition, and may be accompanied by a grasp reflex. The motor disorders rarely progress to paralysis, although some cases of hemiplegia have been reported (Sonan *et al.*, 1988). There is often a characteristic impairment in initiation of movement. Cranial nerve paralysis and peripheral nerve involvement with polyradiculoneuritis are very rare (Van Bogaert and Janssens, 1957). Abnormal movements are consistently observed, although there is considerable interindividual variation. They may be seen as a slight resting and intention tremor, true choreoathetoid movements and buccolingual hyperkinesia. Overall these movements are seen as an incessant gesticulation with instability, grimacing and lack of precision in the execution of movement, which is characteristic of the disease. Isolated zones of myoclonus may also be observed. These dyskinesias vary considerably from one patient to another, both in their outward signs and localization. Disorders of tone are observed mostly as an extrapyramidal hypertonia with increased resistance and very occasionally as hypotonia. Sensory disorders appear early in the course of the condition. The deep hyperaesthesia described by Kerandel is quite characteristic, and any sensory stimulus is perceived as painful.

In the early phases of the disease, there is a complete disruption of the normal circadian sleep wakefulness cycle (Buguet *et al.*, 1989). These disturbances become progressively more severe, and are found in 68% of cases (Boa *et al.*, 1988). The common designation of this disease as sleeping sickness is well deserved, as the disorganization of the normal sleep–waking cycle is a cardinal outward sign. However, these disorders are less common in infestations due to *T. rhodesiense*, which have a more acute course. In the last stages, there is perpetual somnolence, the patient has great difficulty in maintaining attention and immediately falls asleep in the absence of stimulation.

Mental disorders are as common as those of sensation and sleep, although they may not always be readily discriminated from the attentional disorders. The symptomatology is one of behavioural disturbances with agitation and aggression, sometimes accompanied by psychotic episodes, criminal behaviour, fugues and impulsiveness. The psychiatric symptomatology is highly variable, although it is usually observed as indifference, with a circadian cyclothymia in mood. The endocrine disorders seen during the lymphaticohaematological phase increase in severity, with complete loss of libido, and thyroid insufficiency. The constant feeling of cold makes the patient seek the sun.

The terminal phase of the disease is that of a demyelinating encephalitis. By this stage, the lesions are irreversible. Exacerbation of the disorders of consciousness is accompanied by a state of dementia with incoherence, senility, stereotypic behaviour and epileptic fits with marked wasting and somnolent cachexia. The patient is bedridden, expressionless and indifferent, and usually dies of an intercurrent infection.

Clinical Forms

The clinical picture described represents the generally observed scenario, although the duration of each stage can never be determined accurately.

Death may ensue rapidly in the acute and hyperacute forms which are characterized by high fever and a marked alteration in general state with severe myocardial involvement. Other cases evolve slowly with latency periods of several years, which gives a false impression of cure. These 'clinical silences' must be borne in mind, as an abrupt relapse or a deterioration in state of the patient due to an intercurrent infection can occur at any time. Some of these clinical latent periods may arise from the use of drugs which do not cross the blood–brain barrier and thus do not destroy trypanosomes in the brain. There may be an improvement in the general symptomatology without a true cure of the disease.

Some hemiplegic and pseudotumoral forms with raised intracranial pressure and papilloedema may be mistaken for other diseases (Collomb *et al.*, 1968). In children, the clinical expression of the disease is also highly variable. It presents essentially as a neurological disease with disorders of tone, involuntary movements and disorders of sleep with altered consciousness. Minor behavioural disturbances with a change in personality are common, accompanied by a moderate rise in temperature. The child may be infested directly from a bite or via the placenta (Debroise *et al.*, 1968; Burke *et al.*, 1974).

In the disease due to *T. rhodesiense* the infection is generally more severe and pursues a fulminating course; the marked disorders of consciousness and sleep follow a 3–6 month early phase.

DIAGNOSIS

In endemic areas, the diagnosis is readily established from the clinical signs during the neurological phase of the disease. However, whether in endemic regions or elsewhere the diagnosis is less easy to establish in the early phases in the absence of any changes in cerebrospinal fluid (CSF). Even in the presence of CSF changes, isolation of the trypanosome, the only sure basis of the correct diagnosis, is not straightforward. Nevertheless, the high sensitivity of current immunological tests can indicate the diagnosis with a high degree of certainty.

Depending on the phase of the disease, the trypanosome may be isolated in the initial lesions (in very few cases) and then in lymph nodes, blood and CSF. Trypanosomes can be identified from their mobility on direct examination between slide and cover-slip of a centrifuged drop of blood. This may be aided by staining with May–Grunwald–Giemsa solution. The parasite may be more readily identified after triple centrifugation, culture of blood on NNN medium and filtration on cellulose columns followed by further centrifugation. However, direct identification of the trypanosome is often difficult. Inoculation of the blood or CSF to a sensitive animal (white mouse, or laboratory rat after ensuring that there is no infestation with *T. lewisi* which is common in these rodents) may be required.

If the immunological tests are in favour of trypanosomiasis, the parasite must be isolated before treatment. It is extremely uncommon that the trypanosome is not discovered after careful use of the above techniques, although more than one sample may have to be examined. In many cases, large amounts of CSF (60–80 ml) may be required before identifying the trypanosome in the pellet obtained by gentle centrifugation. The CSF must always be examined whatever the clinical phase of the disease. Even in the very early stages there may be a moderate elevation in cell content; this progressively increases without a concomitant increase in protein content which rarely exceeds 1 g l^{-1}. The presence of lymphocytes and sometimes plasmocytes (Mott cells) is highly suggestive of the diagnosis. The cell count rarely exceeds 400 per ml, although this figure may increase slightly after treatment.

The immunological reaction is reflected by an increase in gammaglobulins in both serum and CSF. In serum, both IgM and IgG are raised, but not IgA, IgE and IgD. Four-fold increases in levels of IgM are frequently found. An elevation of this order in endemic regions is a strong indication of a diagnosis of trypanosomiasis. In leukaemia and dysproteinaemia, IgM levels in CSF are generally within normal limits. In trypanosomiasis, however, electrophoresis of protein reveals a marked elevation in gammaglobulins, which exceed 40% of the total protein count. Increases of this magnitude are only rarely found in other diseases; they may, however, be found in tuberculous meningitis, neurosyphilis, or subacute sclerosing panencephalitis. Serological tests can discriminate between these possibilities.

Indirect immunofluorescence at a threshold of 1/160 is highly specific, although cross-reactions with leishmaniasis can occur. The specificity is higher in the CSF. ELISA tests now used routinely have a higher sensitivity for antibodies with a soluble antigen, and can establish the diagnosis in 90% of cases. However, these costly and time-consuming tests are not feasible for screening purposes, for which indirect haemagglutination tests are preferable. The Testrypcatt (agglutination on a slide) is now widely used. Although sensitive, there are numerous cross-reactions, and the test results need to be confirmed with more sensitive methods. This test is useful for early identification. Another indirect haemagglutination test, the Cellognost is more specific and sensitive than both the Testrypcatt and indirect immunofluorescence (Lemesre *et al.*, 1988). Methods for detecting trypanosome antigens in serum or CSF using monoclonal antibodies gives positive reactions in over 93% of cases, and appear to be highly specific (Nantulya, 1988). These methods hold considerable promise, but the results await confirmation in larger series of patients.

None of these antigenic reactions can supplant physical identification of the parasite. The inherent toxicity of the available methods of treatment necessitates absolute certainty of the diagnosis, especially as the serological tests, albeit sensitive, may not have absolute specificity. The major error is missing the diagnosis in the early stages when the neurological signs are too non-specific to demand lumbar puncture. A dysglobulinaemia in a patient who has resided in an endemic area should also evoke a search for trypanosomiasis.

Electroencephalography (EEG) can aid in establishing the diagnosis by demonstrating the characteristic impairment in vigilance at a very early stage of the disease. EEG is also of value for monitoring treatment (Ormerod and Raseroka, 1988). The waking tracings even during the cerebral phase of the disease are not specific, although synchronous symmetrical bursts of delta waves during the normally unaffected background rhythm may be suggestive. In advanced stages, this background rhythm disappears, and the bursts of slow waves tend to come at more regular intervals. In contrast, the sleep waves are much more suggestive as they are markedly altered in the cerebral stage even though the waking traces are only slightly affected. Sleep is superficial with slow deep sleep (stage IV) disrupted by frequent waking. The overall duration of sleep is markedly reduced. The transients during the first stages of sleep are absent, and there is a certain randomness in the tracings which makes it difficult to identify the different stages which tend to merge together. These changes in sleep tracings are observed in the early stages of the disease even before there is clinical evidence of nervous system involvement.

Neuroradiological examinations (CT scan and MRI) have only been used in a limited number of patients. They show diffuse zones of hypodensity indicating demyelination of the centrum semiovale and periventricular regions.

TREATMENT

Treatment of this disease is based on the use of trivalent and pentavalent arsenical drugs of which the most widely used at present is melarsoprol. These drugs are highly toxic and must be used with care as they cause a severe toxic encephalopathy which is often fatal (around 5% mortality). Unfortunately, these are the only effective drugs which cross the blood–brain barrier. Other drugs (pentamidine, suramine, diminazene aceturate) are better tolerated and equally effective, but do not cross the blood–brain barrier. With these drugs, there is, therefore, a considerable risk of progression of the disease to the neurological phase.

The total injected dose of melarsoprol should not exceed 1620 mg with a maximum of 3.6 mg kg^{-1} and a maximum single intravenous dose of 200 mg. Individual titration of the dosage and the schedule of treatment is preferable to the usual fixed regimen of one injection every 10 days for 30 days. Individual dose titration can reduce the risk of an ensuing encephalitis (Dumas *et al.*, 1976). Various regimens have been proposed of combinations with corticosteroids or adrenaline, although there is no firm evidence for a beneficial effect. The risk of encephalitis is always present. However, a combination of melarsoprol with intravenous calcium appears to be of value (Clarkson and Amole, 1982).

Numerous agents have been tried in the treatment of this disease, although the results have generally been disappointing. Derivatives of imidazole show some promise, especially as some of them cross the blood–brain barrier (Bouteille *et al.*, 1988a). Benzonidazole appears to be effective in 80% of acute cases of American trypanosomiasis, but has no lasting action against human African trypanosomiasis. It is also neurotoxic.

A line of research has focused on trypanosome protein metabolism, as the parasite has difficulty in synthesizing purine bases. Among the purine-containing amino acids, ornithine is involved in the production of polyamines which play a role in protein and nucleic acid synthesis in the trypanosome. Difluoromethylornithine (DFMO), an inhibitor of ornithine decarboxylase, the enzyme which transforms ornithine into putrecine (Breton *et al.*, 1988) has been proposed for human use. It is effective, but not infallible, especially in children or towards *T. rhodesiense*. It also has the disadvantage of only being usable at a dose of 400 mg kg^{-1} day^{-1} for 2 weeks via the intravenous route, or at 300 mg kg^{-1} day^{-1} for 1 month via the oral route (Doua *et al.*, 1988). This drug is not currently available for use.

No effective vaccines have yet been developed in spite of the strong antigenic potential of the trypanosome, as this parasite is particularly deft at avoiding the host's immune defences by modifying its own antigenic variants. This camouflage strategy effectively rules out the use of classical vaccines. While further research is undertaken, hopes for future treatment lie in the combination of various agents each having partial activity (Jennings, 1988; Ormerod and Roseroka, 1988). Finally, recent studies in sheep have confirmed the effectiveness of melarsoprol at a reduced dosage, which might lessen the incidence of toxic encephalopathy (Bouteille *et al.*, 1988b).

REFERENCES

Boa YF, Traore MA, Doua F *et al.* (1988) Les différents tableaux cliniques actuels de la trypanosomiase humaine africaine à *T. b. gambiense*. Analyse de 300 dossiers du foyer de Daloa, Côte d'Ivoire. *Bulletin de la Societe de Pathologie Exotique et de ses Filiales* **81**: 427–444.

Bouteille B, Darde Ml, Pestre Alexandre M *et al.* (1988a) Traitement de la trypanosomiase expérimentale du mouton à *Trypanosoma brucei*: recerce d'une dose minima active de mélarsoprol. *Bulletin de la Societe de Pathologie Exotique et de ses Filiales* **81**: 548–554.

Bouteille B, Darde ML, Pestre Alexandre M *et al.* (1988b) Traitement de la trypanosomiase expérimentale du mouton à *Trypanosoma brucei* brucei: efficacité du Ro 15–0216 (derivé 2-nitroimidazolé). *Bulletin de la Societé de Pathologie Exotique et de ses Filiales* **81**: 616–622.

Breton JC, Bouteille B and Sonan T (1988) Le DFMO: alternative thérapeutique de la trypanosomiase humaine africaine. *Bulletin de la Societé de Pathologie Exotique et de ses Filiales* **81**: 571–577.

Buguet A, Gati R, Sevre JP *et al.* (1989) 24 hour polysomnographic evaluation in a patient with sleeping sickness. *Electroencephalography and Clinical Neurophysiology* **72**: 471–478.

Burke JA, Bengosi ME and Diantete NL (1974) Un cas de trypanosomiase africaine (*T. gambiense*) congénitale. *Annales de la Société Belge de Médecine Tropicale* **54**: 1–4.

Clarkson AB and Amole BO (1982) Role of calcium in trypanocidal drug action. *Science* **216**: 1321–1323.

Collomb H, Virieu R, Dumas M and Ayats H (1968) Les formes pseudo-tumorales avec hémiplégie de la trypanosomiase humaine africaine (à propos de quatre observations). *Bulletin de la Societé Médicale d'Afrique Noire de Langue Française* **13**: 734–737.

Debroise A, Debroise-Ballereau C, Satge P and Rey M (1968) La trypanosomiase africaine du jeune enfant. *Archives Francaises de Pédiatrié* **25**: 703–720.

Doua F, Boa YF, Schechter *et al.* (1988) L'alpha-difluorométhylornithine (Eflornithine) dans le traitement de la trypanosomiase humaine africaine à *T. gambiense* au stade tardif: efficacité et tolérance (à propos de 14 cas). *Bulletin de la Societé de Pathologie Exotique et de ses Filiales* **81**: 589–590.

Dumas M, Girard PL and N'Diaye IP (1976) Traitement de la trypanosomiase humaine africaine en milieu hospitalier. *Médecine d'Afrique Noire* **23**: 39–41.

Evans DA and Brightman CAJ (1980) Pleomorphism and the problem of recrudescent parasitaemia following treatment with salicylhydroxamic acid (SHAM) in African trypanosomiasis. *Transactions of the Royal Society of Tropical Medicine and Hygiene* **74**: 601–604.

Hublart M, Lagouche L, Ragadot A *et al.* (1988) Fonction endocrine et trypanosomiase africaine. Bilan de 79 cas. *Bulletin de la Societé de Pathologie Exotique et de ses Filiales* **81**: 468–476.

Jennings FW (1988) Augmentation d'efficacité des arsenicaux avec la difluorméthyl-ornithine: études experimentales dans la trypanosomiase murine. *Bulletin de la Societé de Pathologie Exotique et de ses Filiales* **81**: 595–607.

Jennings FW, Whitelaw DD, Holmes PH *et al.* (1979) The brain as a source of relapsing *Trypanosoma brucei* infection in mice after chemotherpay. *International Journal for Parasitology* **9**: 381–384.

Lemesre JL, Noireau F, Makoundou ML *et al.* (1988) Apport des techniques sérologiques dans l'analyse du liquide céphalo-rachidien de patients congolais atteints de la maladie du sommeil. *Bulletin de la Societé de Pathologie Exotique et de ses Filiales* **81**: 506–510.

Mattern P, Mayer G and Felici M (1972) Existence de formes amastigotes de *Trypanosoma gambiense* dans le tissu plexuel choroidien de la souris infectée expérimentalement. *Comptes Rendus de l'Academie des Sciences (Paris)* **274**: 1513–1515.

Nantulya VM (1988) Immunodiagnostic de la maladie du sommeil à *T. rhodesiense*: détection des antigènes circulants de trypanosomes dans le sérum et le liquide cérébrospinal par immuno-essai enzymatique utilisant un anticorps monoclonal. *Bulletin de la Societé de Pathologie Exotique et de ses Filiales* **81**: 511–512.

Noireau F, Apembet JD and Frezil JL (1988) Revue clinique des troubles endocriniens observés chez l'adulte trypanosomé. *Bulletin de la Societé de Pathologie Exotique et de ses Filiales* **81**: 464–467.

Ormerod WE and Raseroka BH (1988) Criblage de molécules pour un traitement sans rechute de la maladie du sommeil. *Bulletin de la Societé de Pathologie Exotique et de ses Filiales* **81**: 543–547.

Ormerod WE and Venkatesan S (1971) An amastigote phase of the sleeping sickness trypanosome. *Transactions of the Royal Society of Tropical Medicine and Hygiene* **65**: 6–741.

Poltera AA (1985) Pathology of human African trypanosomiasis with reference to experimental African trypanosomiasis and infections of the central nervous system. *British Medical Bulletin* **41**: 169.

Sonan T, Giordano C, Boa F and Dumas M (1988) Formes hémiplégiques de la trypanosomiase humaine africaine. *Bulletin de la Societé de Pathologie Exotique et de ses Filiales* **81**: 459–463.

Van Bogaert L and Janssens P (1957) Contribution à l'étude de la neurologie et neuropathologie de la trypanosomiase humaine. *Annales de la Societé Belge de Médecine Tropicale* **37**: 379–427.

Van Marck EAE, Le Ray D, Beckers A *et al.* (1981) Light and electron microscope studies on extravascular *Trypanosoma brucei gambiense* in the brain of chronically infected rodents. *Annales de la Societé Belge de Médecine Tropicale* **61**: 57–78.

17

American Trypanosomiasis

Antonio Spina-França

Neurology Investigation Centre, Department of Neurology, Faculty of Medicine, The University of Sao Paulo, PO Box 5199, 01051–970 Sao Paulo, Brazil

INTRODUCTION

American trypanosomiasis (AT) is a parasitic disease which was described by Carlos Chagas at the beginning of this century and bears his name. He also identified the aetiologic agent, its biological cycle, vectors and natural reservoirs (Chagas, 1911). The investigations performed by Chagas and his collaborators led to a body of research on AT that continues to this day. Involvement of the central and peripheral nervous systems has been known since the first studies of this disease.

This chapter reviews the essential characteristics of the nervous system involvement in AT. The present state of knowledge of AT (Kirshhoff, 1993), as well as previously published critical evaluations (Spina-França and Mattosinho-França, 1978, 1988) of the reports of nervous system involvement, are also included.

BIOLOGY

Trypanosoma cruzi is the flagellate protozoan causing AT. In its biological cycle, the amastigote form, which is rounded or elliptical, is found inside the host's cells. The trypomastigote form, which is elongated ($20 \times 1 \times 2$ μm), is found in the bloodstream outside the cells. There are several strains of *T. cruzi* and it is those of high virulence that involve the nervous system.

Both vertebrate and invertebrate hosts participate in the *T. cruzi* biological cycle and vertebrates are the permanent hosts. Several wild vertebrates function as natural reservoirs but domestic animals such as cats and dogs can also become permanent hosts. The invertebrate hosts are the vectors for the *T. cruzi* and they are represented by several species of the genus *Triatomina* – the assassin bugs or cone-nosed bugs. These invertebrates are large, flying haematophagous hemipterous insects of the family Reduviidae that feed by stinging vertebrate animals.

T. cruzi is found in the vector's faeces deposited while stinging and enters through broken skin or mucous membrane. The biological cycle for the *T. cruzi* is completed when a *Triatomina* insect becomes infected by stinging and sucking the blood of an infected vertebrate.

Wild assassin bugs perpetuate the *T. cruzi* infection among vertebrate animals that function as natural reservoirs and semiwild *Triatomina* species are the vectors for domestic animals. *Triatomina* adapted to human dwellings are responsible for the transmission of *T. cruzi* to humans and for maintenance of the endemic infection.

HUMAN INFECTION

Humans, particularly children, are stung by the vector on the uncovered skin such as the face. Low socioeconomic status is common in endemic AT areas. The population at risk lives in precariously constructed clay houses with roofs made out of straw. *Triatomina* are usually present in the cracks and fissures of these dwellings. The vector comes out of its shelter at night to feed on blood. Human infection can result from other mechanisms, by placental fetal infection and by blood transfusions (Schmuñiz, 1991).

American trypanosomiasis is endemic only in Latin American between latitudes 25° North and 38° South. It is present independent of climate, temperature and altitude. High prevalence areas exist which are distributed irregularly and are particularly found in regions where vectors have adapted to human dwellings. The non-urban population is mostly affected and extreme variations in the prevalence of the infection are found in different regions. The number of infected subjects living in these areas is about 16 to 18 million. Migrations from rural areas account for the presence of people infected by *T. cruzi* in non-endemic regions of Latin America. In the USA, trypanosomiasis is found in people from Latin American countries where the disease is common (Hagar and Rahimtoola, 1991).

THE HUMAN DISEASE

The disease progresses from an acute to a chronic state. General infectious manifestations predominate in the acute stage. Cells close to the site of inoculation are invaded by *T. cruzi*, giving rise to the amastigote form. The amastigotes proliferate, occupying the host's cell cytoplasm. These infected cells burst releasing numerous parasites which become trypomastigote in form and invade local defence cells to initiate new reproductive cycles. Local lymphatic invasion follows presaging the haematogenous dissemination. From the bloodstream, cells of other tissues are invaded, causing secondary infected sites. Recurrent episodes of haematogenous dissemination occur as infected cells release new trypomastigotes. General infectious symptoms are present in this phase, but are not cyclical. The immune defences progressively reduce the haematogenous spread, which becomes insignificant after the first 2 months when the acute state usually ends. The disease becomes asymptomatic for several years and remains dormant in many individuals for the rest of their lives. In others, it can take more than 10 years before the first signs of the chronic state emerge. Cardiac manifestations predominate due to myocardial infiltration, and gastrointestinal involvement is common, typically with megaoesophagus or megacolon. During the chronic state, any factors modifying the host's immune response may lead to the rupture of clusters of residual amastigotes (pseudocysts); the released trypomastigotes can then, in turn, produce a new acute episode of AT. The most common modifiers of the immune system function are the use of immunosuppressant drugs and the acquired immune deficiency syndrome (AIDS).

T. cruzi causes an immediate cellular and humoral immune response. Specific immunoglobulins can be detected in the serum soon after the onset of the acute infection. Immune responses to organisms released by the infected host cells take place, in addition to hypersensitivity phenomena. These phenomena occur in the chronic phase of AT, and account for some of the clinical manifestations observed in this phase (Tanowitz *et al.*, 1992). These complex chronic phase manifestations can be caused by residual clusters of *T. cruzi* or can result from the different immune responses that have already been mentioned. Tissue damage due to the parasite's activity as well as secondary denervation due to neural damage play an important role.

The demonstration of the parasite in the bloodstream and the detection of anti-*T. cruzi* antibodies by immune diagnostic methods are the basis for the diagnosis of AT (Camargo *et al.*, 1986). Detection of IgM class antibodies is more common in the acute phase of AT. The presence of the parasite in the peripheral blood and/or elevated titres of anti-*T. cruzi* IgM antibodies constitutes the main indications for anti-*T. cruzi* drug therapy (Marr and Docamp, 1986). The drugs of choice at present are niphotimox (Bayer 2502) and benzonidazole (Ro 7–1051). Drug therapy is often unsatisfactory and can cause side-effects, one of which is peripheral neuropathy.

NEUROPATHOLOGY

During the acute phase of AT the nervous system becomes invaded by *T. cruzi*. Several areas of the central nervous system (CNS) can harbour clusters of amastigotes. Inflammatory foci of different magnitude are encountered scattered both in grey and white matter. These foci are usually small and they are made up of cells invaded by the *T. cruzi*. Glial proliferation as well as lymphocytic and plasmacytic cell infiltrates are conspicuous in these sites. Perivascular cell infiltrates can be present near these foci. The leptomeninges may be involved by a predominantly perivascular discontinuous inflammatory reaction.

The general features of this CNS inflammatory reaction correspond to an acute non-suppurative encephalomyelitis. However, there are variations in the extent and intensity of the inflammatory response. In rare circumstances, the CNS inflammatory response takes the form of a localized encephalitis consisting of acute necrotic encephalitic foci or large granulomas that behave like tumours. Similar findings occur in the meningoencephalitis secondary to a reactivation of the acute state that is seen in patients with the chronic form of AT who become infected with the HIV virus (Rocha *et al.*, 1994). An acute inflammatory reaction during the chronic phase is unusual (Pittella *et al.*, 1993). It is transitory and does not lead to scar formation.

An inflammatory reaction can be seen around the neural sheath, in the interfascicular space and in the connective tissue adjacent to the peripheral nerves as demonstrated in experimental laboratory animals. These inflammatory infiltrates are predominantly perivascular. Perineurial and endoneurial cells may harbour clusters of amastigotes. Segmental axonal degeneration of peripheral nerves may be a consequence of chronic parasitism of the Schwann cells (Said *et al.*, 1987). A reduction may also be observed in the number of myelinated fibres as well as paranodal demyelination (Molina *et al.*, 1987).

The invasion of neurones by *T. cruzi* and the multiplication of amastigotes in them occurs in the acute phase. Such neurones containing proliferating amastigotes can be observed in various locations of the nervous system. These two linked phenomena account for the neural damage and secondary neuronal loss, which varies on a region-to-region basis within the nervous system. The neuronal loss is remarkably random and discontinuous as demonstrated in both autopsy and experimental studies by Köberle and colleagues (Köberle, 1968). Axonal degeneration with its ensuing denervation is the main consequence of neuronal loss. Late hypersensitivity phenomena may account for additional neuronal damage in the chronic form of AT.

CLINICAL FEATURES

Meningoencephalitis

Headache is one of the most common manifestations of the acute infectious phase of AT. The pain is usually continuous but not severe. Irritability, sleepiness, mental obtundation and convulsive seizures may occur in a sequential progression. Like the headache, these other clinical manifestations are the consequence of the invasion of the nervous system by *T. cruzi*. Meningoencephalitis is one of the less frequent clinical manifestations of the acute phase of the disease.

The meningoencephalitis is of sudden onset with signs of meningeal irritation, sensory changes and convulsive seizures. Irritability, sleepiness, mental obtundation, stupor and coma occur progressing over 1 to 2 weeks. The meningoencephalitis in infants is more severe and is characterized by early coma and recurrent convulsive seizures. Death often supervenes 24–48 h later. Clear-cut cases of meningoencephalitis produce unmistakable CSF changes with mild to moderate pleocytosis, typically with lymphocytes and monocytes, a mild to moderate increase in protein and occasional elevation of the gammaglobulins. Additionally, it is not uncommon to find *T. cruzi* by light microscopy or its isolation through other means. It is often possible to find anti-*T. cruzi* antibodies in the CSF (Hoff *et al.*, 1978).

Changes in the immunological status during the progression of chronic AT may account for the occurrence of *de novo* acute episodes which may include clinical CNS manifestations. This phenomenon can also be seen in immunosuppressed patients (Leiguarda *et al.*, 1980), and in AIDS. In the latter, meningoencephalitis has been recorded (Gallo *et al.*, 1992; Oddó *et al.*, 1992; Rosemberg *et al.*, 1992) with or without expanding space-occupying cerebral lesions (Del Castillo *et al.*, 1990; Gluckstein *et al.*, 1992; Rocha *et al.*, 1994). The CSF findings are similar to those observed in primary meningoencephalitis of acute AT (Spina-França *et al.*, 1988). A similar picture is seen in subjects infected with *T. cruzi* during the course of an already established AIDS, for instance, following a blood transfusion. Typical acute signs of CNS involvement may occur and are sometimes accompanied by a full-blown meningoencephalitis.

Chronic Encephalopathy

During the chronic form of AT, the occurrence of signs and symptoms typical of well-established neurological syndromes is exceptional. The more commonly found clinical manifestations follow a pattern of minor cerebral dysfunction and specific CSF changes are not detected in the chronic phase of AT (Spina-França, 1988). Hence, the diagnosis of chronic AT encephalitis in endemic areas is not clear-cut. In order to support the diagnosis, other causes for the cerebral changes must be excluded and anti-*T. cruzi* antibodies should be detected in the serum.

Epileptiform electroencephalographic activity is significantly more common in patients with the chronic form of AT than in control subjects (Girardelli, 1969). Anti-*T. cruzi* antibodies are more frequent in epileptic patients than in control subjects (Medrado-Faria *et al.*, 1976). The comparison between epileptic patients with and without detectable titres of anti-*T. cruzi* antibodies showed significant differences: the group of serum-positive anti-*T. cruzi* patients had a higher incidence of partial seizures which were difficult to control (Jardim and Takayanagui, 1981). Cognitive disorders are more frequent in children who had contracted *T. cruzi* meningoencephalitis than controls (Jörg *et al.*, 1972) and memory and attention disorders as well as low IQ are recorded in adults with the chronic form of AT (Mangone *et al.*, 1984). Patients with the chronic form of AT may develop abnormal evoked potentials (Pelli-Noble *et al.*, 1990) but evaluation of the evoked potentials of central myelinated motor pathways shows they are largely spared (Segura *et al.*, 1994).

Peripheral Neuropathy

The peripheral neuropathy of chronic AT is mild and slowly progressive. Motor signs such as absence of deep tendon reflexes predominate in the lower limbs (Benavente *et al.*, 1989). The neuropathy results from neuronal loss in the anterior horn of the spinal cord (DeFaria *et al.*, 1988), but it can also be axonal (Sica *et al.*, 1991) as a consequence of neural infection by the *T. cruzi* and/or from a vasculitis due to the hypersensitivity phenomena mentioned earlier. In the case of axonal aetiology for the neuropathy, chronic motor as well as sensory manifestations can be demonstrated (Nascimento *et al.*, 1991).

Stroke

Chronic Chagas cardiopathy is the most common and serious clinical manifestation of the chronic form of AT, it is also the main cause of death. The involvement is complex, in which different roles are played by the parasite, the host immune responses as well as the neuronal loss (Gea *et al.*, 1993). The complications of cardiopathy are many, including brain damage. Among the most common complications are cerebral atrophy due to chronic and persistent hypoxia, and embolic stroke (Pitella, 1985). The embolic stroke may occur during the progression of the cardiopathy, originating from mural thrombi which are frequently located in the apex of the heart, over fibrous lesions of the endocardium. Mural thrombus fragments in the left ventricle are dislodged and are carried by the bloodstream, causing embolic phenomena in other sites including the distribution of the cerebral arteries. This embolic stroke is clinically indistinguishable from other causes of embolic stroke, and it progresses in the same manner as embolic strokes of other causes. It is a major cause of cerebrovascular disease in endemic AT regions.

FINAL REMARKS

Involvement of the nervous system in AT may frequently be asymptomatic or oligosymptomatic in its clinical manifestations. An exception is the occurrence of an embolic stroke resulting from cardiac mural thrombosis and embolism. Meningoencephalitis is another exception, being one of the most severe complications provoked by the *T. cruzi* infection. Indeed, AT meningoencephalitis has to be considered as one of the major complications of AIDS, not only in the areas of high prevalence of AT, but also in countries admitting immigrants from high AT prevalence areas.

ACKNOWLEDGEMENT

I would like to thank J.A. Livramento, L.R. Machado and L.C. Mattosinho-França for their part in preparing this chapter.

REFERENCES

Benavente OR, Patiño OL, Peña LB *et al.* (1989) Motor unit involvement in acute human acute Chagas disease. *Arquivos de Neuro-Psiquiatria* **47**: 283–286.

Camargo ME, Segura EL, Kagan IG *et al.* (1986) Three years of collaboration on the standardization of Chagas disease serodiagnosis in the Americas: an appraisal. *Bulletin of the Pan American Health Organization* **20**: 233–244.

Chagas C (1911) Nova entidade morbida no homem: resumo geral dos estudos etiolojicos e clinicos. *Memorias do Instituto Oswaldo Cruz* **3**: 219–275.

DeFaria CR, Rezende JM and Rassi A (1988) Estudo da desnervação periférica nas diferentes formas clínicas da doença de Chagas. *Arquivos de Neuro-Psiquiatria* **46**: 225–237.

Del Castillo M, Mendoza G, Oviedo J *et al.* (1990) AIDS and Chagas disease with central nervous system tumor-like lesion. *American Journal of Medicine* **88**: 693–694.

Gallo P, Fabião OM, Neto, Suarez JM and Borba RP (1992) Acute central nervous system infection by *Trypanosoma cruzi* and AIDS. *Arquivos de Neuro-Psiquiatria* **50**: 375–377.

Gea S, Ordonez P, Cerban F *et al.* (1993) Chagas disease cardioneuropathy: association of anti-*Trypanosoma cruzi* and anti-sciatic nerve antibodies. *American Journal of Tropical Medicine and Hygiene* **49**: 581–588.

Girardelli MA (1969) Electroencefalografia y enfermedad de Chagas crónica. *Boletin Chileno de Parasitologia* **24**: 32–35.

Gluckstein D, Ciferri F and Ruskin J (1992) Chagas disease: another cause of cerebral mass in the acquired immunodeficiency syndrome. *American Journal of Medicine* **92**: 429–432.

Hagar JM and Rahimtoola SH (1991) Chagas disease in the United States. *New England Journal of Medicine* **325**: 763–768.

Hoff R, Teixeira RS, Carvalho JS and Mott KE (1978) *Trypanosoma cruzi* in the cerebrospinal fluid during the acute stage of Chagas disease. *New England Journal of Medicine* **298**: 604–606.

Jardim E and Takayanagui OM (1981) Epilepsia e doença de Chagas crônica. *Arquivos de Neuro-Psiquiatria* **39**: 32–41.

Jörg ME, Freire RS, Orlando AS *et al.* (1972) Disfunción cerebral mínima como secuela de meningoencefalitis aguda por *Trypanosoma cruzi*. *Prensa Médica Argentina* **59**: 1658–1669.

Kirchhoff LV (1993) American trypanosomiasis (Chagas disease): a tropical disease now in the United States. *New England Journal of Medicine* **329**: 639–644.

Köberle F (1968) Chagas disease and Chagas syndromes: the pathology of American trypanosomiasis. *Advances in Parasitology* **6**: 63–116.

Leiguarda R, Roncoroni A, Taratuto AL *et al.* (1990) Acute CNS infection by *Trypanosoma cruzi* (Chagas disease) in immunosuppressed patients. *Neurology* **40**: 850–851.

Mangone CA, Sica REP, Pereyra S *et al.* (1994) Cognitive impairment in human chronic Chagas disease. *Arquivos de Neuro-Psiquiatria* **52**: 200–203.

Marr JJ and Docamp R (1986) Chemotherapy for Chagas disease: a perspective of current therapy and considerations for future research. *Reviews of Infectious Diseases* **8**: 884–903.

Medrado-Faria MA, Marques-Assis L, Silva GR and Camargo ME (1976) Infecção chagásica crônica e síndromes epilépticas. *Revista do Instituto de Medicina Tropical de São Paulo* **18**: 173–181.

Molina HA, Cardoni RL and Rimoldi MT (1987) The neuromuscular pathology of experimental Chagas disease. *Journal of the Neurological Sciences* **81**: 287–300.

Nascimento OJM, Freitas MRG and Chimelli L (1991) Polyneuropathie axonale dans la maladie de Chagas. *Revue Neurologique* **147**: 679–681.

Oddó D, Casanova M, Acuña G, Ballesteros J and Morales B (1992) Acute Chagas disease in acquired immunodeficiency syndrome: report of two cases. *Human Pathology* **23**: 41–44.

Pelli-Noble RF, Iguzquiza OD and Riarte EG (1990) Potenciales evocados visuales en la enfermedad de Chagas-Mazza cronica. *Arquivos de Neuro-Psiquiatria* **48**: 315–319.

Pittella JEH (1985) Brain involvement in the chronic cardiac form of Chagas disease. *Journal of Tropical Medicine and Hygiene* **88**: 313–317.

Pittella JEH, Meneguette C and Barbosa AJA (1993) Histopathological and immunohistochemical study of the brain and heart in the chronic cardiac form of Chagas disease. *Arquivos de Neuro-Psiquiatria* **51**: 8–15.

Rocha A, Meneses ACO, Silva AM *et al.* (1994) Pathology of patients with Chagas disease and acquired immunodeficiency syndrome. *American Journal of Tropical Medicine and Hygiene* **50**: 261–268.

Rosemberg S, Chaves CJ, Higuchi ML *et al.* (1992) Fatal meningoencephalitis caused by reactivation of *Trypanosoma cruzi* infection in a patient with AIDS. *Neurology* **42**: 640–642.

Said G, Joskowicz M, Barreira AA and Eisen H (1985) Neuropathy associated with experimental Chagas disease. *Annals of Neurology* **18**: 676–683.

Schmuñiz GA (1991) *Trypanosoma cruzi*, the etiologic agent of Chagas disease: status in the blood supply in endemic and nonendemic countries. *Transfusion* **31**: 547–557.

Segura MJ, Genovese OM, Segura E, Sanz OP and Sica REP (1994) Central motor conduction in chronic human Chagas disease. *Arquivos de Neuro-Psiquiatria* **52**: 29–31.

Sica REP, Genovese OM and Garcia Erro M (1991) Peripheral motor nerve conduction in patients with chronic Chagas disease. *Arquivos de Neuro-Psiquiatria* **49**: 405–408.

Spina-França A and Mattosinho-França LC (1978) American trypanosomiasis (Chagas disease). In: *Handbook of Clinical Neurology*, vol. 35 (eds PJ Vinken and GW Bruyn), pp 85–114. Amsterdam: North Holland Publishers.

Spina-França A and Mattosinho-França LC (1988) South American trypanosomiasis (Chagas disease). In: *Handbook of Clinical Neurology*, vol. 52 (eds PJ Vinken, GW Bruyn and HL Klawans), pp 345–349. Amsterdam: Elsevier.

Spina-França A, Livramento JA, Machado LR and Yasuda N (1988) Anticorpos a *Trypanosoma cruzi* no líquido cefalorraqueano: pesquisa pelas reações de fixação do complemento e de immunofluorescência. *Arquivos de Neuro-Psiquiatria* **46**: 374–378.

Tanowitz HB, Kirchhoff LV, Simon D *et al.* (1992) Chagas disease. *Clinical Microbiology Reviews* **5**: 400–419.

18

Schistosomiasis*

Pierre Louis Alfred Bill

Wentworth Hospital and University of Natal, Durban, South Africa

INTRODUCTION

Schistosomiasis is a trematode infection of man affecting at least 200 million people world-wide (Mahmoud, 1977). The infection is widely distributed in Africa, the Middle and Far East, South America and the Caribbean islands (Bird, 1964; Warren, 1980; Scrimgeour and Gajdusek, 1985; Cosnett and van Dellen, 1986). Three species of schistosome, *Schistosoma mansoni*, *S. haematobium* and *S. japonicum*, are responsible for disease in man. The prevalence of the different species of schistosome is primarily determined by the distribution of the snail hosts. *S. haematobium* is found mainly on the continent of Africa. *S. mansoni* has a similar distribution to *S. haematobium* in Africa but in addition is endemic to South America, the Caribbean islands and the Middle East. *S. japonicum* is found mainly in China, Japan and South-East Asia where in addition to man, dogs, cattle and cats have been reported as primary hosts (Wakefield *et al.*, 1962).

Schistosomiasis is increasing in prevalence as man attempts to use water and land resources more efficiently. Many patients are also now being seen in non-endemic areas as a result of population movements and expansion in international travel.

The prevalence of infection varies from under 10% in some areas to more than 80% in others (Pitchford, 1986). Infection rates of *S. haematobium* are highest in the younger age groups up to about 18 years of age after which the rates fall quite rapidly. Infection rates of *S. mansoni* are very often higher than those of *S. haematobium* and do not fall as rapidly.

LIFE CYCLE

Schistosomes alternate generations between definitive hosts (mammals and birds) in which sexual reproduction takes place and intermediate hosts (snails)

---

*The colour plate appears between p. 236 and p. 237

in which asexual multiplication takes place (Warren, 1978). The worms, known as blood flukes, normally inhabit the portal and mesenteric veins, or the vesical plexuses of the urinary bladder. The tributaries of the internal iliac vein around the bladder are the site of predilection for the adult *S. haematobium* worms. In the case of *S. mansoni* infections approximately 60% of the worms are found in the tributaries of the inferior mesenteric veins around the rectum and the remainder in the portal vein and in the liver. Rectal involvement with *S. haematobium* infection, however, is not uncommon due to aberrations in the distribution of these worms. Forty per cent of *S. japonicum* worms are found in the superior mesenteric veins and the remainder in the portal vein and in the liver. Female schistosome worms lay large numbers of eggs, producing between 300 and 3000 eggs daily, many of which pass through the tissues into the lumen of the intestines or urinary bladder and into the outside environment. More than half the eggs produced remain trapped in the tissues. The laying of clusters of eggs in thousands is a feature of *S. japonicum* infection. On reaching fresh water, miracidia hatch from the eggs and penetrate a susceptible snail species, where they develop into sporocysts. The cercariae which form from the sporocysts, leave the snail and penetrate the skin of the definitive host to become schisto-somula. These then migrate to the liver via the lungs, mature to adult worms, mate and pass to their particular final habitats within 4–13 weeks, where they remain paired for years. The average period from cercarial penetration until the appearance of eggs is 50 days. *S. mansoni* and *S. japonicum* characteristically cause intestinal and hepatosplenic disease, whereas *S. haematobium* affects the urinary tract predominantly. *See* Plate 10.

GENERAL ASPECTS OF SCHISTOSOMAL INFECTION

Although schistosomiasis was described in Egyptian and Babylonian inscriptions, it was Theodore Bilharz who established the relationship between the trematode worm and the disease in 1851. *S. mansoni* was identified by Patrick Manson in 1903. The presentation of schistosomiasis occurs in three stages (Bird, 1978; Boyce, 1990). The first stage is caused by the initial skin penetration by cercariae eliciting a humoral response within 6 hours, and manifests as pruritis and fever. The second stage of the illness (Katayama fever) occurs at the time of ova production and deposition 3–6 weeks later. It is thought to be the result of an allergic response to the ova, and is characterized by fever, eosinophilia, lymphadenopathy, diarrhoea, splenomegaly and urticaria. It is most severe in cases of *S. japonicum* infection, and occasionally occurs with heavy infection by *S. mansoni*. The third stage results from a delayed hypersensitivity reaction to the ova deposited in the tissues and is characterized by granuloma formation over a period of months to years.

PATHOGENESIS OF CENTRAL NERVOUS SYSTEM INFECTION

Involvement of the central nervous system in schistosomiasis is uncommon (Scrimgeour and Gajdusek, 1985; Pittella, 1991). The schistosome eggs, many of which are retained in the host tissues, are the parasite factor responsible for schistosomal disease. The host granulomatous reaction to the eggs is the principal factor in the pathogenesis of schistosomiasis. The final disease is also influenced by the number of eggs reaching the central nervous system. The neurological syndromes depend on the spread and localization of ectopic eggs within the nervous system. Eggs released into the portocaval system are believed to reach the spinal veins via the valveless venous plexus of Batson which joins the deep iliac veins and inferior vena cava with the veins of the spinal cord (Warren, 1978; Liu, 1993). This may occur under conditions of reversed abdominal venous flow with increased intra-abdominal pressure. This would explain the predominant localization of schistosoma eggs to the lower spinal cord. Ova in the brain are more randomly distributed, suggesting embolization via pulmonary or portopulmonary venous shunts (Wakefield, 1962; Bird, 1978; Nash, 1982; Scrimgeour and Gajdusek, 1985). Adult worms may anomalously enter the vertebral venous plexus and ascend to the brain, although reports of adult worms in the central nervous system are extremely rare. In one case an adult *S. mansoni* was observed in the cerebral leptomeningeal vessels, and an adult *S. haematobium* was present in the choroid plexus in another case. The larger size and protruding spines of *S. mansoni* and *S. haematobium* eggs may impede their progress and explain their tendency to lodge in the lower vertebral plexus and spinal cord. Ova of *S. japonicum* are smaller and produced in larger numbers, and this may account for their more distant spread to the cranial cavity. *S. japonicum* has a predilection for ectopic localization in the brain, and almost never involves the spinal cord. *S. mansoni* and *S. haematobium* involve the spinal cord far more frequently than the brain, the lumbar cord being the site of damage more frequently. *S. haematobium* affects the spinal cord almost exclusively, while *S. mansoni* may produce lesions in both brain and spinal cord.

The host immunological response to the ova can vary from an intense granulomatous reaction, sometimes forming space-occupying mass lesions, to minimal reactions. The inflammatory reaction may involve blood vessels with a resultant vasculitis (Pittella, 1985) as well as the parenchyma of the brain and spinal cord.

CEREBRAL SCHISTOSOMIASIS

The first pathological description of an intracerebral granuloma caused by parasitic ova of *S. japonicum* was by Yumagiwa in 1899, in a patient suffering from Jacksonian epilepsy. The majority of reported cerebral schistosomiasis cases result from *S. japonicum* infection. In most reported cases the diagnosis is based on presumptive clinical evidence. *S. mansoni* and *S. haematobium* are occasionally responsible.

Cerebral Involvement with *Schistosoma japonicum*

Cerebral complications occur in up to 2–5% of *S. japonicum* infections (Liu, 1993). The disease may present as a space-occupying lesion or occasionally as a generalized encephalitis. Cerebral schistosomiasis japonicum may appear at any time in the course of infection from the first 3 weeks on.

Acute Cerebral Schistosomiasis

S. japonicum ova have a strong tendency to localize in the brain, including the cortex, subcortex, basal ganglia and internal capsule (Bird, 1978; Liu, 1993). Acute cerebral infection by *S. japonicum* may present as a diffuse encephalitis, meningoencephalitis or encephalomyelitis. Described features include speech and visual disturbances, disorientation, memory loss or coma. Some degree of motor weakness including transient hemiplegia, paraplegia or quadriplegia is common. Headache, neck stiffness, incontinence and ataxia may occur. Other findings include cranial nerve abnormalities, spasticity, rigidity and hyper-reflexia. Abnormalities on EEG are common. Many patients develop generalized or focal seizures. Fever and leukocytosis with eosinophilia is common.

Chronic Cerebral Schistosomiasis

The chronic form results from intracranial granulomas and may present with raised intracranial pressure and localizing signs, simulating a brain tumour (Mahmoud, 1977; Bird, 1978; Bambirra *et al.*, 1984; Warren, 1987). *S. japonicum* is reputed to be an important cause of focal epilepsy in the Far East. Usually the bilharzial nature of the granuloma is established by biopsy.

Laboratory and Radiological Findings

The cerebrospinal fluid may show a pleocytosis and high protein, and eosinophils may be noted in the CSF. Pathological examination of affected areas reveals inflammatory changes around the ova with oedema, parenchymal necrosis, cellular infiltration with giant cells and granuloma formation, and occasional vasculitis (Liu, 1993). Abnormalities on the CT scan include focal contrast enhancing mass lesions, and parenchymal lucencies with or without oedema. Multilobe lucencies and severe oedema may be seen.

Diagnosis and Treatment

Examination of the stool for schistosome eggs is mandatory. EEG and CSF findings may be normal or non-specific. A presumptive clinical diagnosis can be made on the basis of an appropriate epidemiological history, stool ova or systemic signs of hepatosplenic schistosomiasis, characteristic neurological findings, and contrast CT studies showing focal lucencies or masses (schistosomal granulomas). Praziquantel is a safe and effective drug for treating *S. japonicum*. A single dose of therapy results in complete clinical cure with resolution of neurological deficits, and mass lesions and oedema on CT scanning. The recommended dosage is 60 mg kg^{-1} day^{-1} in three doses for 1 day. A therapeutic trial of praziquantel is justifiable before brain biopsy if the clinical index of suspicion for schistosomiasis is high. Steroids are probably helpful as adjunctive therapy for the acute inflammatory lesions and should not worsen the infection.

Differential Diagnosis

Acute schistosomal encephalopathy can be mistaken for viral encephalitis, cerebral malaria or bacterial meningitis. In South-East Asia the differential diagnosis of cerebral mass lesions with eosinophilia includes other helminthic infections including paragonimiasis and cysticercosis. A tissue diagnosis may be necessary to exclude non-parasitic causes of intracranial mass lesions such as gliomas, tuberculomas and HIV-associated opportunistic infections and neoplasms.

Prognosis

The immediate prognosis of acute cerebral *S. japonicum* infection is good. The majority of patients are effectively cured with appropriate chemotherapy. Occasionally residual neurological disturbances occur. Some patients remain with focal or complex partial seizures. Status epilepticus is the most common cause of death.

Cerebral Involvement with *S. mansoni* and *S. haematobium*

Ova are commonly detected in the brain tissue of chronic fatal *S. mansoni* and *S. haematobium* infections but these are usually clinically silent (Gelfand, 1950; Alves, 1958; Pittella and Lana-Peixoto, 1981; Pittella, 1985, 1991; Scrimgeour and Gajdusek, 1985; Liu, 1993). Post-mortem studies have demonstrated ova almost anywhere in the brain but mainly in the cerebral and cerebellar cortex and leptomeninges. Deposition of *S. mansoni* ova in the brain and meninges is more frequent in hepatosplenic schistosomiasis especially with cor pulmonale. Generally, neurological symptoms are infrequent or absent. Acute encephalopathy has been rarely noted as an ectopic complication of these infections. In the few cases described with features of encephalitis, seizures were the commonest presenting symptom with abnormal EEG findings (Bird, 1978; Pittella, 1991; Liu, 1993).

Histopathological changes are variable (Pittella, 1981, 1985; Scrimgeour and Gajdusek, 1985; Khalil *et al.*, 1986; Liu, 1993). Ova may be present with little or no histological reaction, or the tissue reaction may be limited to a few mononuclear cells with some perivascular infiltration. In some cases, a granulomatous response is elicited. Focal or diffuse vasculitis and rarely fibrinoid necrosis may occur, and isolated cases of cerebral and subarachnoid haemorrhage have been reported. Although large granulomatous tumoral masses in the cerebral cortex or cerebellum have been described with *S. mansoni* infections, massive lesions are the exception (Bambirra *et al*, 1984; Scrimgeour and Gajdusek, 1985). Epilepsy has been claimed to be caused by these parasites.

SPINAL SCHISTOSOMIASIS

Spinal schistosomiasis is more prevalent than the cerebral form, and is due almost exclusively to *S. mansoni* and *S. haematobium* (Scrimgeour and Gajdusek, 1985; Cosnett and van Dellen, 1986). Only one case of *S. japonicum*-produced spinal cord disease appears recorded. In endemic areas, spinal cord schistosomiasis is a significant cause of non-traumatic paraplegia and is probably under-reported. World-wide *S. mansoni* is the more frequently reported cause of schistosomal myelopathy, while in Africa *S. haematobium* is more often responsible (Wakefield *et al.*, 1962; Bird, 1964; Scrimgeour and Gajdusek, 1985; Cosnett and van Dellen, 1986). Occasionally, infection with both *S. haematobium* and *S. mansoni* is found. The first report of a case of schistosomal myelopathy from Africa was of an Egyptian who had died of chronic bladder schistosomiasis and paraplegia (Ferguson, 1917). In 1930 *S. mansoni* was identified as a cause of schistosomal myelopathy in a patient who had resided in Brazil (Muller and Stender, 1930). Cases of *S. mansoni* myelopathy are mostly reported from South America. Ova may be present in the spinal cord without clinical features, and the prevalence of asymptomatic ova deposition in the spinal cord has been estimated at between 0.3 and 2% of patients with schistosomiasis (Scrimgeour and Gajdusek, 1985).

Pathology

Schistosomal myelopathy and radiculopathy is the consequence of ectopic schistosome ova with subsequent host reactions and tissue damage (Wakefield *et al.*, 1962; Bird, 1978; Nash, 1982; Scrimgeour and Gajdusek, 1985). The ova are thought to reach the vertebral venous plexus and spinal cord via Batson's plexus, explaining why the conus medullaris is the site of predilection. Possibly a gravid schistosome passes along these anastomoses to gain access to the vertebral venous plexus, although an adult *S. haematobium* has never been recorded in the spinal canal (an adult *S. mansoni* has been reported in the subarachnoid vessels of the spinal medulla) (Cosnett and van Dellen, 1986). The clinical presentation reflects one of two main pathological processes: (a) necrotic or transverse myelitis, or (b) granulomatous masses involving the conus medullaris and cauda equina. A rare syndrome of anterior spinal artery occlusion may also possibly occur but is not pathologically proven (Siddorn, 1978).

In the majority of cases of intramedullary granulomatous mass (Wakefield *et al.*, 1962; Scrimgeour and Gajdusek, 1985; Cosnett and van Dellen, 1986; Haribhai *et al.*, 1991; Liu, 1993), the commonest level of involvement is at T12 to L1. The lumbar cord is enlarged and the leptomeninges may be congested. On gross inspection the intramedullary mass appears as a yellowish or grey, amorphous or rubbery mass. Multiple nodules may be noted on the surface of the cord and the granulomatous reaction may extend along the cauda equina, with congestion and oedema of the nerve roots. A fibrotic reaction may occur over the cauda equina and conus medullaris. Involvement of the cauda equina alone is not described. Compression of the spinal cord by a meningeal granuloma has been recorded. More rarely granulomas are found at higher levels of the thoracic cord or lower cervical cord. Histological examination reveals numerous haemorrhages, venous thrombosis, perivascular cuffing or vasculitis and infiltrates of mononuclear cells and eosinophils. Typical granulomas are scattered in the spinal cord parenchyma (Figure 18.1). In many sections, the schistosome ovum can be identified if a characteristic spine is evident. The types of schistosomal ova are not always easily identified in biopsies obtained at laminectomy or at autopsy. The intraspinal mass lesions may closely resemble a glioma macroscopically and may simulate a spinal cord tumour clinically.

Acute or subacute transverse myelitis is probably under-recognized and under-reported compared with schistosomal mass lesions of the spinal cord as this diagnosis depends essentially on circumstantial evidence (Queiroz *et al.*, 1979; Boyce, 1990; Haribhai *et al.*, 1991; Liu, 1993). In this type, *S. haematobium* or *S. mansoni* produce a more diffuse necrotic myelitis which may also involve leptomeninges and roots (meningoradiculomyelitic form). The clinical presentation resembles acute or subacute transverse myelitis with sudden-onset paraplegia, and destruction, vacuolation and subsequent atrophy of the cord. This may occur in a patient known to have schistosomiasis. It differs from other causes of transverse myelitis in that schistosomal transverse myelitis commonly affects the lower dorsal cord whereas other causes of transverse myelitis commonly affect the mid-thoracic region. Higher levels of the spinal cord may, however, also be affected as shown by Queiroz *et al.* (1979) who demonstrated at autopsy total myelonecrosis below T4 with ova of *S. mansoni* in necrotic cord tissue and leptomeninges. Delayed cell-mediated immunity is an

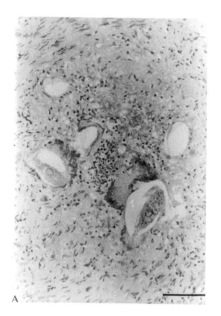
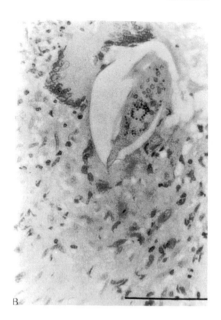
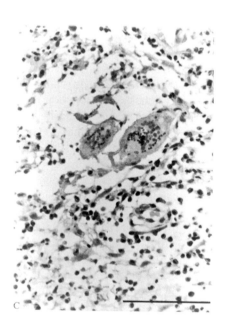

Figure 18.1 (a, b) Granulomata containing ova of *Schistosoma haematobium* with terminal spine, foreign body giant cell reaction and a cellular infiltrate of mononuclear cells and eosinophils. (c) Granuloma containing unidentified bilharzial ova. Bars, 100 μm. From Haribhai *et al.* (1991) with permission.

important factor in the degree of inflammatory response to ova in the CNS. A hypersensitivity reaction to ova in sensitized persons who are rechallenged by further exposure to schistosome antigens may thus account for cases of schistosomal myelopathy presenting with acute paraplegia, the acute immunological reaction being responsible for massive spinal cord necrosis. Another possible mechanism may be schistosoma-induced vascular inflammation leading to infarction of the spinal cord and subsequent necrosis.

Clinical Features

Age and Sex Distribution

Schistosomal myelopathy occurs predominantly in young males living in rural areas, who are more likely to be exposed to schistosome-infected water during childhood or in the course of their work (Molyneux and Galatius-Jensen, 1978; Cosnett and van Dellen, 1986; Joubert *et al.*, 1990). The ratio of male to female cases is approximately 3:1. The reported ages of patients vary from 14 months to 62 years with a mean of 22 years, but most patients are in the age range of 10 to 30 years. The mean age of *S. mansoni* patients is greater than that of *S. haematobium* patients (27 years and 19 years respectively).

Incubation and Onset

The incubation period between exposure to infection and onset of spinal cord dysfunction is difficult to ascertain in most cases but is reported to vary from weeks to months and rarely years (Wakefield *et al.*, 1962; Bird, 1964; Scrimgeour and Gajdusek, 1985; Cosnett and van Dellen, 1986; Liu, 1993). Most patients present with a short history, with symptoms developing over a few days to a few weeks. Paraplegia may also develop within 24 hours. It is occasionally reported to evolve slowly over years, and patients may rarely present with a chronic history of paraplegia. The onset of symptoms tends to be more acute with a shorter incubation period in patients with the myelitic form compared with patients with schistosomal mass lesions, although a rapid onset can also occur in the latter group.

Symptoms and Signs

Patients frequently present with low back pain, sometimes severe and burning, often radiating into the saddle area or lower limbs. This may be accompanied by cramp-like pains and paraesthesiae in the legs. These symptoms may occur in both the myelitic or granulomatous forms, with or without arachnoiditis.

The pain is accompanied by the rapid or subacute onset of paraparesis, impaired sphincter control and sensory abnormalities. All patients present with varying degrees of lower limb weakness which may be symmetrical or asymmetrical. The weakness characteristically progresses over several days or weeks and most patients develop a severe flaccid paraparesis or paraplegia. A few patients retain the ability to walk. Mild muscular wasting, often asymmetric, may be present. Hypotonia is more characteristically found than hypertonia, reflecting the predominant involvement of the conus medullaris and adjacent cauda equina.

The level of the lesion in patients with a granuloma is most commonly T12 to L1, though patients are seen with a level above or below this. Sensory dysfunction is invariably present, although the changes may be subtle and are usually overshadowed by the motor syndrome. Variable and patchy sensory loss in the sacral and lower lumbar dermatomes are the most usual findings. These findings may also be asymmetrical and all modalities of sensation can be involved. Thus, loss of sensation is mostly found in the legs below the knees or at the back of the thighs and perineal region. When higher levels of the spinal cord are involved, the paraplegia is associated with spasticity rather than absent reflexes, and a sensory level is seen. The highest reported sensory level in the granuloma group was at C8 in a quadriplegic patient in whom a large mass was demonstrated radiologically in the cervical canal and disappeared almost completely after treatment (Molyneux and Galatius-Jensen, 1978).

A clear sensory level corresponding to the upper lumbar, lower or mid thoracic and occasionally cervical level is more likely to occur in the myelitic type. Most of our patients with a myelitic presentation had a sensory level at or below T10, although one of our patients presented with a low cervical sensory level and quadriplegia. Some patients are reported with diffuse lesions and signs indicating upper and lower motor neurone dysfunction. Flaccid quadriplegia is a rare presentation of bilharzial myelopathy.

Reflex changes are almost always present with reduced or absent ankle and knee jerks. These changes may also be asymmetrical and occasionally one or other ankle jerk may be brisk and one or both plantar responses extensor. Brisk reflexes are more likely to be found in chronic cases or those presenting with a syndrome of transverse myelitis.

Urinary incontinence and impotence, with a flaccid distended bladder, is found in the majority of patients, and is often accompanied by overflow incontinence. Lesser degrees of bladder disturbance are seen and patients may retain the ability to void urine albeit with difficulty, even when severely paraplegic. The sphincter disturbance usually develops with the progressive paraparesis but occasionally is the presenting symptom.

In summary the physical signs in the granuloma group commonly reflect a patchy, incomplete and often asymmetrical involvement of the conus and cauda equina, with striking motor disturbance and often apparently lesser sensory disturbance. In contrast, the myelitic group is more likely to show a paraplegia with a crisp sensory level. The distinction between these types is, however, not always clear cut.

Investigations

Blood examination often shows eosinophilia, but this is not invariable or specific (Liu, 1993). About one-third of cases of cord schistosomiasis do not have significant eosinophilia at the time of presentation.

Bilharzial ova may be recovered from faeces, urine or rectal biopsy, although not all cases will show ova in the urine or stools (Scrimgeour and Gajdusek, 1985; Cosnett and van Dellen, 1986; Haribhai *et al.*, 1991). In the case of *S. haematobium* the urine is more likely to yield ova especially if centrifuged. Special concentration techniques may be necessary to show ova in the stools. In cases of *S. mansoni* of the cord the most likely source of confirmation of the infection is by biopsy of the rectal mucosa. *S. haematobium* is, however, also frequently found on rectal biopsy. In young children scrapings obtained from the rectal mucosa may identify the ova and are preferable to performing a rectal biopsy. The species can usually be identified by the position in the spine of the ovum, being lateral in *S. mansoni* and terminal in *S. haematobium*. Occasional patients show dual infection with *S. haematobium* and *S. mansoni*. In a country where both parasites are endemic, recovery of one species from urine or faeces does not prove it is the cause of the myelopathy. Occasionally cystoscopy and biopsy of the bladder mucosa is undertaken to demonstrate the ova.

The role of serology in the diagnosis of neuroschistosomiasis is not uniformly accepted. A variety of serological tests have been developed with varying degrees of sensitivity, specificity and cross-reaction with other helminths. The ELISA test using specific antigens derived from the eggs has superseded previous serological tests (Cosnett and van Dellen, 1986; Haribhai *et al.*, 1991; Pammenter *et al.*, 1991). A positive serological response indicates exposure to schistosomes and not necessarily disease. Titres may initially rise following specific medical treatment.

The majority of patients show a CSF pleocytosis with lymphocytic predominance (Scrimgeour and Gajdusek, 1985; Cosnett and van Dellen, 1986; Haribhai *et al.*, 1991; Liu, 1993). The number of cells varies from six to usually less than 100 cells per cubic millimetre. Eosinophils may be present and are highly suggestive of schistosomal or other helminthic parasitic infection. Ova of *S. mansoni* or *S. haematobium* are not detected in the CSF. Most of the patients also show a moderate elevation of CSF protein with values ranging from 0.5 to 1.8 g l^{-1}. Occasionally, xanthochromia has been noted, reflecting a spinal block. The glucose level is usually normal or slightly low. Following medical therapy significant reductions in CSF cell count and protein level are seen and the CSF glucose level may rise slightly. Oligoclonal bands can be demonstrated in the cerebrospinal fluid in many patients (Haribhai *et al.*, 1991). Schistosomal myelopathy patients also show an elevated IgG index, and an increased rate of IgG synthesis within the blood–brain barrier, giving a non-specific indication of the presence of antibodies in the CSF and antibody production within the CNS. Intrathecal IgG synthesis is consistently reduced by medical treatment.

CSF ELISA testing may demonstrate the presence of IgG antibody directed to schistosomal egg antigen in values greater than 3 standard deviations in most patients (Pammenter *et al.*, 1991). This is a moderately sensitive but not entirely specific investigation for the immunodiagnosis of spinal schistosomiasis. Seventy five per cent of patients with proven schistosomal myelopathy develop CSF antischistosomal antibodies by ELISA whereas 7% of patients with non-schistosomal myelopathies are proven positive. The probability of schistosomal myelopathy can thus be reasonably excluded when the test is negative. In cases where other diagnoses can be excluded but the cause of the myelopathy remains obscure, oligoclonal bands in the presence of high antischistosomal antibody titres can be considered as additional evidence of spinal schistosomiasis but not as diagnostic in themselves. In most patients there is no correlation between the raised antischistosome antibody levels in the serum and CSF. Using the ELISA

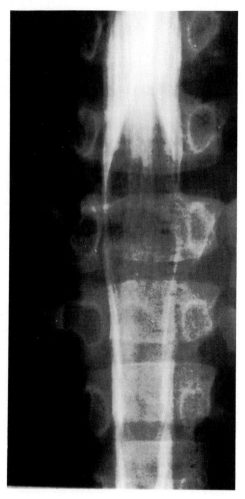

Figure 18.2 Myelogram showing expansion of conus medullaris maximum opposite T11.

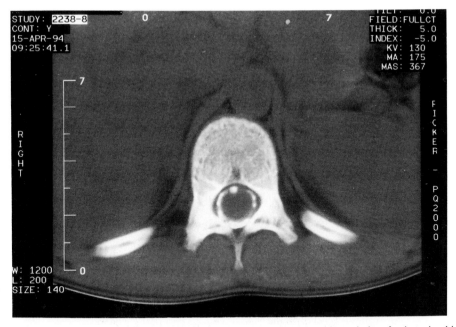

Figure 18.3 CT myelogram showing conus medullaris enlargement and irregularity of subarachnoid contrast material indicating arachnoiditis.

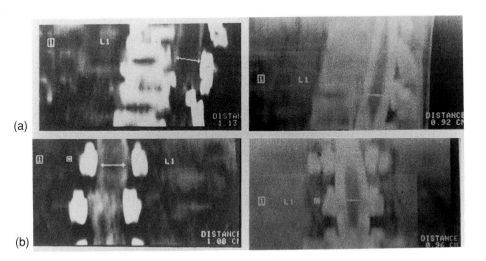

Figure 18.4 Reformatted images of the conus medullaris before and 9 weeks after a 2-week course of praziquantel and corticosteroids. (a) Midline sagittal images showing decrease in anteroposterior cord diameter from 11.3 mm to 9.2 mm. (b) Coronal images showing decrease in transverse cord diameter from 10.8 mm to 9.6 mm. From Haribhai *et al.* (1991) with permission.

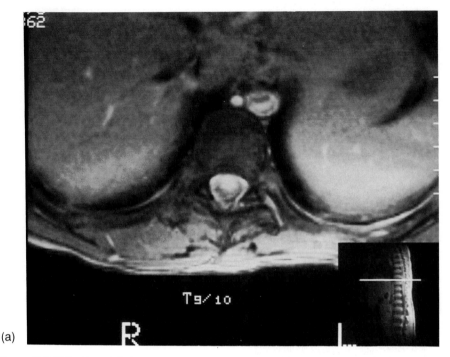

(a)

Figure 18.5 MRI with gadolinium enhancement. (a) Transverse image at level of T9/10 showing anteriorly situated enhancing granuloma.

technique, CSF antischistosome antibody titres are not higher than those in the serum. CSF bilharzia ELISA titres also fall significantly after treatment. Patients who are tested long after treatment may give a negative result.

In patients presenting with a conus medullaris syndrome CT myelography will usually demonstrate expansion of the lower spinal cord or conus region, usually at the T12 to L1 level (Cosnett and van Dellen, 1986; Joubert, 1990; Haribhai *et al.*, 1991) (Figures 18.2 and 18.3). This is often but not necessarily associated with irregularity and matting of the cauda equina roots indicating arachnoiditis. The conus expansion is not usually sufficient to produce a CSF block. Occasionally the conus enlargement is equivocal and the arachnoiditis may appear to be the predominant feature. Cord swelling may appear at a higher level in the dorsal region and there is one report of a presumed granuloma being shown at myelography as high as the eighth cervical vertebra. These radiological abnormalities are found in those cases where the pathology is granulomatous and thus associated with swelling.

When CT myelography is repeated after medical treatment, an impressive decrease in conus size can be shown (Figure 18.4), concomitant with the improvement noted clinically and in the cerebrospinal fluid (Haribhai *et al.*, 1991). A normal myelogram does not exclude the diagnosis as a CT examination may demonstrate spinal cord swelling in such cases. The radiographic appear-

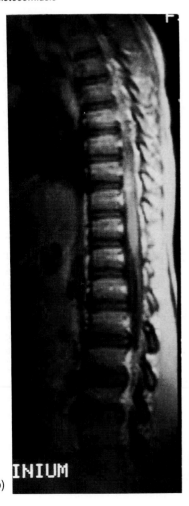

(b)

Figure 18.5(continued) MRI with gadolinium enhancement. (b) Sagittal section showing several intramedullary enhancing granulomas opposite T9/10.

ances on computer-assisted myelography in patients with myelitis are usually normal. Cord atrophy may be demonstrated later in these patients if the radiological examination is repeated.

MRI findings show an enlarged conus medullaris with heterogenous enhancement on T1- and T2-weighted images (Silbergleit, 1992; Blunt *et al.*, 1993) (Figure 18.5). MRI may also show enlargement of the cord extending superiorly well above the more obvious intramedullary lesion of the cord at T12/L1. These findings are relatively non-specific indicators of inflammatory or neoplastic processes.

Diagnosis

Where schistosomiasis is endemic, the condition should be kept in mind in every case developing paraparesis. Spinal schistosomiasis is probably more common than the relatively few cases in the literature would suggest. A history of travel or residence in an endemic area should arouse suspicion. An important clue to the diagnosis is a history of exposure to the parasite. Enquiry should be made about symptoms suggesting infection at different stages of the disease. Five to 15 hours after skin penetration by cercariae some subjects have symptoms of dermatitis. This response is a delayed hypersensitivity reaction in individuals who have been exposed previously, and is characterized by a transient itchy papular rash with round cell invasion of the dermis and epidermis. Later, when the worms have reached maturity, ova may be deposited in the dermis with the formation of granulomas. This is more commonly seen in the skin of the perineum and external genitalia. In two reported cases of spinal schistosomiasis, a clue to the diagnosis was provided by biopsy of papules in the skin of the trunk.

Coinciding with the onset of egg laying is an acute systemic syndrome characterized by fever, chills, anorexia, malaise, sweating, lymphadenopathy, hepatosplenomegaly and pronounced eosinophilia. This syndrome (Katayama fever) is analogous to serum sickness and possibly with immune complex disease. Western travellers are more likely to present acutely with the Katayama syndrome, whereas endemic residents and immigrants from endemic areas may have signs of chronic disease.

Patients may have symptoms of bladder or bowel involvement by bilharzia. It is important to ask about a history of recent or past haematuria. Colonic involvement by *S. mansoni* or *S. haematobium* may cause intestinal symptoms such as dysentery with the passage of blood and mucus in the stools. Other causes of such symptoms are common in the tropics and therefore have little specific diagnostic value.

The simplest and most definitive tests are microscopic examination of urine and stool for schistosome ova. Several consecutive faecal or urine examinations for ova should be performed. In young children, ova may be found in scrapings from perianal skin.

This establishes the diagnosis of visceral schistosomiasis and also the type of fluke. The absence of ova from urine and stool does not exclude the diagnosis. Lumbar puncture may show signs of block or normal dynamics. The CSF may be normal but more usually shows varying degrees of pleocytosis with elevation of protein. Eosinophils may be present.

Without a surgical biopsy a presumptive diagnosis of spinal cord schistosomiasis is based on: (1) evidence of lower thoracic or upper lumbar neurological lesions; (2) demonstration of exposure to schistosomiasis through passive parasitological or serological techniques; (3) exclusion of other causes of transverse myelitis.

Diagnosis of conus granuloma is easier in view of its delineation on computer-assisted myelography. The diagnosis of schistosomal myelitis is circumstantial. Raised levels of specific antischistosomal antibodies can be demonstrated in approximately 75% of patients. Further evidence of the infective nature of the spinal cord disease can be provided by demonstrating intrathecal production of antibodies as shown by an elevated IgG index, increased IgG production rates and the presence of oligoclonal bands in the CSF.

Once schistosomiasis becomes a consideration, physical examination and laboratory tests are directed toward obtaining evidence of acute or chronic schistosomal infection. Tissue biopsy of involved rectal or bladder mucosa during sigmoidoscopy or cystoscopy may be indicated.

Differential Diagnosis

The clinical picture of most cases of schistosomiasis of the spinal cord is so characteristic that if the patient has a history of exposure to the parasite other diagnostic possibilities are few. The differential diagnosis is that of any cause of patchy involvement of the lower cord and cauda equina which has an acute, subacute or chronic history and evidence of a chronic inflammatory reaction in the CSF. Tuberculoma or tuberculous arachnoiditis are possible alternative diagnoses. Cysticercosis may produce CSF changes of chronic inflammation but rarely affects the spinal cord. Transverse myelitis due to syphilis can be excluded by the relevant serological tests. Metastatic neoplasia, lymphoma or an ependymoma in the region of the conus medullaris are other possible diagnoses causing a similar syndrome. In the acute stage the progressive weakness can mimic the Guillain–Barré syndrome.

When the level of the lesion is higher than the lower dorsal spinal cord and when the myelogram is normal, the differential diagnosis becomes broader. Consideration must be given to viral myelitis, idiopathic transverse myelitis, multiple sclerosis and HTLV-I infection. HTLV-I myelopathy is an important differential consideration in patients presenting with spastic paraparesis as it is endemic in some regions where schistosomiasis is found.

Gnathostomiasis, paragonomiasis, echinococcosis, and rarely extradural dracunculiasis are other endemic helminthic infections associated with peripheral eosinophilia that can rarely cause spinal cord disease. Idiopathic adhesive arachnoiditis and lathyrism are other forms of spastic paraplegia found in the tropics.

Treatment

A characteristic clinical picture, together with supportive radiological findings and evidence of systemic schistosomal infection, justify a presumptive diagnosis of CNS schistosomiasis and the institution of therapy (Haribhai *et al.*, 1991). There is good evidence that schistosomiasis of the spinal cord may be effectively treated by medical means alone. Many patients will present in outlying areas of tropical or subtropical countries without the benefit of sophisticated diagnostic techniques. In these cases specific therapy should not be delayed while awaiting the outcome of supportive diagnostic tests. Chemotherapy and chemoprophylaxis also play an important role in containing and preventing the transmission of the disease in endemic areas.

Praziquantel

Praziquantel is a safe, effective and broad-spectrum oral schistosomicidal agent, with few side-effects, and is currently the drug of choice for the treatment of all forms of schistosomiasis (King and Mahmoud, 1989; Chandra Shekhar, 1991; Haribhai *et al.*, 1991). It has been used successfully in schistosomal myelopathy. The drug kills the adult worm by producing paralysis of the parasite musculature, with vacuolation and degeneration of the surface of the worm. This results in a parasitological cure in 71–99% of patients, with a marked reduction in ova production. The clinical response to praziquantel, with or without corticosteroids, in spinal cord schistosomiasis is often quite rapid over several days to weeks. This effect is difficult to explain when the drug is only lethal to adult worms. In experimentally infected animals antischistosomal treatment leads to the rapid resolution of periovular visceral granulomas. It is controversial whether praziquantel is ovicidal or has immunosuppressive or anti-inflammatory actions as well. After oral administration the drug is rapidly and efficiently absorbed from the intestine. Bioavailability is 80–100%. The drug binds reversibly to plasma proteins. A significant proportion of the drug is metabolized during first-pass through the liver. Blood levels of 0.2–2.0 μg ml^{-1} are achieved 1–3 hours after administration (5–7% of ingested drug). The half-life of unaltered drug is 1–1½ hours. Small concentrations of the drug, less than 10–20% of plasma levels, are detected in bile, faeces, CSF and breast milk.

For *S. haematobium* and *S. mansoni* infections, a dose of 40 mg kg^{-1} given in two divided doses 4–6 hours apart is effective, with cure rates ranging between 63 and 100%. *S. japonicum* infections are treated with 60 mg kg^{-1} in three divided doses on one day. There is, however, no consensus regarding the length of treatment necessary for spinal cord bilharzia and treatment regimens using praziquantel have varied in dosage and duration. We have obtained good results using larger doses (50 mg kg^{-1} per day for 14 days), although it is possible that shorter courses may be effective in spinal schistosomiasis.

Other drugs used include oxamniquine and metriphonate, effective against *S. mansoni* and *S. haematobium* respectively. These and other agents have been superseded by praziquantel. The cost of praziquantel remains a limiting factor to its use in developing countries. Most patients show an impressive improvement in motor, sensory and sphincter function within weeks after praziquantel treatment, with or without corticosteroids. The biochemical and radiological abnormalities also respond to therapy, lending support to the diagnosis. Spinal cord disease may occasionally resolve irrespective of the treatment regimen and some patients have improved prior to receiving praziquantel, or following steroid therapy or laminectomy alone without specific anthelminthic chemotherapy.

Praziquantel therapy is well tolerated, and side-effects, if present, are usually mild or transient. The incidence of side-effects is 10–15%. The following have been noted: abdominal pain, nausea, vomiting, anorexia and diarrhoea (rarely with blood). Neurological symptoms include headache, vertigo, dysphoria, dizziness and drowsiness. Fever, urticarial rash and lassitude may occur.

Corticosteroids

The use of corticosteroid therapy in schistosomal myelopathy remains controversial (Scrimgeour and Dajdusek, 1985; Cosnett and van Dellen, 1986; Haribhai *et al.*, 1991; Liu, 1993). Steroids may have therapeutic efficacy by suppressing the inflammatory response and granuloma formation, and halting the tissue destruction. Although there have been no controlled studies, the use of corticosteroids as soon as the diagnosis of spinal schistosomiasis is suspected is probably justified. Rapid, if not complete, improvement following the use of steroids alone has been noted in many cases. It is more usual, however, to administer prednisolone together with praziquantel, in a dose of 60 mg daily for 14 days.

Corticosteroid drugs will also suppress the acute sensitivity state associated with the invasive stage and possibly any hypersensitivity provoked by the death of the adult worms under treatment.

Surgery

Laminectomy is an important adjunct to the management of the patient who develops acute paraplegia with spinal block or who deteriorates despite conservative treatment (Scrimgeour and Gajdusek, 1985; Liu, 1993). When operation is undertaken, the main purposes are biopsy and possibly decompression. At the time of decompression a biopsy should be performed avoiding unnecessary resection of additional granulomatous tissue. Surgical reports usually describe infiltrating yellow-grey lesions in the conus and roots of the cauda equina. Occasionally the lesions are well delineated. Total removal of the lesions is usually not possible. Demonstration of ova in a spinal biopsy remains the definitive proof of schistosomal myelopathy. It has been noted that recovery may occur spontaneously or after laminectomy alone.

Surgical decompression is not urgently required when there is a high index of suspicion, and drug treatment may obviate the need for surgery.

Prognosis

Following treatment with praziquantel and corticosteroids there is usually a rapid onset of clinical improvement, often within a few days, but sometimes delayed for several weeks (Scrimgeour and Gajdusek, 1985; Haribhai *et al.*, 1991). Remarkable improvement occurs in most patients usually by 6 weeks. This is also noted in the laboratory and radiological profiles of patients. There is a parallel improvement in the CSF pleocytosis and chemistry with a decrease in specific antischistosomal antibody titre and intrathecal IgG synthesis. Measurements of spinal cord diameter before and after treatment often show a reduction in cord swelling. Occasionally patients show spontaneous clinical improvement. A poor response may be related to irreversible structural cord damage, or to a delay in diagnosis and treatment, and emphasizes the value of early antischistosomal and corticosteroid therapy.

Previous clinical experience was that about one-third of cases recovered completely, one-third improved with some residual deficit and the remainder were unchanged or deteriorated. The outcome is slightly better in patients with involvement of the conus medullaris and/or cauda equina compared to those presenting with a higher level of spinal cord involvement. Patients with necrotic myelitis have a worse prognosis, although complete recovery is infrequently seen in patients presenting with the myelitic form. The mortality in confirmed cases of schistosoma myelopathy has fallen dramatically (72% prior to 1965 and 11.5% as of 1985) (Scrimgeour and Gajdusek, 1985). With greater awareness of the condition and early commencement of specific therapy a greater proportion of patients can be expected to show improvement on treatment. Recurrence of paraplegia can occur, presumably reflecting reinfection or further deposition of ova with consequent damage to an already compromised spinal cord.

Conclusions

Spinal cord schistosomiasis has a characteristic clinical and investigative profile. This allows a diagnosis to be made confidently using relatively non-invasive tests without resorting to laminectomy and biopsy. Further support for the diagnosis of spinal cord schistosomiasis is the rapid and marked improvement observed in the clinical, laboratory and radiological profiles following antischistosomal drugs used alone or in combination with corticosteroids. Treatment must be instituted early to reduce morbidity due to irreversible neurological damage. This is especially relevant in the management of patients presenting in rural areas of underdeveloped tropical and subtropical countries where sophisticated investigative facilities may not be readily available. When spinal cord schistosomiasis is suspected it is advisable to undertake a therapeutic trial of praziquantel and corticosteroids promptly even without direct proof of diagnosis. The patient should be referred to a neurological centre for more detailed evaluation while treatment is in progress.

REFERENCES

Alves W (1958) The distribution of schistosomal eggs in human tissues. *Bulletin of the World Health Organization* 18: 1092.

Bambirra EA, de Souza Andrade J *et al.* (1984) The tumoural form of schistosomiasis: report of a case with cerebeller involvement. *American Journal of Tropical Medicine and Hygiene* 33(1): 76–79.

Bird AV (1964) Acute spinal schistosomiasis. *Neurology* 14: 647.

Bird AV (1978) Schistosomiasis of the central nervous system. In: *Handbook of Clinical*

Neurology, vol. 35 (eds PJ Vinken and GW Bruyn), pp 231–241. Amsterdam: Elsevier/North-Holland Biomedical Press.

Blunt SB, Boulton J and Wise R (1993) MRI in schistosomiasis of conus medullaris and lumbar spinal cord. *Lancet* **341**: 557.

Boyce TG (1990) Acute transverse myelitis in a 6 year old girl with schistosomiasis. *Paediatric Infectious Disease Journal* **9**: 279–284.

Chandra Shekhar K (1991) Schistosomiasis drug therapy and treatment considerations. *Drugs* **42(3)**: 379–405.

Cosnett JE and van Dellen, JR (1986) Schistosomiasis (bilharzia) of the spinal cord: case reports and clinical profile. *Quarterly Journal of Medicine* **61(236)**: 1131–1139.

Ferguson AR (1917) Some notes on bilharziasis. *Journal of the Royal Army Medical Corps* **29**: 57.

Gelfand M (1950) *Schistosomiasis in South Central Africa: a Clinico-pathological Study*. Cape Town: Juta, pp 194–202.

Haribhai HC, Bhigjee AI, Bill PLA *et al.* (1991) Spinal cord schistosomiasis. *Brain* **114**: 709–726.

Joubert J, Fripp ITH, Hay IT *et al.* (1990) Schistosomiasis of the spinal cord – under-diagnosed in South Africa? *South African Medical Journal* **77**: 297–229.

Khalil HH, Abd El Wahab M, Deeb A *et al.* (1986) Cerebral atrophy: a schistosomiasis manifestation? *American Journal of Tropical Medicine and Hygiene* **35(3)**: 531–535.

King CH and Mahmoud AAF (1989) Drugs five years later; Praziquantel. *Annals of Internal Medicine* **110**: 290–296.

Liu LX (1993) Spinal and cerebral schistosomiasis. *Seminars in Neurology* **13(2)**: 189–200.

Mahmoud AA (1977) Schistosomiasis. *New England Journal of Medicine* **297(24)**: 1329–1331.

Molyneux ME and Galatius-Jensen F (1978) Successful drug treatment of schistosomal myelopathy. *South African Medical Journal* **54**: 871–872.

Müller HR and Stender A (1930) Bilharziose des Ruckenmarkes unter dem Bilde einer Myelitis dorsolumbalis transversa completa. *Archiv für Schiffs- und Tropen-Hygiene, Leipzig* **34**: 527–538.

Nash TE (1982) Schistosome infections in humans: perspectives and recent findings. *Annals of Internal Medicine* **97**: 740–754.

Pammenter MD, Haribhai HC, Epstein SR *et al.* (1991) The value of immunological approaches to the diagnosis of schistosomal myelopathy. *American Journal of Tropical Medicine and Hygiene* **44(3)**: 329–335.

Pitchford RJ (1986) Some aspects of bilharzia in southern Africa. *South African Medical Journal* (Supplement) October: 80–82.

Pittella JEH (1985) Vascular changes in cerebral schistosomiasis mansoni; a histopathological study of fifteen cases. *American Journal of Tropical Medicine and Hygiene* **34(5)**: 898–902.

Pittella JEH (1991) The relation between involvement of the central nervous system in schistosomiasis mansoni and the clinical forms of the parasitosis. A review. *Journal of Tropical Medicine and Hygiene* **94**: 15–21.

Pittella JEH and Lana-Peixoto MA (1981) Brain involvement in hepatosplenic schistosomiasis mansoni. *Brain* **104**: 621–632.

Queiroz L de S, Nucci A, Facure NO and Facure JJ (1979) Massive spinal cord necrosis in schistosomiasis. *Archives of Neurology* **36**: 517–519.

Scrimgeour EM and Gajdusek DC (1985) Involvement of the central nervous system in *Schistosoma mansoni* and *Schistosoma haematobium* infection. *Brain* **108**: 1023–1038.

Siddorn JA (1978) Schistosomiasis and anterior spinal artery occlusion. *American Journal of Tropical Medicine and Hygiene* **27(3)**: 532–534.

Silbergleit R (1992) Schistosomal granuloma of the spinal cord: evaluation with MRI imaging and intraoperative sonography. *American Journal of Radiology* **158**: 1351–1353.

Wakefield GS, Carroll JD and Speed DE (1962). Schistosomiasis of the spinal cord. *Brain* **85**: 535–555.

Warren KS (1978) The pathology, pathobiology and pathogenesis of schistosomiasis. *Nature* **273**: 609–612.

Warren KS (1986) The relevance of schistosomiasis. *New England Journal of Medicine* **303(4)**: 203–206.

Warren KS (1987) Schistosomiasis. In: *Oxford Textbook of Medicine*, 2nd edn (eds DJ Weatherall, JGG Ledingham and DA Warrell). Oxford: Oxford University Press.

19

Other Parasites

Peter K. Newman

Department of Neurology, Middlesbrough General Hospital, Middlesbrough, Cleveland, UK

INTRODUCTION

Parasitic protozoa and helminths are widespread in nature. Human disease follows consumption of contaminated and poorly cooked food, use of contaminated water, as a result of poor hygiene, or inoculation by insect vector. These conditions arise particularly, but not exclusively, in connection with inadequate sanitation and housing. Poverty and ignorance are the twin evils that lead to so many millions of people being afflicted by diseases that are usually preventable. The modern onslaught of AIDS has enabled parasitic diseases to gain access to another group of sufferers both in the developing and developed regions of the world. Intestinal, cutaneous, lymphatic and other system involvement is common, whereas neurological disease is less usual but often devastating when it occurs.

Full accounts are given elsewhere in this book of the neurological complications of infections with *Trypanosoma* species, *Plasmodium falciparum*, *Schistosoma* species and *Taenia solium*. There follows a synopsis of other neurological disorders caused by parasites, in which the more important conditions naturally merit more detailed coverage than the few lines allotted to extremely rare diseases. For the sake of completeness, mention is made of diseases such as toxocariasis and toxoplasmosis which are not predominantly tropical and have a world-wide distribution, but more detailed accounts are to be found in general textbooks of infectious diseases. See Table 19.1 for a summary of parasites causing neurological disease.

PROTOZOA

Cerebral Amoebiasis

Amoebic dysentery and the less common progression to liver or lung amoebic abscess are well-recognized consequences of poor hygiene and inadequate

TABLE 19.1 Parasites and neurological disease

Group	Organism	Neurological features	Main geographical regions
Protozoa	*Plasmodium falciparum*	Cerebral malaria	Throughout the tropics and subtropics
	Trypanosoma brucei (*gambiense* and *rhodesiense*)	African sleeping sickness	Equatorial West and East Africa
	Trypanosoma cruzi	Peripheral neuropathy, myositis, stroke	Central and South America
	Entamoeba histolytica	Meningoencephalitis, cerebral abscess	Throughout the tropics and subtropics
	Free-living amoebae (*Naegleria fowleri* and *Acanthamoeba* sp.)	Meningitis, granulomatous, meningoencephalitis	World-wide (rare)
	Toxoplasma gondii	Encephalitis, cerebral abscess	World-wide
	Sarcocystis sp.	Muscle pain and swelling	World-wide (rare)
	Microsporidiosa	Encephalitis	Japan (case report)
Helminths Nematodes	*Angiostrongylus cantonensis*	Eosinophilic meningoencephalitis	Widespread in tropics, esp. S. East Asia, Pacific Islands
	Gnathostoma spinigerum	Eosinophilic meningoencephalitis	Widespread in tropics, esp. Thailand and Japan
	Trichinella spiralis	Muscle pains, meningoencephalitis	Temperate and tropical areas
	Strongyloides stercoralis	Meningitis, encephalopathy	Patchy in tropics and subtropics
	Toxocara canis	Eosinophilic meningitis, myelitis, encephalitis	World-wide
	Loa loa	Meningoencephalitis	Central and West Africa
	Dracunculus medinensis	Spinal cord compression	Africa and Asia
	Onchocerca volvulus	Optic atrophy, epilepsy	Mainly West Africa, also South America and Middle East
	Wucheria bancrofti	Filariae in CNS	India, widely in tropics and subtropics
	Dipetalonema perstans	Meningoencephalitis	Tropical Africa and America
	Micronema deletrix	Meningoencephalitis	North America (case reports)
Trematodes	*Schistosoma mansoni*	Spinal cord	Africa, Brazil, Arabia
	Schistosoma japonicum	(esp. *S. mansoni*) and cerebral lesions	China, Indonesia, Philippines
	Schistosoma haematobium	(esp. *S. japonicum*)	Africa, Arabia, S. West Asia

TABLE 19.1 Parasites and neurological disease *(Cont.)*

Group	Organism	Neurological features	Main geographical regions
	Paragonimus sp.	Epilepsy, cerebral mass lesion, encephalopathy, cord compression	Widespread in tropics, esp. Far East
Cestodes	*Echinococcus granulosus*	Cerebral or spinal hydatid cysts	World-wide
	Taenia solium	Fits, cerebral mass lesions; neurocysticercosis	Widespread, esp. Latin America, India
	Spirometra sp.	Cerebral and spinal sparganosis (mass lesions)	S. East Asia, East Africa, North America
	Taenia (Multiceps) sp.	Similar to neurocysticercosis	Temperate and tropical areas (rare)
	Diphyllobothrium latum	B_{12} deficiency	Northern temperate areas and world-wide

provision of a clean water supply in tropical countries. Cerebral complications of systemic infection with *Entamoeba histolytica* were first described in 1849 (Morehead) and have been occasionally reported since, usually with a poor outcome and sometimes found at autopsy having been unsuspected in life (Lombardo *et al.*, 1964). The patient typically presents an acute meningoence-phalitis with fever, headache, altered mental state, meningism and often focal neurological features, usually arising in a background of amoebic dysentery and hepatic abscess (Orboson *et al.*, 1951). Amoebic serology is positive and the systemic lesions will be confirmed by abdominal and pulmonary imaging with computed tomography (CT) or ultrasound; the presence of trophozoites or cysts in faecal samples may not be helpful in differential diagnosis in residents or travellers from endemic regions. A CT brain scan will reveal ring enhancing abscesses or more diffuse low-density lesions. Lumbar puncture is not advised and, moreover, the cerebrospinal fluid (CSF) reaction is non-specific and organisms are not found. Aspiration biopsy of a cerebral lesion with direct microscopy of the wet preparation may reveal amoebic trophozoites, and infection has been confirmed using staining or immunofluorescent techniques. Late presentation and diagnosis contributes to the grim prognosis but survivals have been reported with surgical aspiration and removal of infected and necrotic abscess material combined with intravenous metronidazole for up to 3 weeks (Shah *et al.*, 1994). Subsequent colonic elimination of amoebic cysts can be achieved using diloxamide (Cook, 1990).

Primary Amoebic Meningoencephalitis

Human neurological disease caused by infection with the ubiquitous free-living amoebae (FLA) was first recognized in Australia (Fowler and Darter, 1965). Approximately 200 cases have subsequently been described and a very complete account is given by Duma (1991). *Naegleria fowleri* (Figure 19.1) is implicated in an acute meningitis in previously healthy individuals who while swimming have been exposed to infected water, whereas *Acanthamoeba* infection may lead to a granulomatous amoebic meningoencephalitis presenting as subacute or chronic meningitis, or brain abscess, in debilitated immunoincompetent individuals. The former organism is thought to enter via the nose and olfactory apparatus, while the latter originates from a focus of infection outside the nervous system. The CSF in *Naegleria* infection shows an acute pyogenic reaction and specific cultures for FLA will usually be positive; standard CSF stains will not show FLA but direct microscopy of wet preparations may reveal the organisms. In granulomatous amoebic meningoencephalitis the CSF reaction is non-specific but serological tests may be positive for *Acanthamoeba* and CT scanning shows multiple parenchymatous lesions. The diagnosis of FLA infection will probably only be considered when the clinical context is suspicious and investigation for more common conditions is negative.

The prognosis is poor in primary amoebic meningoencephalitis. Only a handful of patients have survived infection with *Naegleria*, in which therapy with amphotericin B is considered essential, possibly augmented by rifampicin,

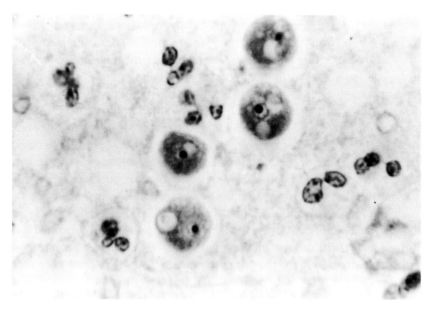

Figure 19.1 *Naegleria fowleri* – olfactory bulb smear stained with haematoxylin. Courtesy of Dr H. Zaiman and Dr E. Clifford Nelson.

miconazole, sulphisoxazole or tetracyclines (Seidel *et al.*, 1982). An interesting report from Western Province, Papua New Guinea (Tucker and Zerk, 1991), suggests a possible higher prevalence in this area, where 6 of 24 cases of meningitis admitted to a health centre in a 2-year period had CSF demonstration of *Naegleria* trophozoites, and survival in one case was achieved with metronidazole and chloroquine treatment. The mortality rate for granulomatous amoebic meningoencephalitis is even more bleak, amphotericin B is not effective, but partial responses have been reported using sulphamethazine (Cleland *et al.*, 1982) and 5-fluorocytosine (Harwood *et al.*, 1988). Other drugs untested in man have been shown to have in-vitro activity against *Acanthamoeba* species (Duma, 1991). Successful treatment of cutaneous *Acanthamoeba* infection before dissemination to the nervous system has occurred has recently been described, using intravenous pentamidine followed by oral itraconazole (Slater *et al.*, 1994).

Sarcocystis

A brief mention only is made of *Sarcocystis* infection of human muscle which has been reported on a few occasions from various parts of the world (Beaver *et al.*, 1979). The protozoal sporocysts are probably acquired by the faecal–oral route in the context of poor hygiene, and there is a reservoir in domestic and wild animals. The consequent appearance in muscle with the formation of characteristic sarcocysts does not generally produce symptoms, although there may be complaints of muscular aches and pains or swellings (Pallis and Lewis, 1988).

Microsporidiosis

This parasitic protozoan has only been documented in a few cases including one instance of central nervous system infection presenting as encephalitis in a Japanese child who had a CSF leukocytosis and microsporidia on direct smear examination (Matsubayashi *et al.*, 1959). *Microsporidia* are being increasingly recognized in patients with AIDS who present with chronic diarrhoea.

Toxoplasmosis

Congenital *Toxoplasma* infection is beyond the scope of this chapter and the acquired condition is only briefly summarized as it is more commonly recognized in a non-tropical environment, particularly in the context of AIDS (see Chapter 4). Man is one of several intermediate hosts for *Toxoplasma gondii*. Infection usually occurs following the ingestion of tainted meat or as a result of poor hygiene where infected cat faeces are present in the soil. In many severe cases of acquired infection the patient is immunocompromised. Acute infection may cause myalgia, fever, lymphadenopathy, rash, neck stiffness and anorexia, but more commonly is not symptomatic. Later there may be more persistent lymphadenopathy and painless retinochoroiditis is common. Encephalitis may be seen in the acute stage, especially in immunodeficient individuals. Seropositivity is widespread indicating a high level of asymptomatic infection in the population at large. In the immunocompromised host, latent cysts are reactivated to produce a subacute encephalopathy often with focal stroke-like deficits. This may occur in those with AIDS or cancer. The CT brain scan shows multiple low-density lesions which are often ring enhancing. The response to treatment with combined pyrimethamine and sulphadizine is generally rapid, and can be used as a diagnostic test for cerebral toxoplasmosis in patients with AIDS (Porter and Sande, 1992).

HELMINTHS

Nematodes

Eosinophilic meningitis or encephalitis due to helminthic infection is familiar to physicians in South-East Asia and other tropical zones. The clinical presentations can be similar in infestations by several organisms, and the diagnosis may depend on the local expectations of the physician supported in some instances by serological tests or by identification of the organism.

Angiostrongyliasis

The rat lungworm *Angiostrongylus cantonensis* (Figure 19.2) is widespread in the tropics, particularly recognized in South-East Asia, Pacific Islands, Papua New Guinea and also Australia. The rat is the definitive host, snails and slugs the intermediate hosts, and man is infected after consuming raw snails or unwashed vegetables contaminated by rat faeces. The contrasting modes of infection are illustrated by an account from Thailand of multiple cases following sharing a common meal containing the local delicacy of raw Pila snails (Vejjajiva, 1978), and a report from Australia where the disease presented in four vegetarians (Fuller *et al.*, 1993). The ingested larva migrates to the brain and spinal cord producing tracks and cavities and an intense CSF pleocytosis with up to 75% eosinophils. There is a meningitic reaction with severe headache and neck stiffness which is usually self-limiting and resolves after a month, but a good prognosis is not invariable and cranial nerve palsies, paraparesis, persisting disability and death may result (Jaroonvesama, 1988; Schmutzard *et al.*, 1988). An ELISA test may be helpful in diagnosis. Treatment is symptomatic as antihelminthics are ineffective and could theoretically produce an even more intense cerebral reaction to killed worms.

Gnathostomiasis

Gnathostoma spinigerum is thought to have been first isolated in 1836 from the stomach of a tiger captive at London Zoo (Vejjajiva, 1978). The parasite (Figure

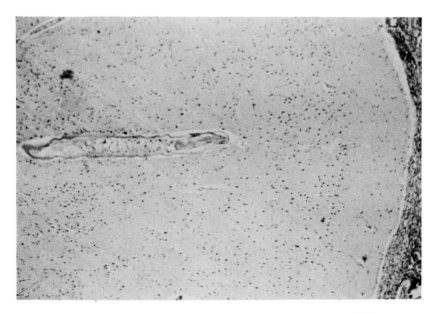

Figure 19.2 *Angiostrongylus cantonensis* – larva in brain. Courtesy of Professor W. Peters and Dr J. Cross.

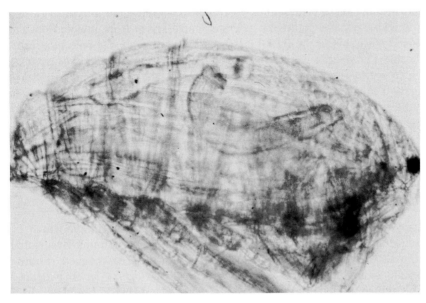

Figure 19.3 *Gnathostoma nipponicum* – 2nd stage larva in a *Cyclops* water flea. Courtesy of Professor W. Peters.

19.3) is widespread in the tropics where, particularly in Thailand, it causes infection following ingestion of freshwater fish or frogs, the second intermediate hosts, or drinking water contaminated by *Cyclops*, the first intermediate host. The migrating immature worm induces cutaneous swellings and peripheral blood eosinophilia but causes havoc when ascending a peripheral nerve and entering the central nervous system. Intense nerve root pain is followed a few days later by sudden paraplegia or cerebral symptoms. The CSF shows a pleocytosis with eosinophilia which is not as intense as in *Angiostrongylus* infection, but the hallmark of *Gnathostoma* is the finding of xanthochromia or red blood cells resulting from the multiple haemorrhages created by the migrating worm. The mortality is at least 12%, survivors have a high residual morbidity and it has been suggested that 22% of haemorrhagic cerebral vascular accidents in Thais may be caused by *Gnathostoma* (Punyagupta *et al.*, 1990). The worm has been recovered at autopsy from brain or spinal cord but is not detected directly in life. Indirect serological tests are not well established but the clinical diagnosis in an endemic area should not pose a problem and the possibility of gnathostomiasis will be suspected in a traveller from an endemic area with typical clinical features and a history suggesting ingestion of the intermediate host. Treatment with albendazole has given encouraging results (Kraivichian *et al.*, 1992) but other accounts are less optimistic.

Trichinosis

Trichinella spiralis infection follows consumption of undercooked meat from diseased domestic or wild animals. Trichinosis is prevalent in temperate as well as tropical areas and outbreaks in France have arisen from infected horsemeat. Muscle invasion after the initial intestinal phase may present with muscle pains, fever and facial oedema. Migration of the larva into the nervous system can produce meningitis, seizures, psychosis, coma and focal deficit. It has been suggested in a recent review that the protean neurological and cardiac features may be due to a secondary hypereosinophilia syndrome, and not primarily to direct tissue infiltration by the worm (Fourestie *et al.*, 1993). Muscle biopsy is often diagnostic and an ELISA test may be helpful. Treatment is with corticosteroids for the acute symptoms as well as with thiabendazole or mebendazole.

Strongyloidiasis

Strongyloides stercoralis is a common cause of gut infestation which in the presence of immunosuppression may lead to an overwhelming hyperinfection syndrome in which the central nervous system may be invaded resulting in pyogenic meningitis due to *Escherichia coli*. This can occur in patients with AIDS, and an association between *S. stercoralis* and HTLV-I infection has also been recognized (Nakada *et al.*, 1984). A greater awareness of the hyperinfection syndrome has been urged by Cook (1987).

Dracontiasis

The guinea worm *Dracunculus medinensis* infects millions with its characteristic subcutaneous lesions and ulcers, but does not usually cause neurological involvement. It is occasionallly reported as an extradural abscess causing spinal cord compression which can be treated surgically as well as with antihelminthic drugs (Reddy *et al.*, 1969).

Filariasis

Human filarial infection also does not generally lead to neurological disease, but *Loa loa* has been implicated in a meningoencephalitis (Vitris *et al.*, 1989) and there is a single remarkable case where Bancroftian filariasis has been reported in association with recurrent Guillain–Barré syndrome (Bhatia and Misra, 1993). The filariae in this condition, as well as in the other filariases, may invade the CNS. The extensive lymphoedema characteristic of Bancroftian filariasis can cause secondary peripheral nerve lesions. Brown and Voge (1982a) refer to cases where *Dipetalonema perstans* has caused encephalitis. The spread of the microfilariae of *Onchocerca volvulus* to the eye is a frequent cause of blindness in endemic areas, and in some cases optic nerve involvement may lead to optic atrophy (Rodger, 1987).

Toxocariasis

Toxocara canis causes ocular larva migrans with the well-known complication, particularly in children, of blindness due to choroidoretinitis. In visceral larva migrans, nervous system involvement has also been reported, resulting in eosinophilic meningitis, transverse myelitis and encephalitis (Sommer *et al.*, 1994).

Micronemiasis

Brown and Voge (1982b) cite two cases where infection with *Micronema deletrix* led to meningoencephalitis, and these are mentioned here for the sake of completion.

Trematodes

Paragonimiasis

Human disease caused by the lung fluke *Paragonimus* (Figure 19.4) is particularly prevalent in the Far East (China, Japan, Korea, Taiwan) but occurs in many other tropical countries. Eggs are shed from pulmonary cysts, develop into miracidia to be taken up by freshwater snails and then crabs, as first and

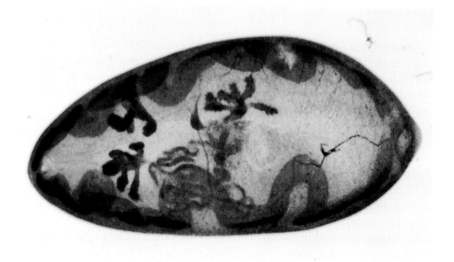

Figure 19.4 *Paragonimus westermani.* Courtesy of Professor W. Peters.

second intermediate hosts, and then the cycle is completed when the human or animal primary host is infected by consuming infested crustacea. Metacercaria then migrate from the gut into the lungs where the mature fluke develops. Pulmonary paragonimiasis is the usual presentation with chronic chest symptoms productive of rusty sputum and associated radiographic abnormalities.

Cerebral paragonimiasis is now rarely reported but it was estimated that there were 5000 active cases in Korea in 1966 (Oh, 1967). It may be suspected as a cause of chronic seizures or cerebral space-occupying lesion in an endemic area, or with a more acute illness of fever, headache, seizures and focal deficit (Toyonaga, 1992). A skull radiograph may show characteristic round or oval calcified lesions, demonstrated with greater precision by CT or magnetic resonance (MR) imaging (Kadota *et al.*, 1989). Even rarer cases of spinal involvement have been recorded. Active paragonimiasis is treated with praziquantel or bithionol; surgical resection in cerebral paragonimiasis fails to improve symptoms.

Cestodes

Hydatid Disease

Infestation by the hydatid larva is an important parasitic disease world-wide, wherever human proximity to sheep and dogs is accompanied by poor hygiene. Dog is the definitive host of *Echinococcus granulosus*, sheep and other domestic

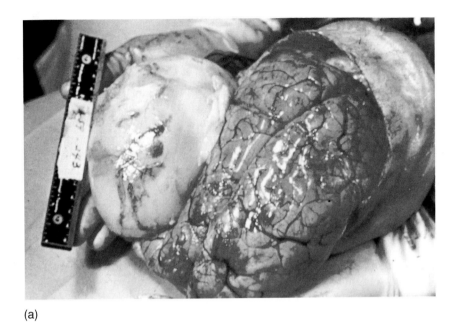

(a)

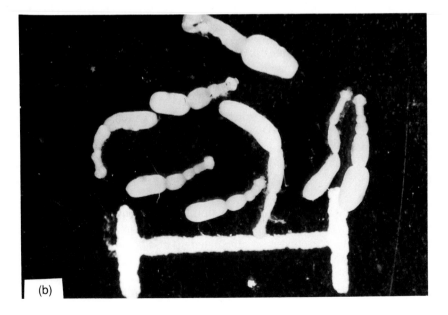

(b)

Figure 19.5 (a) Hydatid cyst in brain. (b) *Echinococcus granulosus* – adults (bar, 1 cm). Courtesy of (a) Dr H. Zaiman and Dr H. Fink and (b) Professor W. Peters.

animals may be intermediate hosts, and transmission of eggs to man occurs by contamination with dog faeces. The viable eggs breach the intestinal mucosa and are carried to viscera where they develop into unilocular cysts. Liver and or lung involvement accounts for most cases, neurological disease due to cerebral or spinal spread occurring in about 2%. Children and young adults are more commonly affected. See Figure 19.5.

Cerebral hydatid disease presents with symptoms and signs of raised intra-cranial pressure, seizures and focal deficits including hemianopia, dysphasia and hemiparesis. Papilloedema is usually present. In children there may be skull radiographic changes but CT brain scanning is the more definitive investigation and will reveal in most cases a single cerebral cyst; second or multiple cysts are seen in a few cases usually when a fertile cyst has ruptured and released sterile scolices into the surrounding brain. Extraneurological disease will be evident in about 20% of cases, but serology may not be positive and skin testing is unhelpful. The treatment of cerebral hydatidosis is surgical, with excision of the entire cyst using the Dowling technique, and carefully avoiding rupture as the cyst is delivered. A large Turkish series found a recurrence rate of 26.6% (Cataltepe et al., 1992) and in a long-term follow-up study from Italy, two-thirds of 12 cases were in good health a mean of 28 years after surgery (Lunardi et al., 1991). Albendazole or praziquantel may be used as adjunctive treatment in selected cases and in those where cyst rupture has occurred spontaneously or during surgery.

Paraplegia is seen when vertebral hydatosis spreads to the extradural space, usually in the thoracic region and leads to spinal cord compression (Pamir et al., 1984). Repeated surgery is often required and an initial aggressive decompression with bone grafting is more likely to be successful than a simple laminectomy. Antihelminthic drugs may be used in conjunction with radical surgery. The prognosis in spinal hydatid disease is guarded (Karray et al., 1990).

Myocardial embolization of hydatid cysts into the brain has been recorded as a very rare cause of acute stroke in young adults in an endemic area (Benomar et al., 1994). Orbital hydatid cysts may present with unilateral proptosis and ophthalmoplegia, and can be successfully removed (Lerner et al., 1991).

Sparganosis

In South-East Asia and North America human infection with the *Spirometra* species of tapeworm is seen when contaminated drinking water is taken. Sparganosis usually presents as a subcutaneous nodule or with conjunctivitis, but cerebral sparganosis occurs and there have also been a few reported instances of spinal cord involvement (see Figure 19.6 a–d). Cerebral sparganosis presents as a mass lesion and can be seen as such on CT or MR imaging; sequential scanning may indicate whether the worm is alive or dead within the granuloma and hence guide the decision regarding surgical intervention (Chang et al., 1992). The differential diagnosis from other causes of granuloma, primary or secondary tumour, may be difficult but can be achieved by stereotactic biopsy

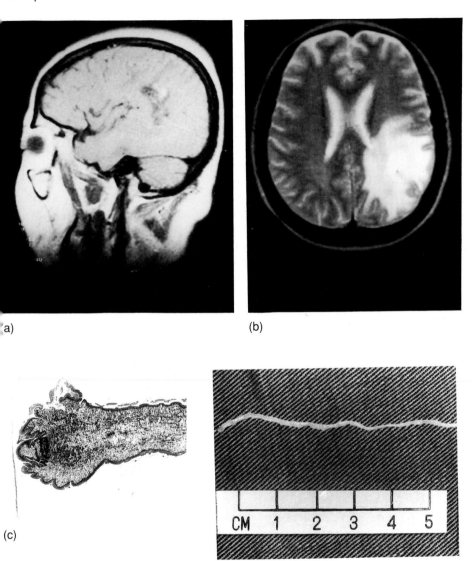

Figure 19.6 Sparganosis. (a) T1-weighted sagittal MRI brain; (b) T2-weighted axial MRI brain; (c) anterior section of worm (H & E × 50); (d) sparganum recovered from central canal of spinal cord. Courtesy of Dr Tsai and Journal of Neurosurgery and Dr Fung and Journal of Neurosurgery.

with removal of the worm leading to a full recovery (Tsai *et al.*, 1993). Spinal granuloma due to sparganosis causing cord compression has also been successfully treated by surgical resection (Cho *et al.*, 1992). The *Spirometra* tapeworm is similar to the fish tapeworm *Diphyllobothrium latum* which can indirectly cause neurological disease by means of malabsorption-induced vitamin B$_{12}$ deficiency.

Coenuriasis

Taenia (Multiceps) species infect sheep as an intermediate host, causing unsteadiness of gait. In man, the parasite has been rarely reported to cause neurocoenuriasis which presents in a similar fashion to neurocysticercosis, although the cyst in the cerebrum, brainstem or spinal cord is usually solitary. Surgical removal and praziquantel are the recommended treatments (McGreevy and Nelson, 1991).

CONCLUSION

A brief summary has been given of protozoal and helminth infestations of the nervous system. Most of these conditions are rare but some are very common. In most cases the disease could be eradicated by public health measures combined with access to treatment. Sadly the prevalence is often increasing rather than decreasing, and the problem of 'worms in the head' as yet shows no sign of disappearing.

REFERENCES

Beaver PC, Gadgil K and Morera P (1979) *Sarcocystis* in man: a review and report of five cases. *American Journal of Tropical Medicine and Hygiene* **28(5)**: 819–844.

Benomar A, Yahyaoui M, Birouk N, Vidailhet M and Chkili T (1994) Cerebral artery occlusion due to hydatid cysts of myocardial and intraventricular cavity cardiac origin. *Stroke* **25**: 886–888.

Bhatia B and Misra S (1993) Recurrent Guillain–Barré syndrome following acute filariasis. *Journal of Neurology, Neurosurgery and Psychiatry* **56**: 1133–1134.

Brown W and Voge M (1982a) *Neuropathology of Parasitic Infections*, pp 197–203. Oxford: Oxford University Press.

Brown W and Voge M (1982b) *Neuropathology of Parasitic Infections*, pp 220–224. Oxford: Oxford University Press.

Cataltepe O, Colak A, Özcan O, Özgen T and Erbang A (1992) Intracranial hydatid cysts: experience with surgical treatment in 120 patients. *Neurochirurgia* **35**: 108–111.

Chang KH, Chi JG, Cho SY *et al.* (1992) Cerebral sparganosis: analysis of 34 cases with emphasis on CT features. *Neuroradiology* **34(1)**: 1–8.

Cho YD, Huh JD, Hwang YS and Kim HK (1992) Sparganosis in the spinal cord with partial block: an uncommon infection. *Neuroradiology* **34**: 241–244.

Cleland PG, Lawande RV and Onyemelukwe G (1982) Chronic amoebic meningoencephalitis. *Archives of Neurology* **39**: 56–57.

Cook GC (1987) *Strongyloides stercoralis* hyperinfection syndrome: how often is it missed? *Quarterly Journal of Medicine* **64**: 625–629.

Cook GC (1990) Colorectal parasitic infections; invasive *Entamoeba histolytica* and its role in colonic and hepatic disease. In: *Parasitic Disease in Clinical Practice*, pp 110–112. London: Springer Verlag.

Duma RJ (1991) Primary amoebic meningoencephalitis: infection by free living amoebae. In: *Infections of the Central Nervous System* (ed. HP Lambert), pp 253–263. London: Edward Arnold.

Fourestie V, Douceron H, Brugieres P *et al.* (1993) Neurotrichinosis. *Brain* **116**: 603–616.

Fowler M and Carter RF (1965) Acute pyogenic meningitis due to *Acanthamoeba* species. *British Medical Journal* **2**: 740–742.

Fuller AJ, Munckhoff W, Kiers L, Ebeling P and Richards MJ (1993) Eosinophilic meningitis due to *Angiostrongylus cantonensis*. *Western Journal of Medicine* **159**: 78–80.

Harwood CR, Rich GE, McAleer R and Cherion G (1988) Isolation of *Acanthamoeba* from a cerebral abscess. *Medical Journal of Australia* **148**: 47–49.

Jaroonvesama N (1988) Differential diagnosis of eosinophilic meningitis. *Parasitology Today* **4**: 262–266.

Karray S, Zlitni M, Fowles JV *et al.* (1990) Vertebral hydatosis and paraplegia. *Journal of Bone and Joint Surgery* **72(1)**: 84–88.

Kodota T, Ishikura R, Tabuchi Y *et al.* (1989) MR imaging of chronic cerebral paragonimiasis. *American Journal of Neuroradiology* **10**: 521–522.

Kraivichian P, Kulkumthorn M, Yingyourd P, Akarabovorn P and Paireepai CC (1992) Albendazole for the treatment of human gnathostomiasis. *Transactions of the Royal Society of Tropical Medicine and Hygiene* **86**: 418–421.

Lerner SF, Morales AG and Croxatto JO (1991) Hydatid cyst of the orbit. *Archives of Opthalmology* **109**: 285.

Lombardo L, Alonso P, Arroyo LS, Brandt H and Mateos JH (1964) Cerebral amoebiasis. Report of 17 cases. *Journal of Neurosurgery* **21**: 704–709.

Lunardi P, Missori P, DiLorenzo N and Fortuna A (1991) Cerebral hydatosis in childhood: a retrospective survey with emphasis on long term follow-up. *Neurosurgery* **29**: 515–517.

Matsubayashi H, Koike T, Mikata I *et al.* (1959) A case of encephalitozoon-like body infection in man. *Archives of Pathology* **67**: 181.

McGreevy PB and Nelson GS (1991) Coenuriasis. In: *Hunter's Tropical Medicine*, 7th edn (ed. GT Strickland), pp 858–859. Philadelphia: WB Saunders.

Morehead C (1849) Notes on the pathology and treatment of diseases of the brain, as observed in the European General Hospital at Bombay. *Trans Med Phys Soc Bombay* **9**: 112–115.

Nakada S, Kohakura M, Komoda H *et al.* (1984) High incidence of HTLV-1 antibody in carriers of *Strongyloides stercoralis*. *Lancet* **i**: 633.

Oh SJ (1967) Cerebral paragonimiasis. *Transactions of the American Neurolological Association* **92**: 275–277.

Orboson JA, Reevers N, Leedham CL and Blumberg JM (1951) Amoebic brain abscess. *Medicine (Baltimore)* **30**: 247–282.

Pamir MN, Akalan N, Özgen T *et al.* (1984) Spinal hydatid cysts. *Surgical Neurology* **21**: 53–57.

Pallis CA and Lewis PD (1988) Involvement of human muscle by parasites. In: *Disorders of Voluntary Muscle*, 5th edn (ed. J Walton), pp 611–615. Edinburgh: Churchill Livingstone.

Porter SB and Sande MA (1992) Toxoplasmosis of the central nervous system in the acquired immunodeficiency syndrome. *New England Journal of Medicine* **327**: 1643–1648.

Punyagupta S, Bunnag T and Jathjudatta P (1990) Eosinophilic meningitis in Thailand: clinical and epidemiological characteristics of 162 patients with myeloencephalitis probably caused by *Gnathostoma spinigerum*. *Journal of the Neurological Sciences* **96**: 241–256.

Reddy CR, Sita Devi C, Reddy M and Reddy NV (1969) Dracontiasis: review of surgical problems and treatment. *International Surgery* **52**: 481–488.

Rodger FC (1987) Onchocerciasis. In: *Manson's Tropical Diseases*, 19th edn (eds PEC Manson-Bahr and DR Bell), pp 1152–1155. London: Ballière Tindall.

Schmutzhard E, Boongird P and Vejjajiva A (1988) Eosinophilic meningitis and radiculomyelitis in Thailand, caused by CNS invasion of *Gnathostoma spinigerum* and *Angiostrongylus cantonensis*. *Journal of Neurology, Neurosurgery and Psychiatry* **51**: 80–87.

Seidel JS, Harmatz P, Visvevara GS *et al.* (1982) Successful treatment of primary amoebic meningoencephalitis. *New England Journal of Medicine* **306**: 346–348.

Shah AA, Shaikh H and Karim M (1994) Amoebic brain abscess: a rare but serious complicaton of *Entamoeba histolytica* infection. *Journal of Neurology, Neurosurgery and Psychiatry* **57**: 240–241.

Slater CA, Sickel JZ, Visvesvara GS, Pabico RC and Gaspari AA (1994) Brief report: successful treatment of disseminated *Acanthamoeba* infection in an immunocompromised patient. *New England Journal of Medicine* **331**: 85–87.

Sommer C, Ringelstein EB, Biniek R and Glöckner WM (1994) Adult *Toxocara canis* encephalitis. *Journal of Neurology, Neurosurgery and Psychiatry* **57**: 229–231.

Toyonaga S, Kurisaka M, Mori K and Suzuki N (1992) Cerebral paragonimiasis: report of five cases. *Neurologia Medico-Chirurgica (Tokyo)* **32**: 157–162.

Tsai M, Chang C, Ho Y and Wang AD (1993) Cerebral sparganosis diagnosed and treated with stereotactic techniques. *Journal of Neurosurgery* **78**: 129–132.

Tucker GS and Zerk G (1991) Primary amoebic meningoencephalitis in the Western Province. *Papua New Guinea Medical Journal* **34**: 87–89.

Vejjajiva A (1978) Parasitic diseases of the nervous system in Thailand. *Proceedings of the Australian Association of Neurology* **15**: 92–97.

Vitris M, Nkam M, Binam F *et al.* (1989) Meningoencephalite filarienne: discussion a propos d'un cas. *Medicine Tropicale* **49**: 293–295.

Section 4
ENVIRONMENTAL CONDITIONS

20

Toxic and Nutritional Disorders

Nimal Senanayake

Department of Medicine, Faculty of Medicine, University of Peradeniya, Peradeniya, Sri Lanka

INTRODUCTION

With the increasing use of vast quantities of chemicals in industry, agriculture and medicine, disorders of toxic aetiology are fast becoming a major health problem all over the world. People in tropical countries are particularly at risk because of the indiscriminate use of toxic chemicals. Naturally occurring toxins of plant and animal origin, and nutritional deficiencies, compound the problem (Senanayake and Roman, 1991, 1992).

The same toxic or nutritional factor may produce different neurological manifestations; conversely, different factors may produce the same manifestation. No part of the nervous system is immune, and any structure from the brain down to the skeletal muscle may be affected (Table 20.1). Peripheral nerves are particularly susceptible, and polyneuropathy with distal axonal degeneration ('dying back' neuropathy) (Cavanagh, 1979) is a common manifestation of toxic disorders. In this condition, long or large nerve fibres are affected, the degeneration beginning in the distal parts. The defect is thought to be an impairment of axonal transport caused by the toxic agent (Griffin and Watson, 1988). Manifestations outside the nervous system may provide a clue to the aetiological agent. Epidemiological studies complement clinical investigations.

Toxic and nutritional factors causing neurological disorders, which are of special relevance to the tropics, are discussed in this review.

HEAVY METALS

Inorganic and organic compounds of a number of heavy metals affect the nervous system, the peripheral nerves in particular.

TABLE 20.1 Toxic and nutritional factors affecting the nervous system

	Principal sites affected								
	EN	BG	CB	ON	SC	PN	NMJ	SM	ANS
Toxic agents									
Heavy metals									
Arsenic						+			
Thallium						+			
Lead	+					+			
Manganese		+							
Mercury	+	+							
Drugs									
Isoniazid, ethionamide						+			
Ethambutol						+			
Nitrofurantoin						+			
Metronidazole						+			
Dapsone						+			
Aromatic diamidines						+			
Chloroquine						+		+	
Clioquinol				+	+	+			
Industrial agents									
Tri-ortho-cresyl phosphate					(+)	+			
Methanol	+	+		+					
Insecticides									
Organophosphorus	+					+	+		+
Organochlorines	+								
Pyrethroids	+					(+)			
Biological agents									
Diphtheria						+			
Cassava					+				
Lathyrus					+				
Gloriosa						+			
Podophyllin						+			
Karwinskia						+			
Cycad	+	+			+				
Ciguatoxin						+			
Shellfish						+			
Tetrodotoxin						+			
Snake venom						+	(+)		
Spider venom						+			+

TABLE 20.1 Toxic and nutritional factors affecting the nervous system (*Cont.*)

	Principal sites affected								
	EN	BG	CB	ON	SC	PN	NMJ	SM	ANS
Nutritional deficiencies									
Thiamin	+					+			
Niacin	+								
Vitamin B_{12}					+	+			
Vitamin D	+							+	
Protein-energy	+					+		+	
Alcohol	+		+			+		+	
Drug abuse	+								

EN, encephalon; BG, basal ganglia; CB, cerebellum; ON, optic nerve; SC, spinal cord; PN, peripheral nerves; NMJ, neuromuscular junction; SM, skeletal muscles; ANS, autonomic nervous system.

Arsenic

Polyneuropathy is the prime feature of acute and chronic arsenic intoxication (Jenkins, 1966; Chuttani *et al.*, 1967). Delay between acute poisoning and neuropathic symptoms is 3 days to 3 weeks. Vomiting, diarrhoea, burning sensation in the eyes, excessive tear secretion, photophobia, nasal congestion, facial swelling and mental confusion, are followed by numbness and weakness of the feet and hands. Burning sensation in the feet, generalized muscle pains, and cramps may be present. The tendon reflexes disappear early. 'Glove-and-stocking' sensory loss is a cardinal feature. Mucocutaneous signs include Mees' lines (transverse white bands across nails), increased pigmentation, patches of hypopigmentation, hyperkeratosis with desquamation of palms and soles, and inflammatory changes of the oral mucosa. 'Rain-drop' pigmentation is not usual in dark-skinned patients (Senanayake *et al.*, 1972).

Electrophysiological abnormalities are characteristic of distal axonal degeneration (Windebank, 1987). Nerve biopsies show degeneration of myelinated fibres into linear rows of myelin ovoids (Le Quesne and McLeod, 1977). The diagnosis is confirmed by demonstrating arsenic in urine, hair and nail-clippings. Improvement may appear in 1 to 4 months, but the severely affected patients may be crippled for life (Senanayake *et al.*, 1972). Dimercaprol (British antilewisite, BAL) or penicillamine is the treatment, which should be given early.

Arsenic added to food, beverages or water, with criminal intent, is the commonest mode of poisoning (Senanayake *et al.*, 1972). Other sources of arsenic in the tropics include illicit liquor (moonshine whiskey) (Gerhardt *et al.*, 1980), ocean fish (Bagchi and Ganguly, 1941), oral abortifacients (Simpson, 1965), opium (Jayasinghe *et al.*, 1983), and traditional remedies (Dean *et al.*, 1984).

Lead

Lead causes encephalopathy in children, and peripheral neuropathy in adults. The former manifests as ataxia, slurred speech, convulsions and coma. Lead neuropathy is an atypical motor paresis, affecting the extensors of the fingers and wrist asymmetrically, with a predilection for the dominant hand. In the lower limbs, the muscles innervated by the peroneal nerve or the 5th lumbar root may be affected. Abdominal colic, punctate basophilia and anaemia help in the diagnosis. Pathological and electrophysiological studies of lead neuropathy suggest an axonopathic process. Ethylenediamine tetra-acetate (EDTA), penicillamine and BAL have been used in the treatment of lead poisoning with varying results.

Refining of jeweller's wastes, reconditioning car batteries for recovery of scrap lead (Mirando and Gomez, 1967), burning lead-containing batteries for cooking or to provide heat (Greengard *et al.*, 1961), illicit liquor distilled using lead pipes or radiators (Whitfield *et al.*, 1972), and lead paint are known causes of lead poisoning.

Thallium

Thallium, a constituent of some rodenticides, causes an acute painful neuropathy following severe gastrointestinal symptoms (Cavanagh *et al.*, 1974). Alopecia is a characteristic feature. Prussian blue (potassium ferric ferrocyanide) is the treatment of choice.

Manganese

Manganese has poisoned miners in many countries. Prolonged exposure causes behavioural changes, and later, parkinsonism due to widespread damage to basal ganglia. Manganese has also been implicated in a type of motor neurone disease with onset in early childhood, and a cerebellar syndrome with oculomotor disturbances in aborigines in Groote Eylandt, Australia (Kilburn, 1987).

Mercury

Mercury vapour, inorganic salts and organomercurials are all potentially toxic. The neurological effects manifest as tremors and personality changes ('Mad

Hatter syndrome'). Ingestion of fish from waters contaminated with methyl mercury discharged from manufacturing plants caused poisoning in Japan (Minamata disease). Widespread poisoning occurred in the Middle East when grain treated with mercury fungicides was inadvertently consumed by farmers.

DRUGS

Many drugs cause adverse neurological manifestations, affecting the nervous system at different points, from cerebral hemisphere to peripheral nerve (Argov and Mastaglia, 1979). Drugs of special relevance in the tropics are discussed next.

Isoniazid

Isoniazid causes a peripheral neuropathy presenting with sensory loss in the limbs associated with burning sensation and muscle tenderness. Those severely affected develop weakness and ataxia. The neuropathy is dose-related, 2% being affected on 300 mg day^{-1}, and 17% on 400 mg day^{-1} (Critchley, 1987). The rate of isoniazid acetylation in the liver is genetically determined and slow acetylation, a recessive inheritance widely distributed among Europeans and Africans, increases the liability to develop neurotoxicity. Ethionamide, a thioamide derivative of isonicotinic acid, may also produce a sensory neuropathy.

Ethambutol

Ethambutol, another antituberculous agent, causes optic neuritis; sensory or sensorimotor neuropathy has also been reported, mostly from Japan. The frequency is about 16/1000 patients (Ando *et al.*, 1970). Symptoms tend to disappear with the cessation of treatment.

Nitrofurantoin

Nitrofurantoin causes a neuropathy, related to the plasma level of the drug and the duration of treatment. Paraesthesia and sensory loss are followed by foot-drop and weakness of hands. Recovery can be slow and incomplete. Histology shows axonal degeneration with changes in dorsal root ganglia and anterior horn cells (Critchley, 1987).

Metronidazole

Metronidazole causes sensory changes during long-term treatment of Crohn's disease (Ursing and Kamme, 1975). Two of our patients developed sensorimotor polyneuropathy on a much lower dose of metronidazole for chronic amoebic colitis (Senanayake and Jayatissa, 1984). One patient recovered completely after discontinuing the drug, but the other succumbed to his intestinal disease. Recovery usually takes 2 or more years (Karlsson and Hamlyn, 1977).

Chloroquine

Chloroquine causes a neuromyopathy after prolonged use in the treatment of rheumatoid arthritis or lupus erythematosus. Symptoms appear 5 to 11 months after starting treatment, and improve when the drug is discontinued (Loftus, 1963). Histology shows vacuolation of muscle fibres, and changes in the terminal axons and Schwann cells (Tegner *et al.*, 1988).

Clioquinol

Clioquinol, used in the treatment of diarrhoea, is the agent of subacute myelo-optico-neuropathy (SMON), observed in Japan in the 1950–60s (Nakae *et al.*, 1973). It is rarely seen outside Japan, except for certain milder forms (Thomas, 1984). It may be mistaken for Devic's disease or multiple sclerosis. With the restrictions on the use of clioquinol, the incidence of SMON has reduced markedly.

Dapsone

Dapsone, used in the treatment of leprosy, may cause a subacute motor neuro-pathy when given in high doses over a long period (Gehlmann *et al.*, 1977).

Aromatic Diamidines

Aromatic diamidines (stilbamidine isetionate, propamidine, pentamidine), used in the treatment of leishmaniasis and trypanosomiasis, have occasionally caused disturbance of sensory function of the trigeminal nerve.

INDUSTRIAL CHEMICALS

Exposure to industrial chemicals may occur at factories and manufacturing plants due to accidents or deficiencies in the exposure-monitoring system. On the other hand, the general public may be affected through air pollution or contamination of water or food.

Tri-*ortho*-cresyl Phosphate (TOCP)

TOCP, an industrial solvent, has caused poisoning in many parts of the world by contamination or adulteration of food, drink or edible oils (Smith and Spalding, 1959; Vora *et al.*, 1962; Morgan and Penovich, 1978). In an outbreak in Sri Lanka, the victims were either teenage girls, or women after childbirth. Gingili oil, given traditionally to women at menarche and postpartum, had been contaminated with TOCP in containers which had previously been used to store mineral oil. Acute distal axonopathy with motor manifestations, followed by pyramidal tract dysfunction were the cardinal effects. Despite pronounced disability in the early stages, these patients made a remarkable recovery (Senanayake and Jeyaratnam, 1981; Senanayake, 1981).

Other industrial chemicals, such as *n*-hexane, methyl-*n*-butyl ketone, carbon disulphide and acrylamide, also cause neurotoxic effects, mostly peripheral neuropathy.

Methanol (Methyl Alcohol)

Methanol (wood alcohol), an industrial solvent, causes inebriation, followed by vomiting, abdominal pain, visual disturbances, shortness of breath, delirium, coma and death. Some may be left with blindness due to degeneration of the optic nerve and retina. Damage to the putamen and cerebral white matter has also been reported (Filley and Kelly, 1993).

INSECTICIDES

Insecticide poisoning is a major health hazard in many tropical agricultural countries. Poisoning occurs due to ingestion with suicidal intent, accidental ingestion and accidents during spraying. Lack of effective measures to control the import and the sale of insecticides, and disregard for safety precautions during handling, have contributed to the increasing incidence of insecticide poisoning in the tropics.

Organophosphorus Insecticides (OPI)

In Central Sri Lanka, OPI account for more than half the hospital admissions due to acute poisoning (Senanayake and Karalliedde, 1988). The muscarinic, nicotinic and central neurotoxic effects of OPI during the acute cholinergic phase are well documented (Heath and Vale, 1992; Senanayake *et al.*, 1993).

A recently recognized complication is the intermediate syndrome, which develops 1 to 4 days after poisoning, affecting cranial, neck flexor, proximal limb and respiratory muscles (Senanayake and Karalliedde, 1987). The respiratory paralysis carries a high risk of death. Electrophysiological studies suggest a postsynaptic defect at the neuromuscular junction (Senanayake and Karalliedde, 1987, 1992; de Wilde *et al.*, 1991).

OP-induced delayed polyneuropathy (OPIDP) develops 2–4 weeks after the initial exposure. The commonest agent causing OPIDP in Sri Lanka is methamidophos (Senanayake and Johnson, 1982; Senanayake, 1985, 1990). Acute weakness of hands and feet preceded by calf pain is the presenting symptom. Ankle jerks are absent. Some patients develop claw-hand deformity, and some develop pyramidal signs. Improvement may appear about 2 weeks after the onset, but complete recovery can take up to 2 years.

OPIDP is related to the phosphorylation of 'neurotoxic or neuropathy target esterase' (NTE) in nervous tissue (Johnson, 1975, 1990). An essential second step is the 'ageing' of the enzyme, which depends on the chemical structure of the OP. Phosphinates and carbamates are not capable of ageing, hence not neuropathic. In fact, when pretreated, these provide a protective effect against OPIDP, by blocking the receptor (Johnson and Lauwerys, 1969).

Recurrent laryngeal nerve palsy, presumably related to OPIDP, has been reported recently (de Silva *et al.*, 1994). Extrapyramidal signs, namely, rest tremor, cog-wheel rigidity, dystonic movements, athetosis and choreiform movements, have also been observed after OPI poisoning. Inhibition of acetyl cholinesterase in the basal ganglia is suggested as the underlying mechanism (Senanayake and Sanmuganathan, 1995).

Behavioural abnormalities, both transient and persistent, have been associated with OP toxicity. These include depression, irritability, confusion and emotional lability. Most symptoms resolve within a year (Heath and Vale, 1992). Neuropsychological testing is used in the evaluation of suspected OP-induced psychopathology (Rosenstock *et al.*, 1991).

Organochlorines

Organochlorine insecticides, which include dichlorodiphenyltrichlorethane (DDT), aldrin, dieldrin, endrin and lindane, are neurotoxic to man. Acute or subacute poisoning with DDT causes paraesthesia of the tongue, lips and face, apprehension, hypersusceptibility to stimuli, irritability, dizziness, disturbed equilibrium, tremor and convulsions. There is little pathological change seen in the brain, but evidence indicates that DDT is capable of altering the transport of sodium and potassium ions across axonal membranes (Murphy, 1975).

In India, epidemics of poisoning had been attributed to benzene hexachloride (BHC) used mistakenly as a food grain preservative. Recurrent convulsive seizures preceded by auditory and visual aura, headache, confusion and memory lapses, impaired vision and staggering gait were the common symptoms. Some patients presented in status epilepticus (Khare *et al.*, 1977; Nag *et al.*, 1977).

Pyrethrum

Pyrethrum extract is used in many household insecticides because of its rapid knock-down action. In man, massive doses cause convulsions leading to paralysis and muscle fibrillation. Death occurs due to respiratory failure (Murphy, 1975).

BACTERIAL TOXINS

Diphtheria

A neuropathy develops in about 20% of patients following diphtheria (McDonald and Kocen, 1984). Palatal palsy is the initial feature, manifesting 3–4 weeks after the throat infection, followed by impairment of ocular accommodation. Paralysis of pharynx, larynx and respiratory muscles may prove fatal. A sensorimotor polyneuropathy develops about 8–12 weeks later. Histologically, the nerves show segmental demyelination. There is complete recovery in those who survive.

Tetanus is dealt with in Chapter 12.

PLANT POISONS

Chronic cyanide intoxication from dietary cassava has been associated with the pathogenesis of tropical ataxic neuropathy. Lathyrism, caused by the excessive consumption of peas of the *Lathyrus* genus, causes a progressive spastic paraparesis (see Chapters 21 and 22).

Gloriosa superba

Gloriosa superba (climbing lily, glory lily) is a poisonous, tuberous-rooted plant of the *Liliaceae*, the lily family, native to tropical Africa and Asia. Poisoning occurs when the tubers are eaten accidentally, or deliberately with suicidal intent. The manifestations include gastroenteritis, alopecia, aplastic anaemia and polyneuropathy, attributed to colchicine (Angunawela and Fernando, 1971).

Podophyllin

Podophyllin, derived from the dried rhizomes and roots of a mandrake or mayapple (*Podophyllum pelatum*), has been used as a laxative. The resin is used topically for warts and condylomata. Podophyllin poisoning, after ingestion of the Chinese herbal broth guijiu, has caused encephalopathy and sensorimotor polyneuropathy (Ng *et al.*, 1991).

Karwinskia humboldtiana

Karsinskia humboldtiana (tullidora, wild cherry, coyotillo) is a poisonous shrub of the buckthorn family which grows in central and northern Mexico, Texas and New Mexico. Ingestion of the fruit causes a progressive polyneuropathy, sometimes ending with respiratory and bulbar paralysis. The neurotoxicity is attributed to a substance in the endocarp of the drupe, affecting axoplasmic transport (Heath *et al.*, 1982).

Cycas circinalis

Consumption of the cycad seed has been related to the high incidence of motor neurone disease in the Kii peninsula of Honshu Island, Japan and amyotrophic lateral sclerosis and parkinsonism-dementia in the Mariana Islands. Animal experiments, using β-*N*-methylamino-L-alanine present in the cycad seed, support this hypothesis (Spencer, 1987).

ANIMAL POISONS

Ciguatoxicity, paralytic shellfish poisoning (PSP) and tetrodotoxicity are common neurological syndromes caused by the ingestion of toxic crustacea, molluscs and fish from the tropical seas. Ciguatoxic fish such as barracuda, grouper, red snapper and amberjack, contain the dinoflagellate, *Gambierdiscus toxicus* (Morris *et al.*, 1982). PSP is due to bivalve molluscs such as mussels, clams, scallops and oysters that have ingested dinoflagellates of the *Protogonyaulax* genus containing saxitoxin and its derivatives (Rodrigue *et al.*, 1990). A similar syndrome has been reported following the ingestion of certain toxic crustaceans such as horseshoe or king crabs. Tetrodotoxicity occurs by eating Tetrodontiform fish such as pufferfish, a delicacy (fugu) in Japan (Suenaga and Kotoku, 1980). Tetrodotoxin has also been discovered in certain species of crabs, shellfish, starfish and in the venom of blue-banded octopus. The symptomatology includes paraesthesia, and paralysis involving external ocular, masticatory, facial, palatal, tongue and distal limb muscles. Respiratory paralysis may cause death.

The venom of marine snails of the genus *Conus* contains neurotoxic peptides, conotoxins. Careless handling of the cone has resulted in human fatalities. Numbness at the site of the sting, blurring of vision, impaired speech and muscle weakness precede death due to respiratory paralysis (Clench and Kondo, 1943).

Most of these toxins inhibit sodium channels of excitable membranes, blocking the propagation of nerve and skeletal muscle action potentials (Catterall, 1980; Cameron *et al.*, 1991). Conotoxins, in addition, cause inhibition of acetylcholine receptors at the postsynaptic membrane, and calcium channels at the nerve endings (McManus and Musick, 1985).

Snake and spider bites are discussed in Chapter 23.

NUTRITIONAL DISORDERS

Thiamin Deficiency

Thiamin deficiency (beriberi) causes three types of neurological manifestations, namely, peripheral neuropathy, Wernicke's encephalopathy and Korsakoff syndrome. The neuropathy is a mixed polyneuropathy with dominant sensory features, affecting the distal parts of the limbs. The histology shows non-inflammatory degeneration of myelin sheaths.

Wernicke's encephalopathy presents with vomiting, nystagmus, ophthalmoplegia, fever and progressive mental deterioration resulting in a global confusional state which may progress to coma and death. Improvement occurs after treatment with thiamin, but Korsakoff syndrome may supervene. The latter consists of retrograde amnesia, impaired ability to learn and confabulation. The patient is usually alert and responsive, showing no serious abnormality in behaviour. Recovery can be expected only in about 50%. Patients who die in the acute stages of Wernicke–Korsakoff disease show symmetrical necrotic lesions in the paraventricular regions of the thalamus and hypothalamus, mammillary bodies, periaqueductal region of the midbrain, floor of the 4th ventricle and anterior-superior folia of the cerebellum.

Thiamin should be administered promptly when beriberi is diagnosed or suspected. The recommended dose is 50 mg day^{-1} i.m. for several days, followed by 2.5–5 mg day^{-1} orally.

Niacin Deficiency (Pellagra)

Diarrhoea, dermatitis and dementia are the triad of manifestations associated with pellagra. The diarrhoea is due to widespread inflammation of the mucosa, and is associated with glossitis, stomatitis and vaginitis. The dermatitis is bilateral, symmetrical and photosensitive. Fatigue, insomnia and apathy precede the development of the encephalopathy which is characterized by confusion, disorientation, hallucination, loss of memory and, eventually, frank organic psychosis. The mental changes are considered to be associated with diminished conversion of tryptophan to serotonin. The pathological changes are most noticeable in the large Betz cells of the motor cortex. The course is progressive over several years, and death is usually due to secondary complications. The diagnosis must be based on suspicion and response to replacement therapy.

Nutritional Amblyopia

Also referred to as tobacco-alcohol amblyopia, nutritional retrobulbar neuropathy and nutritional optic neuropathy, this disorder presents with impairment of vision progressing over several weeks. Examination shows bilateral symmetrical central or centrocecal scotomas. Pallor of the temporal portion of the optic disc is seen in some cases. The pathological change consists of bilaterally symmetrical loss of myelinated fibres in the central parts of the optic nerves, chiasm and optic tracts. Treatment with B vitamins and adequate nutrition are usually followed by improvement. Untreated, it progresses to irreversible optic atrophy.

Amblyopia may accompany other neurological syndromes believed to have a nutritional cause, such as Strachan's syndrome, which is essentially a disorder of peripheral and optic nerves.

Vitamin B$_{12}$ Deficiency

Insufficient absorption of vitamin B$_{12}$ from the gastrointestinal tract can result in subacute degeneration of the spinal cord, and to a lesser extent, of the optic nerves, cerebral white matter and peripheral nerves. The disorder is encountered in association with pernicious anaemia, and only rarely secondary to vitamin B$_{12}$ deficiency as may occur in infestation with fish tapeworm, sprue, vegetarianism or gastrointestinal surgery. The presenting symptoms are general weakness, and paraesthesia in the distal parts of the limbs. As the illness progresses, the gait becomes unsteady. Later in the course, impaired posterior column sensations and bilateral pyramidal signs occur. Prompt treatment with cyanocobalamine can reverse the early neurological manifestations rapidly and completely.

Vitamin D Deficiency

Dietary factors, multiple closely spaced pregnancies, prolonged lactation and wearing of purdhas by women, are important causes of vitamin D deficiency in the tropics. In adults, osteomalacia causes a myopathy, presenting with weakness of proximal muscles and waddling gait. In childhood, rickets causes mental subnormality. Hypocalcaemia may cause seizures.

Protein-energy (Calorie) Malnutrition (PEM)

The developing nervous system of a child is particularly vulnerable to deprivations in nurture. PEM affects the central nervous system, especially the neuropsychological functions, in a lasting manner. Learning deficits, behavioural problems and manual dexterity are the most obtrusive features. Peripheral nerve and muscle derangements are clinically evident by weakness, hypotonia and hyperreflexia, in accordance with the severity and duration of PEM. Nerve conduction studies show abnormalities which correlate with grades of PEM. The histology is characterized by persistence of small myelinated nerve fibres, failure of internodal elongation and segmental demyelination. Muscle pathology comprises obliteration of cross-striations, streaming of Z bands, increased interfibrillary spaces, mitochondriomegaly and small-for-age fibres.

Rehabilitation leads to almost complete restoration of nervous system function, although certain derangements remain partially unimproved (Chopra and Sharma, 1992).

Chronic Alcoholism

The most frequent neurological disorders, in a recent study of 641 chronic alcoholics, were cerebellar degeneration (38%), peripheral neuropathy (34%) and seizures (14%). Other manifestations included Korsakoff's psychosis (8%), Wernicke's encephalopathy (4%), dementia (4%) and hepatic encephalopathy (2%). The most frequent cognitive disorders were frontal lobe dysfunction (58%) and short-term memory loss (32%) (Tuck and Jackson, 1991). Some of these syndromes are attributed to coexistent nutritional deficiency (see earlier).

Cerebellar cortical degeneration usually manifests over several weeks or months, and affects stance and gait predominantly. Nystagmus and dysarthria are less frequent. The pathological changes consist of degeneration of the vermis and adjacent parts of the anterior lobes of the cerebellum.

Central pontine myelinolysis is a relatively rare disorder characterized by demyelination of the central portion of the pons. It has also been encountered in non-alcoholic patients who are nutritionally deprived. The principal neurological abnormalities are progressive weakness of facial muscles and tongue causing impairment of speech and deglutition. Other features include sensory impairment over the face, absent corneal reflex, pseudobulbar palsy and flaccid quadriplegia with extensor plantar responses. Progression is rapid, ending in coma and death, over 2 to 3 weeks.

Marchiafava–Bignami disease was originally assumed to occur exclusively in males of Italian descent who consumed excessive amounts of crude red wine, but it has since been encountered in others. The patients are agitated and confused having hallucinations, disturbance of memory, negativism and progressive dementia, suggestive of frontal lobe disease. Symmetrical zones of demyelination are seen in the central corpus callosum. These changes have also been encountered in conjunction with Wernicke's disease and nutritional amblyopia, as well as in malnourished, non-alcoholic patients.

Excessive alcohol consumption has also been reported to cause acute rhabdomyolysis and chronic alcoholic myopathy (Freilich and Byrne, 1992).

Drug Abuse

Drugs of abuse, such as cannabis, lysergic acid diethylamine, mescaline and cocaine, produce hallucinatory and other psychic effects, and subsequently, withdrawal symptoms. Cocaine abuse has recently been associated with neuropsychological abnormalities, stroke, cerebral atrophy and dystonia. Much of the information is anecdotal or retrospective, and well-designed prospective studies are essential to study this area more fully (Freilich and Byrne, 1992).

REFERENCES

Ando K, Ohashi T, Matsuoka Y *et al.* (1970) Neuropathies due to antituberculous drugs. *Saishin Igaku* **25**: 901–915.

Angunawela RM and Fernando HA (1971) Acute ascending polyneuropathy and dermatitis following poisoning by tubers of *Gloriosa superba. Ceylon Medical Journal* **16**: 233–235.

Argov Z and Mastaglia FL (1979) Drug-induced peripheral neuropathies. *British Medical Journal* i: 663–666.

Bagchi RBKN and Ganguly HD (1941) Arsenic in food. *Indian Medical Gazette* **76**: 720–722.

Cameron J, Flowers AE and Capra MF (1991) Electrophysiological studies on ciguatera poisoning in man (Part II). *Journal of the Neurological Sciences* **101**: 93–97.

Catterall WA (1980) Neurotoxins that act on voltage-sensitive sodium channels in excitable membranes. *Annual Review of Pharmacology and Toxicology* **20**: 15–43.

Cavanagh JB (1979) The 'dying back' process – a common denominator in many naturally occurring and toxic neuropathies. *Archives of Pathology and Laboratory Medicine* **103**: 659–664.

Cavanagh JB, Fuller NH, Johnson HRM and Rudge P (1974) The effects of thallium salts with particular reference to the nervous system changes. *Quarterly Journal of Medicine* **43**: 293–319.

Chopra JS and Sharma A (1992) Protein energy malnutrition and the nervous system. *Journal of the Neurological Sciences* **110**: 8–20.

Chuttani PN, Chawla LS and Sharma TB (1967) Arsenical neuropathy. *Neurology (Minneapolis)* **17**: 269–274.

Clench WJ and Kondo Y (1943) The poison cone shell. *American Journal of Tropical Medicine* **23**: 105–120.

Critchley EMR (1987) Neuropathies due to drugs. In: *Handbook of Clinical Neurology,* vol. 7(51), *Neuropathies* (ed. WB Matthews), pp 293–314. Amsterdam: Elsevier.

de Silva HJ, Sanmuganathan PS and Senanayake N (1994) Isolated bilateral recurrent laryngeal nerve paralysis: a delayed complication of organophosphorus poisoning. *Human and Experimental Toxicology* **13**: 171–173.

de Wilde V, Vogelares D, Colardyn F *et al.* (1991) Postsynaptic neuromuscular dysfunction in organophosphate induced intermediate syndrome. *Klinische Wochenschrift* **69**: 177–183.

Dean AG, Washburn JW and Briesemeister K (1984) Update: arsenic poisoning in Hmong patients. *Minnesota Department of Health Disease Control News Letter* **11**: 69.

Filley CM and Kelly JP (1993) Alcohol- and drug-related neurotoxicity. *Current Opinion in Neurology and Neurosurgery* **6**: 443–447.

Freilich RJ and Byrne E (1992) Alcohol and drug abuse. *Current Opinion in Neurology and Neurosurgery* **5**: 391–395.

Gehlmann LK, Koller WC and Malkinson FD (1977) Dapsone-induced neuropathy. *Archives of Dermatology* **113**: 845–846.

Gerhardt RE, Crecelius EA and Hudson JB (1980) Moonshine-related arsenic poisoning. *Archives of Internal Medicine* **140**: 211–213.

Greengard J, Rowley W, Elam H and Perlstein M (1961) Lead encephalopathy in children: intravenous use of urea and its management. *New England Journal of Medicine* **264**: 1027–1030.

Griffin JW and Watson DF (1988) Axonal transport in neurological disease. *Annals of Neurology* **23**: 3–13.

Heath AJW and Vale JA (1992) Clinical presentation and diagnosis of acute organophosphorus insecticide and carbamate poisoning. In: *Clinical and Experimental Toxicology of Organophosphates and Carbamates* (eds B Ballantyne and TC Mars), pp 513–519. Oxford: Butterworth-Heinemann.

Heath JW, Ueda S, Bornstein MB, Daves GD Jr and Raine CS (1982) Buckthorn neuropathy in vitro: evidence for a primary neuronal effect. *Journal of Neuropathology and Experimental Neurology* **41**: 204–220.

Jayasinghe KSA, Misbah SA, Soosainathan S *et al.* (1983) Contaminated opium as a source of chronic arsenic poisoning in Sri Lanka. *Ceylon Medical Journal* **28**: 22–27.

Jenkins RB (1966) Inorganic arsenic and the nervous system. *Brain* **89**: 479–498.

Johnson MK (1975) The delayed neuropathy caused by some organophosphorus esters: mechanism and challenge. *CRC Critical Reviews in Toxicology* **3**: 289–316.

Johnson MK (1990) Organophosphates and delayed neuropathy – is NTE alive and well? *Toxicology and Applied Pharmacology* **102**: 385–899.

Johnson MK and Lauwerys R (1969) Protection by some carbamates against the delayed neurotoxic effects of di-isopropyl phosphorofluoridate. *Nature* **222**: 1066–1067.

Karlsson IJ and Hamlyn AN (1977) Metronidazole neuropathy. *British Medical Journal* **ii**: 832.

Khare SB, Rizvi AG, Shukla OP *et al.* (1977) Epidemic outbreak of neuromuscular manifestations due to chronic BHC poisoning. *Journal of the Association of Physicians in India* **25**: 215–222.

Kilburn CJ (1987) Manganese, malformations and motor disorders: findings in a manganese exposed population. *Neurotoxicology* **8**: 421–430.

Le Quesne PM and McLeod JG (1977) Peripheral neuropathy following a single exposure to arsenic. *Journal of the Neurological Sciences* **32**: 437–451.

Loftus LR (1963) Peripheral neuropathy following chloroquine therapy. *Canadian Medical Association Journal* **89**: 917–920.

McDonald WI and Kocen RS (1984) Diphtheritic neuropathy. In: *Peripheral Neuropathy* (eds PH Dyck, PK Thomas, EH Lambert and R Bunge), pp 2010–2017. Philadelphia: WB Saunders.

McManus OB and Musick JR (1985) Postsynaptic block of frog neuromuscular transmission by conotoxin. *Journal of Neuroscience* 5: 110–116.

Mirando EH and Gomez M (1967) Lead poisoning in childhood in Ceylon. *Archives of the Diseases in Children* 42: 579–582.

Morgan JP and Penovich P (1978) Jamaica ginger paralysis. *Archives of Neurology* 35: 530–532.

Morris JG Jr, Lewin P, Hargrett NT *et al.* (1982) Clinical features of ciguatera fish poisoning: a study of the disease in the U.S. Virgin Islands. *Archives of Internal Medicine* 142: 1090–1092.

Murphy SD (1975) Pesticides. In: *Toxicology* (eds LJ Casarett and J Doull), pp 408–453. New York: Macmillan.

Nag D, Singh GC and Sanong S (1977) Epilepsy epidemic due to benzahexachlorine. *Tropical and Geographical Medicine* 29: 229–232.

Nakae K, Yamamoto S, Shigematsu I and Kono R (1973) Relation between subacute myelooptic neuropathy (SMON) and clioquinol: a nationwide survey. *Lancet* i: 171–174.

Ng THK, Chan YW, Yu YL *et al.* (1991) Encephalopathy and neuropathy following ingestion of a Chinese herbal broth containing podophyllin. *Journal of the Neurological Sciences* 101: 107–113.

Rodrigue DC, Etzel RA, Hall S *et al.* (1990) Lethal paralytic shellfish poisoning in Guatemala. *American Journal of Tropical Medicine and Hygine* 42: 267–271.

Rosenstock L, Keifer M, Daniel WE *et al.* (1991) Chronic central nervous system effects of acute organophosphate pesticide intoxication. *Lancet* 338: 223–227.

Senanayake N (1981) Tri-cresyl phosphate neuropathy in Sri Lanka: a clinical and neurophysiological study with a three year follow up. *Journal of Neurology, Neurosurgery and Psychiatry* 44: 775–780.

Senanayake N (1985) Polyneuropathy following insecticide poisoning: a clinical and electrophysiological study. *Journal of Neurology* 232 (supplement): 203.

Senanayake N (1990) Toxic polyneuropathies. *Ceylon Medical Journal* 35: 45–55.

Senanayake N and Jayatissa SK (1984) Sensori-motor polyneuropathy due to metronidazole. *Ceylon Medical Journal* 29: 153–156.

Senanayake N and Jeyaratnam J (1981) Toxic polyneuropathy due to gingili oil contaminated with tri-cresyl phosphate affecting adolescent girls in Sri Lanka. *Lancet* i: 88–89.

Senanayake N and Johnson MK (1982) Acute polyneuropathy after poisoning by a new organophosphate insecticide. *New England Journal of Medicine* 306: 155–156.

Senanayake N and Karalliedde L (1987) Neurotoxic effects of organophosphorus insecticides: an intermediate syndrome. *New England Journal of Medicine* 316: 761–763.

Senanayake N and Karalliedde LD (1988) Pattern of acute poisoning in a medical unit in Central Sri Lanka. *Forensic Science International* 36: 101–104.

Senanayake N and Karalliedde L (1992) Intermediate syndrome in anticholinesterase neurotoxicity. In: *Clinical and Experimental Toxicology of Organophosphates and Carbamates* (eds B Ballantyne and TC Mars), pp 126–132. Oxford: Butterworth–Heinemann.

Senanayake N and Roman GC (1991) Toxic neuropathies in the tropics. *Journal of Tropical and Geographical Neurology* 1: 3–15.

Senanayake N and Roman GC (1992) Disorders of neuromuscular transmission due to natural environmental toxins. *Journal of the Neurological Sciences* **107**: 1–13.

Senanayake N and Sanmuganathan PS (1995) Extrapyramidal manifestations complicating organophosphorus insecticide poisoning. *Human and Experimental Toxicology* (in press).

Senanayake N, de Silva WAS and Salgado MSL (1972) Arsenical polyneuropathy: a clinical study. *Ceylon Medical Journal* **17**: 195–203.

Senanayake N, de Silva HJ and Karalliedde L (1993) A scale to assess severity in organophosphorus intoxication: POP Scale. *Human and Experimental Toxicology* **12**: 297–299.

Simpson K (1965) *Taylor's Principles and Practice of Medical Jurisprudence*, vol. 2. London: Churchill.

Smith HV and Spalding JMK (1959) Outbreak of paralysis in Morocco due to ortho-cresyl phosphate. *Lancet* **ii**: 1019–1021.

Spencer PS (1987) Guam ALS/Parkinsonism-Dementia: a long-latency neurotoxic disorder caused by slow toxin(s) in food? *Canadian Journal of Neuroscience* **14**: 347–357.

Suenaga K and Kotoku S (1980) Detection of tetrodotoxin in autopsy material by gas chromatography. *Archives of Toxicology* **44**: 291–297.

Tegner R, Tome FMS, Godeau P, Lhermitte F and Fardeau M (1988) Morphological study of peripheral nerve changes induced by chloroquine treatment. *Acta Neuropathologica* **75**: 253–260.

Thomas PK (1984) Neurotoxicity of halogenated hydroxyquinoles: Non-Japanese cases. *Acta Neurologica Scandinavica* **70** (supplement 100): 155–158.

Tuck RR and Jackson M (1991) Social, neurological and cognitive disorders in alcoholics. *Medical Journal of Australia* **155**: 225–229.

Ursing B and Kamme C (1975) Metronidazole for Crohn's disease. *Lancet* **i**: 775–777.

Vora DD, Dastur DK, Braganca BM *et al.* (1962) Toxic polyneuritis in Bombay due to ortho-cresyl-phosphate poisoning. *Journal of Neurology, Neurosurgery and Psychiatry* **25**: 234–242.

Whitfield CL, Chien LT and Whitehead JD (1972) Lead encephalopathy in adults. *American Journal of Medicine* **52**: 289–298.

Windebank AJ (1987) Peripheral neuropathy due to chemical and industrial exposure. In: *Handbook of Clinical Neurology*, vol. 7(51), *Neuropathies* (ed. WB Matthews), pp 263–292. Amsterdam: Elsevier.

21

Konzo

Hans Rosling and Thorkild Tylleskär

Unit for International Child Health, University Hospital, S-751 85 Uppsala, Sweden

INTRODUCTION

In 1938 Trolli published a report on an epidemic spastic paraparesis observed in the southern part of Bandundu region in present Zaire. This is to our knowledge the first description of the disease entity that we have chosen to name konzo, the local designation used among the population studied by Trolli (1938). Konzo is a yaka word (van der Beken, 1993) that means 'tied legs' which is a good description of the spastic gait resulting from the disease (Figure 21.1). The onset is abrupt and konzo mainly affects women and children in rural areas of

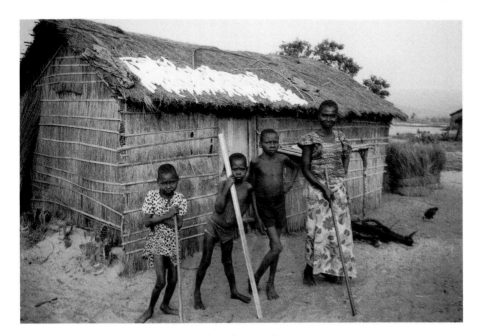

Figure 21.1 Patients affected with konzo of varying severity.

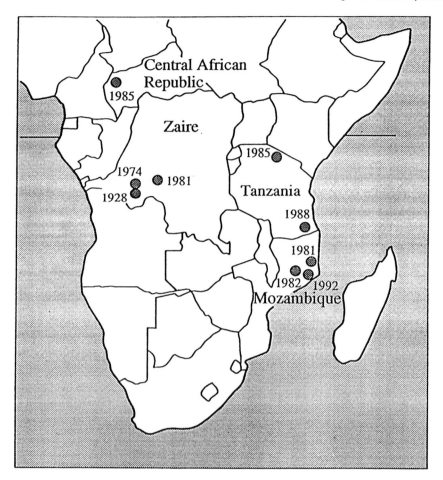

Figure 21.2 Reported occurrence of konzo in Africa with year of first known outbreak.

Africa with severe agroecological problems. Epidemic outbreaks with totally about 4000 cases have been reported from remote rural areas of Mozambique, Tanzania, Zaire and Central African Republic (Tylleskär *et al.*, 1994) (Figure 21.2). An infectious cause was first suspected (Trolli, 1938; Carton *et al.*, 1986) but recent studies indicate that konzo is caused by dietary cyanide exposure from insufficiently processed roots of bitter cassava (Figure 21.3).

Cassava is a high-yielding staple crop for 400 million people in the tropics (Figure 21.4). The bitter varieties contain high amounts of the cyanogenic glucoside linamarin but are preferred in many areas with low agricultural suitability because they provide the best food security. However, roots from these potentially toxic varieties can be rendered safe by effective processing methods that in two steps remove cyanogenic substances from the roots. First, disintegration of plant cells by mechanical grating or fermentation will bring

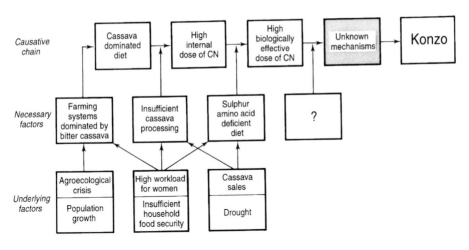

Figure 21.3 A conceptual framework of the present understanding of the causation of konzo.

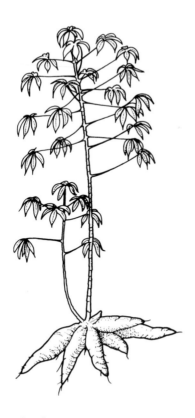

Figure 21.4 Cassava (*Manihot esculenta*).

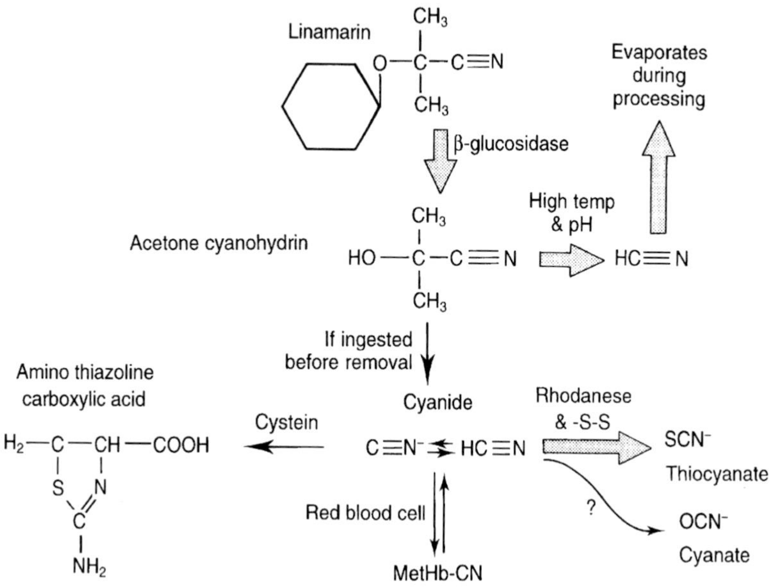

Figure 21.5 Cyanogenesis of cassava and cyanide detoxification in the human body.

linamarin in contact with an endogenous glucosidase to break it down to glucose and acetone cyanohydrin. In a second step, drying or heating will break down cyanohydrin to yield hydrogen cyanide that evaporates into the air at 27°C (Figure 21.5).

This chapter reviews the studies that identified konzo as a distinct disease entity and the strong, but not conclusive, evidence for an aetiological role of dietary cyanide. We also discuss the relationship between konzo and tropical ataxic neuropathy that is clinically different but also has been attributed to cyanide exposure from cassava.

A Distinct Clinical Entity

Carton et al. (1986) studied epidemic spastic paraparesis in the same parts of Bandundu region as Trolli (1938) and concluded that the disease was identical to the epidemic spastic paraparesis reported from Mozambique (Ministry of Health Mozambique, 1984a, b; Cliff et al., 1985). Reporting a similar outbreak in northern Tanzania, Howlett et al. (1990) stated that this spastic paraparesis is a distinct disease entity that is best named konzo, the local name mentioned in the title of Trolli's (1938) first report.

The diagnostic criteria used for konzo are:

1. A visible symmetrical spastic abnormality of gait while walking or running.
2. A history of onset in less than one week followed by a non-progressive course in a formerly healthy person.
3. Bilaterally exaggerated knee or ankle jerks without signs of disease of the spine.

The first and third criteria will be fulfilled by several types of spastic paraparesis, but the history of a rapid onset and non-progressive course by very few beside lathyrism (Spencer, *et al.*, 1986). It is thus necessary to exclude consumption of *Lathyrus sativus* but konzo can be clinically distinguished from other tropical myeloneuropathies. Konzo should not be considered as an HTLV-I negative form of tropical spastic paraparesis, since this has gradual onset, progressive course and different epidemiological behaviour. Neither should konzo be included with tropical ataxic neuropathy as two different expressions of the same neurotoxic effect of cassava as an aetiological role of cassava is yet to be proven for both these conditions. We consequently separate the discussion of konzo into functional, anatomical and aetiological diagnoses (Tylleskär, 1994).

FUNCTIONAL DIAGNOSIS

The clinical picture of konzo can be summarized based on 250 patients in seven case series reported from epidemic outbreaks in Mozambique, Tanzania and Zaire (Trolli, 1938; Lucasse, 1952; Ministry of Health Mozambique, 1984a; Carton *et al.*, 1986; Howlett *et al.*, 1990; Tylleskär *et al.*, 1991, 1993; Banea *et al.*, 1992a).

The onset of konzo is sudden; in 90% of the cases it occurs in one day and often in less than an hour. The initial symptoms are described as trembling or 'cramping' in the legs, heaviness or weakness of the legs, a tendency to fall or an inability to stand. Spasticity is present immediately, without any initial phase of flaccidity. Initially patients experience generalized weakness and are usually in bed for some days before trying to walk. Some 10–20% of patients complain of blurred vision at onset and some have persistent visual problems. About one-third of the patients have initial speech difficulties which typically clear during the first month, except in severely affected patients who may remain with a spastic dysarthria. After the initial weeks of functional improvement the disability remains unchanged over the years. The exception is that about 10% of patients in some series have suffered a second, aggravating episode, identical to the first onset. We interpret these aggravating episodes as new 'onsets' and patients run a ten-fold increased risk of a new onset compared with the risk for the general population of having a first onset of the disease (Tylleskär *et al.*, 1991).

The striking finding is a symmetric spastic paraparesis, ranging from hyper-reflexia in the legs to severe spastic paraparesis with associated weakness of the trunk. Severe cases have a tetraparesis with spasticity, hyperreflexia and occasionally also clonus in the arms. The increase in muscle tone in the hip and knee flexors sometimes leads to contractures in flexion. In moderately affected patients, the arms are apparently unaffected but impaired fine movements in the arms can be found as a sign of an affection of the corticospinal tracts (Tylleskär *et al.*, 1993). The severity varies from patient to patient but the longest upper motor neurones are always more affected than the shorter ones (Howlett *et al*, 1990). The reflexes of the lower limbs are exaggerated in all cases, but due to contractures they might be impossible to elicit in some patients. Extensor plantar responses can be elicited in most moderate and severe cases. Coordination is intact and there is no ataxia or other signs of cerebellar dysfunction.

Cranial or bulbar symptoms are only seen in severe cases that may have disturbances of vision, eye movements and speech. Visual disturbances reported by patients may be due to bilateral central visual field defects (Tylleskär *et al.*, 1993). When eye movements are examined in field studies, slowing of smooth pursuit can be demonstrated in severe cases. Konzo patients have generally no sensory deficits and there is no urinary, bowel or sexual dysfunction. Higher intellectual functions show no apparent deficit.

Lucasse (1952) classified the disease into a *mild form* where the patients are not using walking aids, a *moderate form* where the patients regularly use stick(s) or crutches and a *severe form* where the patients are unable to walk. In Zaire we found 65%, 20–25% and 10–15% of patients to have a mild, moderate and severe form respectively (Tylleskär *et al.*, 1991; Banea *et al.*, 1992a). Community-based rehabilitation providing walking aids and access to primary school is of great importance with a major impact on the life of affected individuals.

The major diagnostic difficulty is not to distinguish konzo from other paralytic disorders but to distinguish individuals with mild forms of konzo from non-affected subjects. In high-prevalence communities many persons give a history of mild konzo but on examination they walk and run without visible signs of spasticity. Most of those persons had exaggerated knee or ankle jerks (Tylleskär *et al.*, 1991). In Mozambique a high frequency of ankle clonus was found in apparently healthy children in a konzo-affected population (Cliff *et al.*, 1986). It seems reasonable to assume that these subjects are subclinical cases.

ANATOMICAL DIAGNOSIS

The spinal cords were reported as normal in the only two autopsies on presumed konzo patients (Trolli, 1938). The scarce medical facilities available explains the absence of further pathological studies. The selective character of the clinical impairment points to a focal lesion at cellular level and this is supported by normal MRI recently found in two konzo patients that were invited from Tanzania to Sweden for examination. A presynaptic cortical lesion is favoured by the fact that transcranial magnetic stimulation failed completely in these patients with severe konzo (Tylleskär *et al.*, 1993).

Konzo may also be caused by a lesion of cell bodies of the upper motor neurones or a subpopulation of such cells in the motor cortex. A third possibility is a conduction block in the motor axons of the motor neurones and a fourth possibility is a synaptic failure in the spinal cord. Konzo can thus not be regarded as a 'myelopathy' until further studies have elucidated the site of the lesion.

AETIOLOGICAL DIAGNOSIS

The epidemic occurrence, familial clustering and some evidence of transmission to secondary cases were regarded as support for an infectious aetiology (Trolli, 1938; Carton *et al.*, 1986). However, konzo patients do not show any signs of infection and laboratory tests for infection as well as virus isolation have been negative. Konzo patients are seronegative to HTLV-I and other retroviruses (Rosling *et al.*, 1988; Howlett *et al.*, 1990; Tylleskär *et al.*, 1993). Furthermore, the outbreaks of konzo remain restricted to rural areas with no secondary cases in neighbouring townships or along major roads used by frequent travellers from affected areas. Other peculiarities in the epidemiological pattern such as sparing of all breast-fed children and a ten-fold increased risk of a second attack among cases also argue against infection but are compatible with the toxic-nutritional hypothesis presented later.

The Cyanide Hypothesis

So far, konzo has only been reported from cassava-growing areas but affected populations only constitute some few per cent of the total cassava-eating populations in the tropics, thus factors other than simply eating cassava are important in causing konzo. Our concept for the social and biomedical causation of konzo (Figure 21.3) illustrates how we think it is induced by cyanide exposure from insufficiently processed cassava in combination with a sulphur amino acid deficient diet. It should be noted that Georgiades, one of Trolli's (1938) colleagues was the first to suggest that konzo may be caused by cyanide exposure from cassava. The following evidence now supports this hypothesis.

A strong association has been found between the geographical distribution of konzo and the chain of events leading to a high cyanide and low sulphur intake. The cumulative incidence of konzo may vary from zero to more than 20 per 1000 inhabitants over a distance of 20 kilometres. All affected populations cultivate bitter cassava varieties as their almost exclusive staple food because no other crop can provide food security on the marginal land available. In contrast, neighbouring unaffected populations have had access to more fertile land (Banea *et al.*, 1992a) or a more varied diet due to fishing (Cliff *et al.*, 1985, 1986; Howlett *et al.*, 1992). Shortcuts in traditional cassava processing due to food shortage or intensive sales of the better processed roots have meant more frequent consumption of insufficiently processed cassava resulting in high cyanide intake (Banea *et al.*, 1992b) as indicated by higher serum and urinary thiocyanate levels in affected populations (Ministry of Health Mozambique, 1984a,b; Tylleskär *et al.*, 1992; Mlingi *et al.*, 1993). A simultaneous lower intake of protein-rich food providing sulphur for cyanide detoxification has been documented by both dietary interviews and demonstration of lower urinary levels of inorganic sulphate (Cliff *et al.*, 1985; Mlingi *et al.*, 1993). A strong argument for a causal role of this chain of events is its consistent association with konzo in several widely separated geographical clusters in ecologically different areas across the African continent (Figure 21.2).

An equally strong temporal association has been documented between konzo outbreaks and monotonous consumption of insufficiently processed cassava. During epidemics the affected populations have higher cyanide intake than before and after (Casadei *et al.*, 1990; Essers *et al.*, 1992; Mlingi *et al.*, 1993). An additional argument for a causal role is that the same special diet during the outbreaks have been induced by different mechanisms, drought in East Africa and a sudden increase in commercialization of cassava in Zaire.

The peculiar age and sex distribution of konzo with higher incidence among women and children, apart from those breast-fed, has two possible explanations. It may reflect higher vulnerability to cyanide due to higher metabolic demand for sulphur in growth and pregnancy. Women and children may also be more exposed to high cyanide and low sulphur intake as they are less privileged with regard to food. The fact that breast-fed children are spared supports the cyanide hypothesis, since they eat the least cassava and have the highest sulphur amino acid intake in affected communities.

The associations mentioned above were demonstrated by ecological study design using comparisons on an aggregated level. An association has also been found on the individual level between high blood cyanide and the onset of konzo (Tylleskär *et al.*, 1992). During 2 months search in remote villages in Zaire we identified three konzo patients at the time of onset. Estimation of the combined effect of high cyanide intake and decreased conversion rate was obtained by measuring blood cyanide (Figure 21.5) which was close to lethal levels. The 23 controls from the same communities also had increased but significantly lower blood cyanide. In contrast, serum thiocyanate was equal in cases and controls (Tylleskär *et al.*, 1992), which can be explained by a decreased cyanide to thiocyanate conversion rate due to low intake of sulphur amino acids providing the substrate for formation of thiocyanate. Another case-control study in Zaire found an association on the individual level between reduced soaking time for cassava and konzo (Tylleskär *et al.*, 1995) and a dose–response relationship which further strengthens the argument.

The fact that the konzo-affected population in Bandundu region in Zaire only consume soaked cassava roots was regarded as an argument against the cyanide hypothesis as soaking is known as an effective processing method (Carton *et al.*, 1986). However, we found that the traditional soaking method had been shortened as a response to intensive commercialization following construction of a new tarmac road to the capital Kinshasa. Food chemistry experiments performed in affected communities revealed that cassava flour from short-soaked roots contained high remaining amounts of acetone cyanohydrin that disappeared after 2 weeks storage (Tylleskär *et al.*, 1992). This can explain why no cyanide exposure or konzo case has been reported from Kinshasa. Apparently minor differences in length and sequence of short-cuts in the traditional soaking methods resulted in considerable variation in remaining cyanogens in the flour used to make the staple porridge. The cause of cyanide consumption is thus not the consumption of cassava per se but the inability of poor populations to adhere to the effective traditional processing methods (Banea *et al.*, 1992b).

Tropical Ataxic Neuropathy and Konzo

Tropical ataxic neuropathy (TAN) reported from Nigeria differs clinically from konzo as it has a gradual onset of a progressive polyneuropathy with various sensory deficits. Osuntokun (1981) found an association between TAN and cassava consumption resulting in moderate cyanide intake as supported by slightly increased serum thiocyanate levels. Serum thiocyanate varies with the diet and was found to be 0–77 μmol 1^{-1} in non-smoking adults in Sweden (Tylleskär, 1994). Mean ($\pm$SD) serum thiocyanate in cases of TAN were 114 $\pm$ 39 μmol 1^{-1} ($n = 375$) (Osuntokun, 1981). This corresponds to the levels found in smokers but is considerably lower than both cases and controls in konzo-affected populations that have mean serum thiocyanate above 300 μmol 1^{-1} (Tylleskär *et al.*, 1992). Mean ($\pm$SD) blood cyanide in TAN cases was 1 $\pm$ 0.4 μmol 1^{-1} ($n = 108$) (Osuntokun, 1973), which is comparable to smokers and to the control subjects in a konzo-affected population (Tylleskär *et al.*, 1992). Blood cyanide in konzo cases at onset was 20 times higher. TAN cases are thus exposed to low cyanide levels during longer periods. The contradiction may be explained if different dose-rates cause the different neurological patterns. One would thus expect TAN to appear in konzo-affected populations but this has not yet been verified. Another explanation is that cyanide exposure is a contributory but not an essential factor in one or both of the conditions.

PATHOGENIC MECHANISMS

A valid argument against the cyanide hypothesis is that cyanide from other sources has not caused a similar disease in humans. On the contrary survivors of single high doses of cyanide have acquired a parkinsonian-like syndrome. This may be explained by the pattern of blood cyanide that will result from the high cyanide and low sulphur intake associated to konzo that will not result from other forms of cyanide exposure. The ingestion of porridge rich in cyanogenic glucosides and cyanohydrin will result in a gradual release of cyanide in the gut. Simultaneously decreased detoxification rate, due to low sulphur availability, will result in increased but relatively stable blood cyanide levels that will create a special metabolic situation (Tylleskär *et al.*, 1993). A direct cyanide effect is therefore not a plausible pathogenic mechanism for konzo but the deranged metabolism may produce a metabolite causing overexcitation of the neurones (Bitner et al., 1985). This is analogous to the association of an excitatory amino acid β-N-oxalylamino-L-alanine, BOAA or β-ODAP) in the grass pea and lathyrism (Spencer et al., 1986). These almost identical diseases may thus have common final causative steps.

Another possibility is that the specific toxicity in konzo arises from a cyanide to cyanate conversion due to decreased cyanide to thiocyanate conversion. Cyanate (OCN) is a carbamylating agent and its administration to primates over several weeks has resulted in an upper motor neurone damage identical to that of konzo (Shaw et al., 1974). Confirmation of an aetiological role of cyanide in konzo may be produced by an experimental animal model or a quasiexperimental preventive intervention. It may be speculated that vitamin deficiencies, toxic effects of consumed wild plants or a cassava toxin other than cyanide may be aetiological factors in konzo. Quite apart from public health aspects, the elucidation of the pathogenic mechanisms in konzo is a challenge to basic neuroscience since the results may yield new understandings of neurodegenerative mechanisms (Tylleskär, 1994).

KONZO AND THE PPE SPIRAL

Konzo is a challenge to public health since the underlying factors result from the vicious circle of poverty, population growth and environmental deterioration known as the PPE spiral (Grant, 1994) which creates social collapse and human misery in several parts of Africa. It should be noted that the toxic varieties of cassava that are implicated in the causation of konzo also gave agricultural advantages that saved many more people from starvation in the affected populations. Elucidation of the social and biological role of cassava cyanogenesis is now given high priority in agricultural research (Bokanga et al., 1994). Konzo epidemics should be regarded as a warning for a special type of agroecological crisis with declining soil fertility and increased population pressure on marginal land that is becoming more common in Africa and elsewhere. Although evidence for the cyanide hypothesis is not conclusive we consider it strong enough to urge prevention. A first option is the promotion of effective processing of cassava roots. A second is to introduce cassava varieties with lower levels of linamarin. However, such varieties must first be proven to yield well under the harsh local conditions in the areas concerned.

REFERENCES

Banea M, Bikangi N, Nahimana G et al. (1992a) Haute prévalence de konzo associée à une crise agro-alimentaire dans la région de Bandundu au Zaïre. Annales de la Société Belge de Médecine Tropicale **72**: 295–309.

Banea M, Poulter N and Rosling H (1992b) Shortcuts in cassava processing and risk of dietary cyanide exposure in Zaire. *Food and Nutrition Bulletin* **14**: 137–143.

Bitner RS, Kanthasamy A, Isom GE, Yim GKW (1995) Seizures and selective CA-1 hippocampal lesions induced by an excitotoxic cyanide metabolite, 2-iminothiozolidine-4-carboxylic acid. *Neurotoxicology* **16**: 115–122.

Bokanga M, Essers S, Poulter N, Rosling H and Tewe O (1994) International workshop on Cassava Safety. *Acta Horticulture* **375**: 7–19.

Carton H, Kazadi K, Kabeya *et al.* (1986) Epidemic spastic paraparesis in Bandundu (Zaire). *Journal of Neurology, Neurosurgery and Psychiatry* **49**: 620–627.

Casadei E, Cliff J and Neves J (1990) Surveillance of urinary thiocyanate concentration after epidemic spastic paraparesis in Mozambique. *Journal of Tropical Medicine and Hygiene* **93**: 257–261.

Cliff J, Lundquist P, Mårtensson J, Rosling H and Sörbo B (1985) Association of high cyanide and low sulphur intake in cassava-induced spastic paraparesis. *Lancet* **ii**: 1211–1213.

Cliff J, Essers S and Rosling H (1986) Ankle clonus correlating with cyanide intake from cassava in rural children from Mozambique. *Journal of Tropical Pediatrics* **32**: 186–189.

Essers AJA, Alsén P and Rosling H (1992) Insufficient processing of cassava induced acute intoxications and the paralytic disease konzo in a rural area of Mozambique. *Ecology of Food and Nutrition* **27**: 17–27.

Grant J (1994) *The State of the World's Children*. New York: Oxford University Press.

Howlett WP, Brubaker GR, Mlingi N and Rosling H (1990) Konzo, an epidemic upper motor neuron disease studied in Tanzania. *Brain* **113**: 223–235.

Howlett WP, Brubaker G, Mlingi N and Rosling H (1992) A geographical cluster of konzo in northern Tanzania. *Journal of Tropical and Geographical Neurology* **2**: 102–108.

Lucasse C (1952) La 'kitondjii', synonyme le 'konzo', une paralysie spastique. *Annales de la Société Belge de Médecine Tropicale* **33**: 393–401.

Ministry of Health Mozambique (1984a) Mantakassa: an epidemic of spastic paraparesis associated with chronic cyanide intoxication in a cassava staple area of Mozambique. 1. Epidemiology and clinical and laboratory findings in patients. *Bulletin of the World Health Organization* **62**: 477–484.

Ministry of Health Mozambique (1984b) Mantakassa: an epidemic of spastic paraparesis associated with chronic cyanide intoxication in a cassava staple area in Mozambique. 2. Nutritional factors and hydrocyanic content of cassava products. *Bulletin of the World Health Organization* **62**: 485–492.

Mlingi NV, Assey V, Swai A *et al.* (1993) Determinants of cyanide exposure from cassava in a konzo-affected population in northern Tanzania. *International Journal of Food Sciences and Nutrition* **44**: 137–144.

Osuntokun BO (1981) Cassava diet, chronic cyanide intoxication and neuropathy in Nigerian Africans. *World Review of Nutrition and Dietetics* **36**: 141–173.

Rosling H, Gessain A, de Thé G *et al.* (1988) Tropical and epidemic spastic parapareses are different. *Lancet* **ii**: 1223–1224.

Shaw CM, Papayannopoulu T, Stamotoyannopoulos G (1974) Neuropathology of cyanate toxicity in Rhesus monkeys. *Pharmacology* **12**: 166–176.

Spencer P, Roy D, Ludolph A *et al.* (1986) Lathyrism: evidence for role of the neuroexcitatory aminoacid BOAA. *Lancet* **ii**: 1066–1067.

Trolli G (1938) Paraplégie spastique épidémique, Konzo des indigènes du Kwango. In:

Résumé des observations réunies, au Kwango, au sujet de deux affections d'origine indéterminée (ed. G Trolli), pp 1–36. Brussels: Fonds Reine Elisabeth.

Tylleskär T (1994) The causation of konzo. Studies on a paralytic disease in Africa. PhD thesis Uppsala University.

Tylleskär T, Banea M, Bikangi N *et al.* (1991) Epidemiological evidence from Zaire for a dietary aetiology of konzo, an upper motor neuron disease. *Bulletin of the World Health Organization* **69**: 581–590.

Tylleskär T, Banea M, Bikangi N *et al.* (1992) Cassava cyanogens and konzo, an upper motoneuron disease found in Africa. *Lancet* **339**: 208–211.

Tylleskär T, Howlett W, Rwiza H *et al.* (1993) Konzo: a distinct disease entity with selective upper motoneuron damage. *Journal of Neurology, Neurosurgery and Psychiatry* **56**: 638–643.

Tylleskär T, Légué F, Peterson S, Kpizingui E and Stecker P (1994) Konzo in the Central African Republic. *Neurology* **44**: 959–961.

Tylleskär T, Banea M, Bikangi N *et al.* (1995) Dietary and socio-economic determinants for konzo: a case-referent study in a high incidence area in Zaire. *International Journal of Epidemiology*, in press.

van der Beken A (1993) *Proverbes yaka du Zaire.* Paris: Editions Karthala.

22

Lathyrism

Redda Tekle-Haimanot

Department of Internal Medicine, Faculty of Medicine, Addis Ababa University, PO Box 4147, Addis Ababa, Ethiopia

INTRODUCTION

The term 'lathyrismus' was coined by Cantani (1873) after the legume, *Lathyrus sativus*, the cause of the disabling disease. Lathyrism has been known since the time of Hippocrates (460–377 BC). In his work on epidemics Hippocrates wrote 'At Ainos, all men and women who ate peas continuously became impotent in the legs and that state persisted' (Selye, 1957). The description is consistent with human lathyrism as we now recognize it.

The toxic properties of *Lathyrus* flour were recognized in Europe as early as 1671 when Duke George of Wurthemberg issued an edict banning the sale of *Lathyrus* flour because of its paralysing effects on the legs (Buchanan, 1927). There is historical evidence that the disease was widespread with outbreaks and epidemics reported in parts of Europe, Russia, North Africa, the Middle East and Asia. Although living victims of lathyrism exist in Israel, Spain, Greece and France (Spencer *et al.*, 1986), the disease is now endemic only in Ethiopia (Tekle-Haimanot, 1989), India (Dwivedi, 1989) and Bangladesh (Haque and Mannan, 1989). The prevalence of the disease in these endemic regions ranges between 0.1 and 3%. A great number of reports have appeared this century from India on the epidemiology and clinical characteristics of lathyrism. An earlier work was that of General Sleeman (1844) who, although not medically trained, gave an accurate description of lathyrism in his book *Rambles and Recollections of an Indian Official*. Acton (1922) presented a detailed scientific review of the disease including results of some of his animal experiments.

Subsequent careful and detailed epidemiological and clinical investigations performed in India (Dwivedi and Prasad, 1964; Kulkarni *et al.*, 1977; Attal *et al.*, 1978) have confirmed the observations of earlier workers that the crippling disease is caused by excessive consumption of *Lathyrus sativus* (chickling pea, vetch or grass pea). The disease occurs mainly among the poor who consume the legume in excess, as a staple or during times of food shortages. It affects predominantly young males. The peak months for disease onset are the rainy seasons (especially July) which is probably related to depletion of stored grain (Acton, 1922; Ganapathy and Dwivedi, 1961; Tekle-Haimanot *et al.*, 1990).

AETIOLOGY

Lathyrus sativus (Chickling Pea, Grass Pea or Vetch)

This legume is a hardy crop which is drought and water-logging resistant and can withstand pest and weeds. It has rapid growth potential with a high per hectare yield and provides a nourishing diet of high-quality protein (about 25%) and carbohydrate (about 60%) and yields of 350 cal/100 g. With a low requirement for water, the pulse is a survival food during times of food shortages in lathyrism endemic areas. The disadvantage of this nutritious legume is its potential toxicity (Spencer *et al.*, 1986a). It is commonly consumed boiled or roasted and its flour is used to make bread. It may provide the entire diet during periods of food shortage. In times of plenty it is mixed with other cereals like wheat or rice. The seeds and fodder of grass pea are also used as animal feed.

Neurotoxicity

The most direct confirmation that *Lathyrus sativus* was responsible for human lathyrism came from the unfortunate experience of Romanian Jews interned in a German forced labour camp in the Ukraine. They developed the disease after being maintained on a daily diet of 400 g of grass pea cooked in salt water with bread made of barley and straw in a 4:1 proportion (Kessler, 1947). Prisoners who consumed less of the grass pea (200 g day^{-1}) did not develop the disease. The emergence of new cases ceased with the discontinuation of the grass pea diet in the camp. From the same camp there was also indirect evidence that malnutrition did not significantly contribute to the manifestation of the disease. It appears that excessive consumption plays a major role in toxicity.

Murti *et al.* (1964) and Rao *et al.* (1964) independently isolated the neurotoxic amino acid, β-*N*-oxalyl-α,β-diaminopropionic acid (ODAP) or β-*N*-oxalylamino-L-alanine (BOAA), the suspected culprit of neurolathyrism.

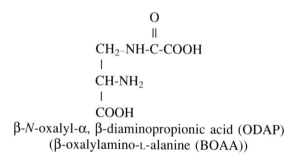

$$
\begin{array}{c}
\text{O} \\
\parallel \\
\text{CH}_2\text{-NH-C-COOH} \\
| \\
\text{CH-NH}_2 \\
| \\
\text{COOH}
\end{array}
$$

β-*N*-oxalyl-α, β-diaminopropionic acid (ODAP)
(β-oxalylamino-L-alanine (BOAA))

There is experimental evidence from primate studies that β-ODAP is the neurotoxic amino acid involved in the aetiology and pathogenesis of lathyrism (Spencer and Schaumburg, 1983).

Epidemiological studies have shown that most people developed lathyrism after consuming grass pea consisting of over 30% of their daily diet for more than 3 months (Acton, 1922; Ganapathy and Dwivedi, 1964; Gebre-Ab *et al.*, 1978). There are reports of cases contracting the disease after consumption of the legume for less than one month (Ganapathy and Dwivedi, 1961; Attal *et al.*, 1978), but this may well be related to an increased intake, as observed by Kessler (1947), or to other factors such as nutritional deficiencies and individual susceptibility to the neurotoxin.

PATHOGENESIS AND PATHOLOGY

Knowledge of the neuropathology of lathyrism is rather limited. Very few postmortem examinations have been performed on cases of lathyrism because most patients are poor and die at home in remote regions and in endemic countries there are religious and cultural prohibitions on postmortems. The few published reports indicate that the neuropathological findings of human lathyrism are dominated by symmetrical axonal degeneration and crossed and uncrossed pyramidal tracts in the thoracic, lumbar and sacral spinal cord (Buzzard and Greenfield, 1921; Sachdev *et al.*, 1969; Streifler *et al.*, 1977). Additionally, loss of pyramidal cells in the region of the motor cortex controlling the leg is noted in an early study of the pathology of the brain in human lathyrism (Filimonoff, 1926). Primary neuronal degeneration, with secondary loss of cortical motor axons, is consistent with the neurotoxic action of ODAP, the culpable agent in grass pea.

Laboratory studies show that ODAP mimics the depolarizing action of the neurotransmitters glutamate and aspartate, and that micromolar concentrations rapidly trigger postsynaptic dendritic oedema followed by neuronal degeneration, in mouse cortical tissue in culture (Ross *et al.*, 1987). Since the primary molecular recognition site for ODAP (in rodent synaptic membranes) appears to be the quisqualate receptor (Ross *et al.*, 1989), it is possible that the dendritic arbor of pyramidal cells of the human motor cortex are endowed with a particularly heavy concentration of quisqualate receptors. Furthermore, if the dendritic expanse of Betz cells is proportional to axon length, those with projection to the lumbosacral cord might respond to the excitatory and excitotoxic (neuronotoxic) action of ODAP before motor neurones innervating the cervical cord. This hypothesis provides a possible molecular and cellular explanation for the clinical manifestations of lathyrism. Critical study of this hypothesis requires an animal model of human lathyrism.

There have been many failed attempts to induce irreversible spastic paraparesis in animals fed with *Lathyrus sativus* seed or its components (Spencer and Schaumberg, 1983). A recent study with carefully nourished macaques fed

L. sativus or ODAP reported the delayed onset of clinical (extensor posturing, increased tone and muscle cramping of hind limbs) and electrophysiological changes consistent with the initial, reversible signs of human lathyrism (Spencer *et al.*, 1986b). The primate neurological signs were also reversible, and neuropathological changes in cortex and cord were lacking. Further studies are therefore required to find a more complete animal model of human lathyrism, and to determine the role of malnutrition and other possible susceptibility factors (such as exercise) for the neurotoxic action of ODAP (Spencer *et al.*, 1988).

CLINICAL FEATURES

Mode of Onset

The widely accepted mode of presentation of lathyrism is that proposed by Ganapathy and Dwivedi (1961) who described three patterns. The most common is the *sudden onset* in which the affected individual complains of heavy, weakened legs after falling down or awakening from sleep. Acton (1921) quoted the description of a victim as follows: '. . . whilst ploughing I suddenly noticed that my legs were weak, there was no pain, but I had difficulties in sitting and getting up from a squatting position, I did not know I was paralyzed . . .'. In the *subacute onset* there are 10–15 days of prodromal symptoms of rheumatic pains, cramping and stiffness at the waist before the manifestation of the paralysis. In the very rare form of *insidious onset* the spastic paraparesis progresses over a period of months with associated dull aching pain in the lumbosacral region and back of the thigh. The patient may or may not give a history of myospasm and is invariably told by others about his ungainly gait.

   In the very mild form the disability might not be obvious. The leg stiffness is detected only during running. Such cases have been referred to as 'latent lathyrism' (Dwivedi and Prasad, 1961). Recognized precipitating factors include such factors as manual labour, febrile illness and diarrhoea.

Age and Sex Distribution

All age groups are affected by lathyrism but around 80% are below the age of 40 when most are physically active. Males are affected more commonly (2.5:1) and more severely than females, although crude estimate of food intake suggested no substantial differences in *L. sativus* consumption. Contrary to the view of Acton (1921), who suggested that women eat less in order to save food for their husbands and children, there is evidence for other susceptibility factors, perhaps hormonal, to account for the gender difference in the levels of affliction. This view is consistent with the epidemiological findings that women of child-bearing age are less severely affected by the disease (Dwivedi and Prasad, 1964; Tekle-Haimanot *et al.*, 1990).

More than one member of the same family may be affected by lathyrism. The extent of *Lathyrus* consumption, the sex and other susceptibility factors may be involved in determining the number of family members that exhibit the disease.

Clinical Signs

The picture of classical spastic paraparesis due to lathyrism is stereotypic. Mental status, speech and cranial nerve function are intact. Cerebellar signs are not detected. Spastic paraparesis of different degrees is manifested associated with adductor spasm in the worse affected cases, as well as exaggerated deep tendon reflexes, extensor plantar response and ankle clonus. Distal lower limb objective sensory deficits to pin-prick and light touch are uncommon. Reversible urinary frequency and urgency, nocturnal erection and ejaculation have been reported in victims of lathyrism. These symptoms and muscle cramping are commonly encountered early in the clinical manifestation of lathyrism, suggesting that *Lathyrus* consumption can result in diffuse and transitory CNS excitation of somatic motor and autonomic function (Ludoph *et al.*, 1987). The spastic paraparesis and the subsequent disabilities are permanent once the disease is manifested. The condition is reversible only if the consumption of grass pea is discontinued at the very early prodromal stage of myospasm. Established cases walk on their toes with an unsteady gait and show scissoring of the legs. With time, in those severely affected, muscle atrophies and contractures in the legs develop.

The staging of the resulting disability is presented in Figure 22.1. The classification is based on walking disability and the need for physical support (Acton, 1922). The majority (90%) of cases fall into stages 1 and 2. About 10% are classified as stages 3 and 4. Females tend to have milder involvement than males. Figure 22.2 shows Ethiopian lathyrism victims with stages 1, 2 and 3 of neurolathyrism.

Differential Diagnosis

Two important myelopathies come into the differential diagnosis of lathyrism. Tropical spastic paraparesis (TSP) is a slowly progressive spastic paraparesis with an insidious onset (see Chapter 3). Unlike lathyrism, cases of TSP commonly complain of sensory and autonomic disturbances including incontinence and impotence (Gessain and Gout, 1992). However, it may sometimes be difficult to differentiate between early TSP and lathyrism, particularly in localities where the two conditions coexist. The mode of onset, sensory symptoms and progression of the spastic paraparesis will assist in the differential

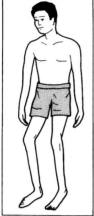

Stage 1:
Mild spastic gait with no use
of a stick; increased stiffness
and exaggerated deep tendon
reflexes (DTR); ankle clonus
present; Babinski's sign absent.

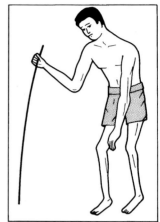

Stage 2:
Spastic gait, with use of one stick;
increased stiffness; mild rigidity;
exaggerated DTR; ankle clonus
present; Babinski's sign present

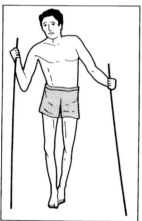

Stage 3:
Spastic gait; with use of two
sticks; crossed adductor gait;
exaggerated DTR; ankle
clonus present; Babinski's
sign present

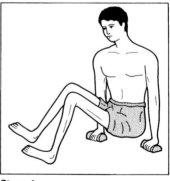

Stage 4:
Crawling or bedridden state; loss
of leg use, with contractures;
arms strong; and pyramidal signs
present.

Figure 22.1 Pictorial representation of the stages of disability in human neurolathyrism.

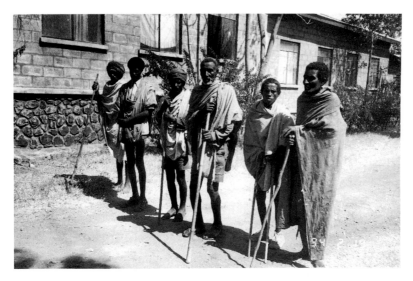

Figure 22.2 Ethiopian lathyrism victims with stages 1, 2 and 3 of disability.

diagnosis. Lack of excessive grass pea consumption will rule out lathyrism in doubtful cases.

The other spastic paraparesis which has very similar clinical setting and manifestations is konzo, caused by excessive and exclusive consumption of insufficiently processed cassava (*Manihot esculenta*) (see Chapter 21). The dietary history helps differentiate between konzo and lathyrism and the two conditions exist in different geographical isolates. However, the clinical and pathogenetic similarities of the two diseases present an investigatory challenge in neurotoxicology.

Additional conditions to be considered in the differential diagnosis are motor neurone disease (amyotrophic lateral sclerosis), cord compression and other myelopathies including those caused by human immunodeficiency virus (HIV).

There are no specific investigations for lathyrism. A detailed dietary history and the exclusion of other conditions mentioned above are the hallmarks of the diagnosis.

TREATMENT

There are no known cures for lathyrism once it is established. Symptomatic treatments have not been successful in alleviating the disabling spasticity. The reported clinical improvement in a small percentage of those affected is presumably not related to traditional treatment or to low-dose vitamin supplements that the patients have received and probably represents a spontaneous feature of the disease, in which improvements have been reported in the early stages (Ludolph *et al.*, 1987).

PREVENTION

Lathyrism is a very serious social problem because it cripples the young and productive age group. The following measures will be appropriate and feasible in the countries where the disease is endemic.

The public should be educated on the toxicity of grass pea, and instructed in ways of processing it to help reduce the toxicity. It is now well documented that soaking or boiling and discarding the excess water reduces the toxic ODAP in the seed. Easy home-based methods of detoxifying the grass pea during food preparation have been found to be effective (Mohan *et al.*, 1966; Tekle-Haimanot *et al.*, 1993). During poor harvest and famine situations communities in lathyrus-growing areas should receive external assistance. The banning of the sale and consumption of *L. sativus* has been found impractical if not impossible.

Recently, interests and hopes have been raised by a more effective and far-reaching approach to solving the lathyrism problem, involving the development of low-ODAP varieties of grass pea. Extensive germplasm collections of grass pea with low-ODAP content exist and plant breeding programmes are under way in endemic countries and elsewhere to develop a safe strain of *L. sativus* by breeding out the neurotoxic element (Palmer *et al.*, 1989). These efforts aim to give farmers a hardy, high-protein crop for home consumption and for use as fodder. This is part of an international collaborative effort to improve *L. sativus* and eradicate lathyrism.

Monitoring thiocyanate levels in populations at risk for neurotoxicity from consumption of bitter cassava has been successfully employed in the prevention of konzo in Mozambique (Casadei *et al.*, 1990). A comparable approach in lathyrism would be to monitor blood or urine levels of ODAP.

REFERENCES

Acton HW (1922) An investigation into the causation of lathyrism in man. *Indian Medical Gazette* **57**: 241–247.

Attal HC, Kulkarni SW, Choubey BS *et al.* (1978) A field study of lathyrism – some clinical aspects. *Indian Journal of Medical Research* **67**: 608–615.

Buchanan A (1927) Report on lathyrism in Central Provinces in 1896–1902. *Government Press*, Nagpur, pp 1–71.

Buzzard EF and Greenfield JG (1921) *Pathology of the Nervous System.* London: Constable, p 232.

Cantani A (1873) Latirismo (Lathyrismus) illustrata de tre casi clinici II. *Morgagni* **15**: 745.

Casadei E *et al.* (1990) Surveillance of urinary thiocyanate concentration after epidemic spastic paraparesis in Mozambique. *Journal of Tropical Medicine and Hygiene* **93**: 257–261.

Dwivedi MP (1989) Epidemiological aspects of lathyrism in India – a changing scenario. In: *Grass-pea: Threat and Promise* (ed. PS Spencer), pp 1–26. New York: Third World Medical Reseach Foundation.

Dwivedi MP and Prasad VG (1964) An epidemiological study of lathyrism in the district of Rewa, Madhya Pradesh. *Indian Medical Research* **52**: 81–114.

Filimonoff IN (1926) Zur pathologisch-anatomischen charakteristik des Lathyrismus. *Zeitschreift fur die Gesamte Neurologie und Psychiatrie* **105**: 75–92.

Ganapathy KT and Dwivedi MP (1961) Studies on clinical epidemiology of lathyrism. Lathyrism Enquiry Field Unit. *Indian Council of Medical Research Ghandi Memorial Hospital, Rewa, Madhya Pradesh*, pp 1–55.

Gebre-Ab T, Wolde-Gabriel Z, Maffi M *et al.* (1978) Neurolathyrism – a review and a report of an epidemic. *Ethiopian Medical Journal* **16**: 1–11.

Gessain A and Gout O (1992) Chronic myelopathy associated with human T-lymphotropic virus type I (HTLV-I). *Annals of Internal Medicine* **117**: 933–946.

Haque A and Mannan MA (1989) The problems of lathyrism in Bangladesh. In: *Grasspea: Threat and Promise* (ed. PS Spencer), pp 27–35. New York: Third World Medical Research Foundation.

Kessler A (1947) Lathyrismus. *Monatschrift Psychiatric und Neurologie* **113**: 345–376.

Kulkarni SW *et al.* (1977) An epidemiologic study of lathyrism in Amgaon Block, Bahandra district. *Indian Medical Research Journal* **66**: 602–610.

Ludolph AC, Hugon J, Dwivedi MP *et al.* (1987) Studies on the aetiology and pathogenesis of motor neuron disease. Lathyrism: clinical findings in established cases. *Brain* **110**: 149–165.

Mohan VS *et al.* (1966) Simple practical procedures for the removal of toxic factors in *Lathyrus sativus* (Khesari dal). *Indian Medical Research Journal* **54**: 410–419.

Murti VVS *et al.* (1964) Neurotoxic compounds of seeds of *Lathyrus sativus*. *Phytochemistry* **3**: 73–78.

Palmer VS *et al.* (1989) International network for the improvement of *Lathyrus sativus* and the eradication of lathyrism (INILSEL): a TWMRF initiative. In: *Grass-pea: Threat and Promise* (ed. PS Spencer), pp 218–233. New York: Third World Medical Research Foundation.

Rao SLN *et al.* (1964) Isolation and characterization of β-oxalyl-L-α, β-diaminopropionic acid. A neurotoxin from the seeds of *Lathyrus sativus*. *Biochemistry* **3**: 432–436.

Ross SM *et al.* (1987) Specific antagonism of excitotoxic action of 'uncommon' amino acids assayed in organotypic mouse cortical cultures. *Brain Research* **425**: 120–127.

Ross SM *et al.* (1989) β-N-oxalylamino-L-alanine action on glutamate receptors. *Journal of Neurochemistry* **53**: 710–715.

Sachdev S *et al.* (1969) Morphological study in a case of lathyrism. *Journal of the Indian Medical Association* **52**: 320–322.

Selye H (1957) Lathyrism. *Revue Candiene de Biologie* **16**: 1–82.

Sleeman WH (1844) *Rambles and Recollections of an Indian Official*, vol. 1. London: Hatchard and Sons.

Spencer PS and Schaumburg HH (1983) Lathyrism: a neurotoxic disease. *Neurobehavioral Toxicology and Teratology* **5**: 625–629.

Spencer PS, Roy D, Ludolph A *et al.* (1986a) Lathyrism: evidence for role of the neuroexcitatory amino acid BOAA. *Lancet* **ii**: 1066–1067.

Spencer PS *et al.* (1986b) *L. sativus*. The need for a strain lacking human and animal neurotoxic properties. In: *Lathyrus and Lathyrism* (eds AK Kaul and D Combes), pp 297–305. New York: Third World Medical Research Foundation.

Spencer PS, Roy DN, Ludolph A *et al.* (1988) Primate model of lathyrism: a human pyramidal disorder. In: *Neurodegenerative Disorder: The Role Played by Endotoxins and Xenobiotics* (eds Guiseppe Nappe *et al.*), pp 231–238. New York: Raven Press.

Streifler M *et al.* (1977) The central nervous system in a case of neurolathyrism. *Neurology* **27**: 1176–1178.

Tekle-Haimanot R (1989) Lathyrism in Ethiopia. In: *Grass-pea: Threat and Promise* (ed. PS Spencer), pp 36–40. New York: Third World Medical Research Foundation.

Tekle-Haimanot R, Yemane K, Elthabeth W *et al.* (1990) Lathyrism in rural central Ethiopia: a highly prevalent neurotoxic disorder. *International Journal of Epidemiology* **19**: 664–672.

Tekle-Haimanot R, Berhanu AM, Elizabeth W *et al.* (1993) Pattern of *Lathyrus sativus* (grass pea) consumption and beta-*N*-oxalyl-α-β-diaminopropionic acid (β-ODAP) content of food samples in the lathyrism endemic region of northwest Ethiopia. *Nutrition Research* **13**: 113–1126.

23

Bites and Stings: Poisoning by Venomous Animals

John B. Harris

Regional Neurosciences Centre, Newcastle General Hospital,
Newcastle-upon-Tyne NE4 6BE, UK

INTRODUCTION

Clinically significant poisoning following bites and stings by venomous animals is not a particularly serious problem in most temperate countries. In many tropical and subtropical countries, however, poisoning by envenomation is the cause of high levels of morbidity and mortality.

The available statistics relating to poisoning by envenomation are of highly variable reliability. Those data collected from major teaching hospitals in developing countries are unreliable indicators of the true incidence of poisoning because in most cases the teaching hospitals are available to a minority, urban population. This segment of society is least likely to come into contact with envenoming species. Data collected as a result of extensive field work involve setting up robust recording systems in remote clinics, and persuading local people to use the clinics rather than traditional healers. As a result of the logistic difficulties involved in such work, data gathered may be accurate but represent a strictly local view of the problem. Detailed studies, however, provide estimates of morbidity/mortality that are unexpectedly high. For example, up to 10% of hospital beds in Savanna regions of Nigeria are occupied by victims of snake bites; 1000 deaths per year from snake bite in Sri Lanka (population 10 million); 1000 deaths per year from scorpion sting in Mexico, mostly involving children.

The epidemiological evidence, imperfect though it is, suggests that the incidence of severe poisoning is changing in many parts of the world. Since the pioneering work of Reid (Reid and Lim, 1957), the fishing population around the coast of north-west Malaya has been considered to be at rather high risk from sea-snake bite. Anecdotal evidence now suggests that sea-snake bite in Malaya is relatively uncommon. The reasons are probably multifactorial – Dr Reid collected his data during the 1950s and 1960s and he had a passionate interest in snake bite; fishing patterns have changed dramatically over the past four decades; the snake population may well have declined. In other areas, increased contact with venomous species as a result of urban spread or expansion of food production into previously virgin land results in an increasing incidence of envenomation. The important point to note is that data on envenomation need to be continually updated. Old data are not particularly reliable.

VENOMOUS ANIMALS OF MAJOR SIGNIFICANCE

Snakes are typically associated most directly with incidents of envenomation. The venom of a snake is elaborated and stored in the venom gland, a structure situated in the head but frequently extending into the body of the animal. The venom is usually delivered via a hollow or grooved venom fang. Inoculation of venom appears to be partially under voluntary control and is achieved by the contraction of the muscular coat surrounding the gland. Snakes do not always envenom when they bite and many bites appear to be defensive in nature. It is important to understand the implications of this habit – a bite by a venomous snake is not synonymous with envenomation.

Spitting snakes exhale powerfully as the jaw is opened and the venom is sprayed 2–3 feet from the fang. Spitting cobras are the most talented 'spitters'.

There are numerous claims for the 'most poisonous' or 'most dangerous' snake. If a judgement is made on overall significance in terms of human poisoning, the small, aggressive saw-scaled viper, *Echis* sp. probably causes more morbidity and mortality than any other (Warrell and Arnett, 1976). It is common, it is small, fast and aggressive, its venom is potent and it inhabits a huge, though discontinuous range, from East Africa, though North Africa and west to the Indian subcontinent. Russell's viper (Figure 23.1) also has a large and discontinuous range that is still not properly defined but extends from mainland

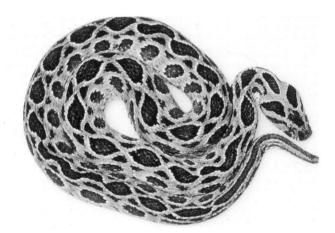

Figure 23.1 *Vipera russelli siamenis,* also known as *Daboia r. s.* and Russell's viper of Burma; a dangerous snake with many relatives throughout South-East Asia. (Reproduced courtesy of David Warrell.)

China to the Philippines and into India and Sri Lanka (Warrell, 1986). The taipan is an exceedingly dangerous Australian snake whose bite is considered deadly unless treated rapidly. It could be said to be one of the most dangerous of all snakes, but it causes few serious incidents of poisoning because its range does not bring it into contact with humans. The global numbers of deaths caused by snake bite are difficult to calculate with accuracy, but by using data from a number of sources, it is clear that it is measured in terms of tens of thousands.

By comparison with morbidity and mortality caused by snake bite, scorpion stings are relatively much less serious. There are, however, areas where they are important – Mexico, Central America, Brazil, Trinidad and possibly North Africa and the Middle East – and cause significant mortality. Elsewhere, scorpion stings cause considerable demand on 'clinic time', even though mortality rates are low. In India, for example, scorpion stings are common even in densely populated city locations where snake bite is rare.

Spider bites are responsible for relatively few deaths, although they feature in popular mythology because so many people loathe spiders. Few species are truly dangerous. The funnel-web spiders of Australia, Papua New Guinea and the Solomon Islands (*Atrax* sp.) are extremely dangerous, but the greatly feared Sydney funnel-web spider has a small distribution and is carefully avoided and its relatives in the rural areas are rarely involved in bites. The armed spider (*Phoneutria* sp.) of Brazil is also involved in lethal bites but is not a widespread spider. *Loxosceles* (the brown recluse spiders) and *Latrodectus* (the black widow spiders) are also widespread, dangerous species and a significant public health problem.

Ticks are close relatives of spiders and many ticks are implicated in the transmission of infectious disease. A few ticks are of neurological importance and they too are considered here.

SNAKE BITE

The world's 3000 species of snake are usually classified into 13 families. Only 10–15% of the snakes are venomous, and all of the venomous species belong to one of five families – Elapidae, Hydrophidae, Viperidae, Crotalidae and Colubridae (or six if the Atractaspidae – the burrowing or mole vipers – are included as a separate family). The Colubridae are, in the main, non-venomous, but the family is important because of a few particularly interesting dangerous species such as the boomslang and bird snake of Southern Africa.

The most significant neurological problem caused by snake bite is neuromuscular paralysis. The typical presentation is of relatively rapid onset neuromuscular weakness, dysphagia and ptosis. This form of paralysis is particularly common following bites by elapid snakes (e.g. cobras, mambas, kraits, all poisonous Australian snakes and coral snakes). It is less common following bites by vipers and pit-vipers, but there are some notable exceptions – the South American rattlesnake, *Crotalus durissus terrificus* causes severe neuromuscular

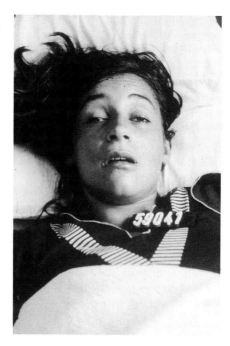

Figure 23.2 Young Brazilian woman with ptosis and neuromuscular weakness after having been bitten by a South American rattlesnake. (Reproduced by courtesy of J-L. Cardoso.)

paralysis (Figure 23.2) (Azevedo-Marques *et al.*, 1987). Neuromuscular paralysis is most commonly caused by the presence in the venom of small polypeptides of 60–70 amino acids (α-neurotoxins). These toxins bind to acetylcholine (ACh) receptors on the postsynaptic face of the neuromuscular junction. The binding of the toxins prevents access to the receptor for ACh released by the nerve terminal. Treatment is specific – the use of an appropriate antiserum which not only inactivates unbound toxin but possibly aids the dissociation of toxin-receptor complex (Gatineau *et al.*, 1988).

Many snakes also elaborate a number of toxic phospholipases. These venom constituents are usually neurotoxic but unlike the α-neurotoxins, the phospholipase toxins (sometimes known as β-neurotoxins) inhibit transmitter release from the motor-nerve terminal. These are found in the venoms of many elapid snakes (although not usually in venoms of cobras), some pit vipers (e.g. *Crotalus durissus terrificus*) and some true vipers (e.g. Russell's viper, especially in the subspecies *pulchella*, found in Sri Lanka). The venoms of kraits (*Bungarus* sp.) and of the elapid snakes of Australia are particularly rich sources of such toxins. Victims of krait bites may be paralysed for a considerable time, and require ventilatory support. One reported case of probable krait bite required ventilatory support for 21 days after the bite (Pearn, 1971) and paralysis is not always reversed by anticholinesterases (Warrell *et al.*, 1983).

The toxic phospholipases are also important because many of them are potent myotoxins. The late Alistair Reid first drew attention to myalgia, muscle necrosis and myoglobinurea following sea-snake bite (Reid and Lim, 1957, 1961). He speculated that since Australian elapid snakes are phylogenic cousins of sea-snakes, muscle damage may be a feature of poisoning by Australian snakes. He was absolutely right (Sutherland, 1981). It is now clear that the venoms of many elapid and crotalid snakes contain such toxins. Particularly important with respect to human envenoming are the tiger snake (*Notechis* sp.), the mulga (*Pseudechis australia*) and the taipan (*Oxyuranus scutellatus* of Australia), the South American rattlesnake (*Crotalus durissus terrificus*), the prairie rattlesnake of North America (*Crotalus viridis viridis*), the canebrake rattlesnake (*Crotalus horridus atricaudatus*) and the true viper (*Bothrops asper*) (for more detail and original sources, see Harris and Cullen, 1990). The damage caused to the muscle can be severe and widespread, giving rise to myoglobinuria and, in many cases, fatal renal failure. Recovery is slow since it requires the regeneration of the muscle. Damage to skeletal muscle is occasionally seen following bites by other species, but is not commonly life-threatening. A routine estimate of serum creatine kinase activity and examination of dark urine for the presence of myoglobin are simple, but necessary tests for muscle damage, because myalgia is not an invariable consequence of muscle damage.

Particular attention needs to be paid to victims of bites by snakes causing both soft-tissue necrosis and haemorrhage. This combination is usually seen following bites by viperid snakes, and in this regard Russell's viper (*Daboia* or *Vipera russelli*) is particularly important, as are snakes of the genus *Bothrops*. The reason that envenoming by these snakes is so important is that regeneration of the muscle may begin at a time when the local circulation is severely damaged. This can lead to the formation of large anoxic foci in regenerating muscles, abscess formation and long-term complications.

Russell's viper is responsible for a very uncommon problem – pituitary haemorrhage, acute adrenal/pituitary dysfunction and panhypopituitarism. Little is known of the mechanisms giving rise to these problems, but it is important to be aware that victims may present with symptoms of panhypopituitarism many months and even years after the bite. The data relating to this issue have been summarized and reviewed by Warrell (1986).

The neurological complications of snake bite identified earlier will, of course, never occur in isolation. Virtually all victims of an envenoming bite will be highly anxious, frightened and sometimes euphoric, many will experience pain, some will complain of numbness and 'tingling', a metallic taste in the mouth, headache and nausea. Almost all will exhibit abnormalities of blood clotting. It is important, however, not to delay the examination of neurological abnormalities.

SCORPION STINGS

Scorpions are widespread animals with a reputation for indiscriminate stinging. The sting is a part of the terminal segment of the tail (the telson) and is supplied by a pair of venom glands both contained within the telson.

Of the many hundreds of known species of scorpions, relatively few are serious risks to man. A large number of them will, however, cause an extremely painful reaction that will last for a few hours. The majority of dangerous scorpions belong the the family Buthidae genera *Centruroides*, *Tityus*, *Androctonus*, *Buthus* (or *Buthotus*). The common symptom of scorpion sting is intense pain, followed by neurotoxic signs such as tachycardia, tachypnoea, salivation, lacrimation, restlessness, fasciculation of skeletal muscle and muscular weakness. The symptoms are variable because scorpion venoms contain small polypeptide neurotoxins that cause the depolarization of excitable membranes (and hence transmitter release and repetitive firing of axons), cardiotoxins that cause severe cardiac arrhythmias, and small transmitters and neuromodulators such as noradrenaline and serotonin. The induced release of catecholamines is particularly important, and gives rise to the concept of 'autonomic storm'.

Treatment of neurotoxic signs is symptomatic, combined with antivenom and pain relief. The major areas of significant levels of poisoning are the Middle East, North Africa, Trinidad (mainly cardiac abnormalities caused by *Tityus trinitatus*), Mexico and South America. Keegan (1980) has prepared a good introduction to scorpions and their medical importance.

BITES BY SPIDERS

Apart from one or two insignificant groups of spiders, all spiders are venomous. The vast majority are too small or weak to inflict a significant bite on man. There is no doubt, however, that bites by spiders are extremely common. Most spider bites are of no great consequence but a few species are particularly important.

The funnel-web spiders (genus *Atrax*) are found in Australia, Papua New Guinea and the Solomon Islands. They are notorious and have been responsible for many deaths. The Sydney funnel-web spider *Atrax robustus* is a species with a natural range of 50 km around the centre of Sydney and seems to be responsible for most serious bites (Figure 23.3). A closely related spider, *Atrax formidibalis*, has also been responsible for human deaths. Both male and female spiders are large and aggressive. The male is especially troublesome. The fangs of the spider are large, the venom potent and the bite aggressive. Envenomation is painful and results in the widespread release of neurotransmitters from nerve terminals leading to salivation, lacrimation, fasciculation of skeletal muscle, and a complex sequence of an initial hypertension, brief return to normal and then a slow and insidious, irreversible decline in blood pressure. The neurological syndrome can be treated symptomatically but the treatment of first resort is antivenom.

Similar symptoms occur following bites by several other spiders, including the black widow (genus *Latrodectus*). Numerous species of this genus exist all over the world and are variously known as button spiders, redback spiders and katipo. Black widow spiders have inflicted fatal bites to many victims (see Ori, 1984 for review). The very large and very aggressive Brazilian armed spider, *Phoneutria*,

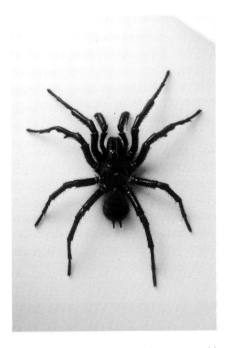

Figure 23.3 Funnel-web spider (male), *Atrax robustus*; a dangerous spider of Sydney with relatives distributed elsewhere in New South Wales, Papua New Guinea and possibly Solomon Islands. (Photograph V. Draffin; reproduced by courtesy of S. Sutherland.)

is also dangerous and has inflicted fatal bites, but there are few epidemiological studies available. There is no universal pattern to spider bites. Most victims of the funnel-web spiders are bitten in or around the home; victims of bites by *Latrodectus* may be bitten as they sort lumber rooms and garages where these small spiders nest (a typical pattern of bites in Australia and USA) or farm workers (in southern Europe for example), where the spiders infest fields and grain stacks. Sugar-cane cutters in Brazil are at risk of bites by *Phoneutria* where the spider occupies a relatively small region around São Paulo.

The toxins found in spider venoms causing neurological problems in man are almost always small polypeptides. As with snake bite, victims need to be carefully watched, since neurological symptoms may be overshadowed by severe pain (both localized and generalized), and the anxiety and horror experienced by many victims of the large spiders in particular.

TICKS

Ticks are close relatives of spiders. There are three stages to the life-cycle of the ticks – larva, nymph and adult – and all are parasitic. The female deposits eggs in ground litter. On hatching, the larvae infest shrubs and bushes and attach themselves to passing mammals. After a maturation period the larvae return to the ground to progress to the nymph stage when they attach themselves once more to a passing host. The cycle is repeated as the adult tick emerges to attach itself once more to the host.

Of approximately 800 known species of tick, 30–40 are believed to be implicated in the neurotoxic poisoning of man (see review by Stone, 1986). These species are very widely spread throughout southern Europe, former USSR, USA, Africa, Asia and Australasia.

The two species most frequently reported as being implicated in human poisoning are the hard tick *Ixodes holocyclus* of Australia and the North American ticks *Dermacentor andersoni* and *D. variabilis*. Ataxia and generalized weakness are the first symptoms of poisoning, and it is estimated that this usually occurs 4–5 days after the tick attaches itself. In severe cases, swallowing and respiration are weakened, and localized palsy may occur (Figure 23.4) (Pearn, 1977). The toxins, and their mode of action have not been formally

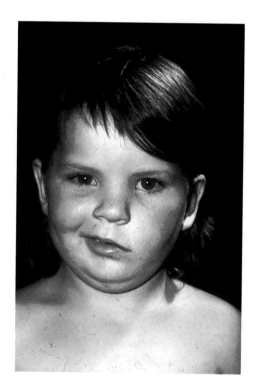

Figure 23.4 A six-year-old girl with a left-sided Bell's palsy. An adult female scrub tick, *Ixodes holocyclus*, had been embedded behind the left ear for several days. The left side of the face and the left-sided peri-ocular muscles are paralysed. (Reproduced with permission from Pearn J (ed.) (1981) *Animal Toxins & Man.* Brisbane: Queensland Department of Health.)

identified, but it is suspected that infestation results in both presynaptic failure of transmission and a block of nerve conduction.

Treatment revolves primarily around removal of the ticks, and symptomatic treatment of any local or systemic allergic or inflammatory reaction. Since a single tick may be involved, careful searching of the body is essential if a tick is suspected as the cause of otherwise inexplicable neurotoxic symptoms. It is an important practical note that although paralysis is rapidly resolved following removal of *Dermacentor* sp., paralysis may take several days to resolve when the infesting species is *Ixodes holocyclus*.

MANAGEMENT OF ENVENOMATION

The following procedure is recommended for management of envenomation:

1. Calm the patient.
2. Do not cut, suck or wash the site of the bite (venom on the skin may be important to identify the snake).
3. Immobilize the limb and apply a broad, firm bandage over the bite site. Do not apply an arterial tourniquet.
4. Transport the patient to medical care.
5. Carry out detailed clinical examination for shock, hypoxia, bleeding, coagulation defects, renal function, neurological signs, somnolence.
6. Carry out detailed laboratory examination: urine, blood, serum enzymes, coagulation defects, ECG.
7. Prepare for intubation/ventilation.
8. Identify source of venom: has the victim captured the animal?; use ELISA for identification of venom on swabs from bite/sting site.
9. Administer antivenom if there is evidence of systemic poisoning; secondary/symptomatic treatment if needed.

Note: Do not release pressure bandage too soon; inadequate or inappropriate antivenom is counterproductive – identification of envenoming species is therefore essential; relapse may be rapid – constant vigilance is necessary.

These guidelines are derived from Sutherland (1976).

REFERENCES

Azevedo-Marques MM, Hering SE and Cupo P (1987) Evidence that *Crotalus durissus terrificus* (South American Rattlesnake) envenomation in humans causes myolysis rather than haemolysis. *Toxicon* **25**: 1163–1168.

Gatineau E, Lee CY, Fromageot P and Menez A (1988) Reversal of snake neurotoxin binding to mammalian acetylcholine receptor by specific antiserum. *European Journal of Biochemistry* **171**: 535–539.

Harris JB and Cullen MJ (1990) Muscle necrosis caused by snake venoms and toxins. *Electron Microscopy Reviews* **3**: 183–211.

Keegan HL (1980) *Scorpions of Medical Importance.* Jackson: University Press of Mississippi.

Ori M (1984) Biology of and poisonings by spiders. In: *Handbook of Natural Toxins*, vol. 2 (ed. AT Tu), pp 397–440. New York: Marcel Decker.

Pearn JH (1971) Survival after snake-bite with prolonged neurotoxic envenomation. *Medical Journal of Australia* **2**: 259–261.

Pearn J (1977) Neuromuscular paralysis caused by tick envenomation. *Journal of the Neurological Sciences* **34**: 37–42.

Reid HA and Lim KJ (1957) Sea-snake bite. A survey of fishing villages in north west Malaya. *British Medical Journal* **2**: 1266–1272.

Reid HA and Lim KJ (1961) Myoglobinuria and sea-snake poisoning. *British Medical Journal* **1**: 1284–1289.

Stone BF (1986) Toxicoses induced by ticks and reptiles in domestic animals. In: *Natural Toxins Animal, Plant and Microbial* (ed. JB Harris), pp 56–71. Oxford: Clarendon Press.

Sutherland SK (1976) Treatment of snakebite in Australia and Papua New Guinea (revised and reprinted December 1978). *Australian Family Physician* **5**: 272–282.

Sutherland SK (1981) Treatment of snake bite in Australia and New Guinea. In: *Animal Toxins and Man* (ed. J Pearn), pp 112–122. Brisbane: Queensland Health Department.

Warrell DA (1986) Tropical snake bite: clinical studies in south east Asia. In: *Natural Toxins Animal, Plant and Microbial* (ed. JB Harris), pp 25–45. Oxford: Clarendon Press.

Warrell DA and Arnett C (1976) The importance of bites by the saw-scaled or carpet viper (*Echis carinatus*), *Acta Tropica* **33**: 307–341.

Warrell DA, Looareesuwan S, White NJ, Theakston RDG, Warrell MJ, Kosarkan W and Reid HA (1983) Severe neurotoxic envenoming by the Malayan krait *Bungarus candidus* (Lin.): response to antivenom and anticholinesterase. *British Medical Journal* **286**: 678–680.

24

Heat Stroke

Mustafa Khogali and Samir Atweh

Faculty of Medicine, American University of Beirut, Beirut-Lebanon

INTRODUCTION

Man is a tropical mammal able to tolerate and adapt to heat better than to cold stress. Despite this ability, he has suffered heat-induced and heat-related illnesses (HRI) throughout recorded history. The effects of heat, including vivid descriptions of heat stroke, have been mentioned in the Old Testament. The Arabs described a disease 'siriasis', which accompanies the dog star Sirius. Many old military campaigns have been lost due to heat illnesses. A Roman army was annihilated by heat in 24 BC. King Edward and his crusaders lost the final battle of the Holy Land because of heat illnesses. The ancient scourge is still prevalent. Modern military organizations still encounter heat illnesses when unacclimatized recruits are subject to heavy physical exercise or combat in a hot environment. Athletes and workers performing heavy work are also prone to develop heat illnesses. Heat stroke is third only to head and spinal injuries and heart failure as a cause of death among American athletes (Knochel, 1989).

When environmental heat stress is maximal, heat illness occurs without strenuous exercise. Cases of heat stroke were reported following a Turkish or sauna bath and among individuals left enclosed in hot areas. The potential effect of heat on the body and its systems is catastrophically demonstrated in large populations by hyperpyrexia found in heat waves. During the heat wave in Peking (14–25 July 1743) 11 000 people died from the heat. In more recent times, reports have reflected the high mortality from heat waves in the United States where, indirectly, heat effects may contribute to as many as 4000 deaths per year (Caldroney, 1986). Thousands of persons, mostly elderly, died during the heat wave in Greece and Italy in the summer of 1987.

Many cases of HRI are encountered during the Makkah pilgrimage in Saudi Arabia when it occurs during the hot weather. Every year, 2 million people from all over the world travel to Makkah for the pilgrimage. The number of cases seen during the years 1980–1986, and for a period of 3 weeks in each year, were 6778 heat stroke cases and approximately 40 000 cases of heat exhaustion. These were the cases that could arrive at the heat stroke treatment centres or hospitals along the pilgrimage route. However, hundreds have died before they could reach heat illness treatment centres.

THERMOREGULATION

Survival depends upon the maintenance of thermal equilibrium around 37°C. To keep the body in thermal equilibrium the amount of heat gained must be equal to the amount of heat lost. This relationship is affected by two physiological mechanisms, the cardiopulmonary system and the sweating mechanism. Changes in blood flow alter the conductance between the core and the skin, while sweating promotes loss of heat from the skin surface. Both central and peripheral mechanisms cause sweating when the skin temperature is elevated. Changes in core temperature seem quantitatively more important and have been estimated to be ten times more potent in producing a heat-dissipating response than are skin temperature changes.

THE SET POINT CONCEPT

The centre controlling the physiological process involved in thermoregulation is situated in the hypothalamus. This thermoregulatory centre comprises two anatomically distinct subcentres, one for heat conservation by cutaneous vaso-constriction and shivering, and the other for heat dissipation by cutaneous vasodilatation and sweating. The central nervous system (CNS) interprets infor-mation received from thermosensors through different pathways, and accordingly instructs thermoregulatory effectors. The thermoregulatory system is operating around an apparent 'set point', i.e. equivalent combinations of skin and core temperature at which heat production and evaporative heat-dissipating mechan-isms simultaneously attain minimum values. Thus, the set point is thermally determined by a dynamic balance between signals from two types of sensors which have opposite temperature response characteristics. The concept of a 'set point' provides a conceptual framework which fits a variety of clinical situations.

HEAT ILLNESS

The inability of humans to adapt to severe heat stress has been well documented. The clinical syndromes vary from heat syncope, to heat cramps, to heat exhaus-tion and to heat stroke (Khogali, 1983a; Yarbrough and Hubbard, 1989; Knochel, 1989).

Heat syncope can occur when an individual experiences orthostatic dizziness or fainting following exposure to a high environmental temperature. It is precipitated by long hours of standing, postural changes or physical activity in hot weather which leads to volume depletion and syncope. It has been described all over the world, among labourers in the Persian Gulf, Indian and African miners and European servicemen. It is a self-limiting condition, since rest in a cool surrounding in a horizontal position with head down is the cure.

Heat cramps are painful muscle contractions following strenuous exercise in individuals whose level of physical fitness will permit sustained physical exertion. Miners, sugar-cane cutters and boiler operators are among the most commonly reported victims. The cramps tend to occur when the person stops work and is relaxing and differs from those experienced during physical exercise which tend to last for short periods and resolve spontaneously. Heat cramp is different from hyperventilation tetany which may occur during heat exhaustion. Muscular cramps occur as a result of salt depletion and patients may exhibit hyponatraemia, hypochloraemia, and low urinary sodium and chloride levels. The treatment is cessation of activity, rest in a cool environment and replacement of fluids and electrolytes.

Heat exhaustion is the most common clinical disorder resulting from work or physical activity in a hot environment and the term is used to describe a number of syndromes leading to collapse (Khogali, 1983b). The common feature is cardiovascular insufficiency brought about predominantly by dehydration and insufficient water intake, salt depletion, or a mixture of both when great losses of sweat have occurred. Heat exhaustion is characterized clinically by weakness, fatigue, frontal headache, impaired judgement, vertigo, thirst, nausea and vomiting and occasionally muscle cramps. The core temperature is usually only moderately elevated (less than 40°C). The early detection of heat exhaustion is of paramount importance in conditions of high ambient temperature. Lind (1983) postulates that heat exhaustion may be part of a series of events leading to heat stroke and it can be regarded as incipient heat stroke. Hales *et al.* (1987) proposed that an increase in both muscle and skin blood flow occurs, with decreases in the gut, kidney and fat. This leads ultimately to decreased central venous volume and pressure which in turns elicits constriction of cutaneous veins and arterioles. Thus cutaneous heat loss is reduced and body core temperature rises further precipitating heat stroke.

Heat stroke is a complex clinical disorder characterized by the triad of disturbance of the nervous system, generalized anhydrosis and a rectal temperature of above 40.6°C (105°F) (Khogali, 1983c; Khogali and Mustafa, 1984; Knochel, 1989). There are three forms:

(a) exertional heat stroke which occurs in healthy individuals following extreme physical activity during environmental thermal stress;
(b) classic heat stroke which occurs in sedentary individuals with compromised homoeostatic mechanisms exposed to high environmental heat;
(c) heat stroke observed among Makkah pilgrims, which has a mixed picture of both the exertional and the classic forms.

A wide variety of factors predispose to heat stroke (Table 24.1). The lack of acclimatization is perhaps the most common predisposing factor among young

TABLE 24.1 Host factors reported to increase risk of heat stroke

Behaviour	Predisposing diseases	Drugs
Lack of acclimatization	Cardiovascular diseases	Anticholinergics
Dehydration	Diabetes mellitus	Antiparkinsonians
Fatigue	Febrile illness	Antihistamines
Inappropriate clothing	Endocrine disorders	Cyclic antidepressants
Alcoholism	Autonomic neuropathies	Diuretics
	Parkinsonism	MAO inhibitants
	Psychosis	Phenothiazines
	Impaired sweat production	Sympathomimetics
	Prior heat injury	
	Skin diseases	

healthy persons. During heat waves elderly individuals and those with pre-existing chronic diseases, especially cardiovascular disease, are at greater risk (Kilbourne *et al.*, 1982; Zhi-Cheng and Yi-tang, 1991). Virtually any chronic disabling disease increases the risk of developing heat stroke.

PATHOPHYSIOLOGY

Since the temperature of all organs is elevated, the degree of insult to the different organs and tissues (Figure 24.1) is related to the absolute rise in the body core temperature and to the duration of critical levels of that temperature and the associated metabolic acidosis and hypoxia. Hales (personal communication, 1994) postulates that there are three phases during progressive heat stress.

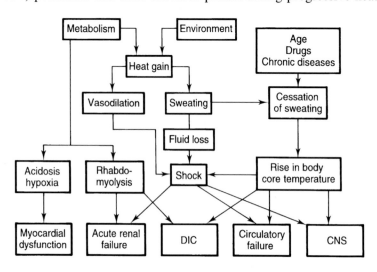

Figure 24.1 Interacting mechanism and the outcome in heat stroke patients.

First, below 40°C, changes in body fluids, electrolytes and cardiovascular activity are the major contributors to morbidity. Secondly, at core temperature between 40°C and 42.5°C, lipopolysaccharide (LPS) toxicity and the overwhelming cardiovascular demands cause morbidity and mortality. Recent studies have indicated that LPS contributes to the pathophysiology of heat stroke (Brock-Utne and Gaffin, 1989) and it has been suggested that anti-LPS might be an appropriate therapy or prophylaxis for heat stroke (Lancet, 1989). This level of core temperature is also dangerous because it causes irreversible tissue damage and mortality (Brinnel *et al.*, 1987). Thirdly, when the core temperature exceeds 42.5°C thermal damage becomes critical, oxidative phosphorylation becomes uncoupled and enzyme systems are affected. Energy metabolism and heat production as a byproduct of membrane-bound ATPase activity would be driven by heat, neuromuscular activity and acidosis. Eventually temperature control mechanisms fail and hyperthermia accelerates leading to dysfunction and failure of organ systems (Figure 24.1).

Damage to the CNS is a hallmark of heat stroke. Brain oedema is universal in heat stroke (Chao, 1987) and is usually accompanied by patchy congestion and petechial haemorrhages. The hypothalamus is generally spared (Knochel, 1989) but the cerebellum often shows marked deterioration and disappearance of Purkinje's cells. In experimental studies, generalized oedematous dilatation was observed in the subarachnoid space of dogs when cerebral temperature exceeded 42°C (Thrall *et al.*, 1986).

DIAGNOSIS

Acute neurological disability is the key to the diagnosis of heat stroke which should be suspected in any patient presenting with mental abnormalities and/or other signs of dysfunction of the CNS along with elevated body core temperature and a history of exposure to heat stress.

Rectal temperature measurement is confused and hyperactive heat stroke victims require the insertion of a thermistor probe with a scale reaching beyond the upper limit of 41°C of the standard clinical thermometer. Heat stroke patients present with an extremely high temperature and 75% of our patients (Al Khawashki *et al.*, 1983) had rectal temperatures greater than 42°C (range 40–44°C). Slovis *et al.* (1982) reported a patient whose rectal temperature was 46.5°C and who survived without sequelae. Measurement of body temperature using an oesophageal or tympanic probe has been advocated but in our experience it is difficult to apply in emergency situations.

CLINICAL PRESENTATIONS

Since heat stroke presents different clinical pictures, physicians may fail to recognize and treat it promptly. It may produce neurological, cardiovascular, respiratory, haematological, renal and hepatic complications.

Central Nervous System

Signs of severe CNS dysfunction dominate the early course of heat stroke. It is preceded by a short prodrome of confusion, irrational or aggressive behaviour, vivid hallucinations, lack of concentration and poor judgement. Headache, dizziness, lethargy and other general weakness are also reported.

Among our patients, 85% in Makkah arrived in coma, and of these 69% had constricted pupils. Other workers reported that the pupils were widely dilated, irregular and unresponsive to light (Knochel, 1989) but this does not indicate cerebral death since these abnormalities may disappear after appropriate cooling. Convulsions occurred both early and late. Survivors may recover completely or suffer chronic disabilities in the form of cerebellar ataxia, dysarthria, aphasia, hemiparesis or dementia.

Cardiopulmonary

The cardiovascular system is usually in a hyperdynamic state, with high cardiac output, and peripheral vasodilatation, unless limited by pre-existing disease. In our patients, 25% presented with hypotension and small volume rapid pulse. Since tachycardia is present in the majority of heat stroke patients, the electrocardiogram may also show branch block, ST and T wave changes and prolonged QT interval. Such changes do not necessarily indicate structural damage to the heart and are usually transient. Owing to the association of hypokalaemia, digitalis and calcium salts have to be used with caution.

Tachypnoea is the rule in heat stroke. Prolonged hyperventilation in conditions of hyperthermia leads to respiratory alkalosis but since the metabolic demands are not met patients may present with compensated metabolic acidosis. Pulmonary oedema can be severe and fatal if it presents as adult respiratory distress syndrome (Soliman et al., 1983; El Kassimi et al., 1986).

Haematological System

Bleeding diathesis in the form of petechial haemorrhages, ecchymoses, epistaxis and haematemesis are quite common during the clinical course. Evidence for disseminated intravascular coagulation (DIC) in heat stroke is supported by the findings of thrombocytopenia, increased levels of fibrin degradation products, hypofibrinogenaemia and prolonged prothrombin time (Strother et al., 1986). Our heat stroke patients showed platelet function abnormalities, fibrinolysis and low levels of factors II, V, VII and X (Mustafa et al., 1985). The high mortality among patients with DIC urges early diagnosis and prompt institution of preventive measures.

Gastrointestinal System

Nausea, diarrhoea, colonic spasm and vomiting start in the early stages and continue, especially in patients who have recently eaten. The diarrhoea in many cases is profuse but stops at the start of cooling.

Hepatic injury with elevated levels of liver enzymes is such a consistent feature of heat stroke that its absence should cast doubt on the diagnosis. Patients who survive longer than 36 hours may develop jaundice and other manifestations of liver disease. The jaundice becomes intense in patients with exertion-induced heat stroke and in our series was more common among Nigerians and Indonesians who are known to perform the rites of pilgrimage in a physically demanding way. The liver is extremely sensitive to thermal injury but hepatic damage may also result from the shock, congestive heart failure and hypoxaemia which so often accompany heat stroke (Rubel, 1984).

Renal System and Electrolyte Status

The majority of cases will show proteinuria and pigmented granular casts in the first specimen of urine. The exertion-induced heat stroke cases may show rhabdomyolysis, haemoglobinuria and myoglobinuria. In our series, acute renal insufficiency occurred only in 3% of cases, but in pure exertion-induced heat stroke the incidence is nearly 20% (Kains *et al.*, 1983).

In the absence of renal failure, most heat stroke patients are hypokalaemic. A number of patients are initially normokalaemic but on rehydration and cooling develop marked hypokalaemia (Khogali and Mustafa, 1984). Hypocalcaemia, hypophosphataemia and hypomagnesaemia have all been reported (Bouchama *et al.*, 1991).

Laboratory Investigations

Assuming availability, the investigations shown in Table 24.2 (a, b, c, d) should be performed immediately. If the patient is in deep coma, in severe shock, with core temperature > 42°C, or bleeding, coagulation studies should also be carried out (Table 24.2e). A computed tomographic brain scan and cerebrospinal fluid analysis are indicated if intracranial bleeding or infection are considered (Table 24.2f).

DIFFERENTIAL DIAGNOSIS

The recognition of heat stroke is not difficult when a patient presents with the triad of hyperpyrexia, altered mental status and hot dry skin in conditions suggestive of heat stress. The agitated, confused and convulsive patient may

TABLE 24.2 Recommended laboratory investigations

(a) Biochemical	(d) Haematological
Aspartate transminase (AST)	Haemoglobin
Alanine transminase (ALT)	Haematocrit
Creatine phosphokinase (CPK)	Leukocytes
Lactic dehydrogenase	total/diff
Blood glucose	Platelets
Blood urea	Prothrombin time
Serum potassium	Bleeding time
Serum creatinine	
Serum chloride	(e) Coagulation
Serum calcium	Active partial thromboplastin time (APTT)
Serum phosphorus	Fibrin degradation product (FDP)
Serum uric acid	Fibrinogen
	Plasminogen
(b) Acid–base balance	Factor V
pH, PO_2, PCO_2, HCO_3	Factor VII
	Factor X
(c)	
Chest radiograph	(f)
Electrocardiogram	CT brain scan

be mistakenly diagnosed as hysterical or epileptic and the body temperature is not taken. A patient with alcohol withdrawal symptoms can present like a case of heat stroke. Prolonged status epilepticus may cause hyperthermia due to muscular heat production. Other disorders in which there is increased muscular tone or activity may mimic heat illness, e.g. discontinuance of antiparkinsonian therapy, acute dystonias and some psychoses (Tek and Olshaker, 1992).

Meningococcal meningitis, tetanus, septic shock and malaria may resemble heat stroke. Ideally, all patients with fever and altered mental status in whom the diagnosis is not certain should have computed tomography and cerebrospinal fluid examination, which is usually normal in heat stroke. Patients coming from endemic areas should be screened for malaria. Other causes of coma such as trauma, diabetes or cerebrovascular accident should be considered. Heat stroke can be easily mistaken for head injury in sports such as baseball and rugby football (Savadie et al., 1991). Some endocrine diseases may cause hyperthermia with altered mental status. Among these are thyroid storm, pheochromocytoma storm and a diabetic ketoacidosis with concomitant sepsis (Tek and Olshaker, 1992).

Drug-induced syndromes of hyperthermia with mental status changes should be considered because specific therapy may be needed (Table 24.1): Clark and Lipton (1991) have reviewed the different aspects of drug-related heat stroke. Neuroleptic drugs are known to cause the neuroleptic malignant syndrome which is a potentially fatal disorder characterized by mental status changes, muscle rigidity, hyperthermia and autonomic dysfunction (Velamoor *et al.*, 1994). Certain patients undergoing general anaesthesia, especially with halothane combined with succinylcholine may develop malignant hyperthermia, characterized by muscular rigidity, severe hyperthermia and acidosis. Recently, Hopkins *et al.* (1991) postulated a relationship between exertional heat stroke and malignant hyperthermia and suggested that dantrolene should be administered as treatment, but there is no further evidence to support this notion. These two entities are differentiated from heat stroke by the muscular rigidity and clinical setting.

Heat stroke may occur in infants who are excessively wrapped or warmed during an infection, who are left locked in cars in hot weather (King *et al.*, 1981), or in the obese active child exercising in a hot environment. Clinicians should consider the possibility of heat stroke in babies who present with shock and encephalopathy, should inquire carefully about clothing and heating, and should anticipate the development of cerebral oedema, renal failure and DIC.

SPECIFIC TREATMENT (COOLING)

The corner-stone of treatment of the heat stroke patient is its early recognition, followed by rapid physiologically effective cooling, with simultaneous stabilization of the oxygen delivery mechanism, i.e. air way, ventilation and circulation. Mortality increases significantly when cooling is delayed.

COOLING MODALITIES

A number of cooling modalities have been reported to be useful in lowering body temperature in heat stroke: ice-water immersion, evaporation cooling using large circulating fans and skin wetting, ice packs, peritoneal lavage, rectal lavage, gastric lavage, alcohol sponge bath and cardiopulmonary bypass.

An alternative method of cooling has been developed by Khogali and associates (Khogali and Weiner, 1980) which utilizes evaporative cooling from the warm skin. In the Makkah body cooling unit (MBCU), the patient lies suspended on a wet surface, while being sprayed with atomized 15°C water from above and below. Air warmed at 45–48°C is blown over the surface of the skin at 3 m min^{-1} (Khogali, 1983d). The MBCU is designed to maximize evaporative cooling by cutaneous vasodilation and avoid shivering, while all other critical management procedures are being carried out smoothly. Mortality rate of patients treated dropped to 8% as compared to 80% before the use of MBCU (Khogali, 1983d).

In support of the MBCU, Khogali (1983a) cites seven objections to the time-honoured method of ice-water immersion: intense peripheral vasoconstriction shunting blood away from the skin and perhaps causing a paradoxical increase in core temperature; induction of shivering may increase heat production significantly above basal level; extreme discomfort to the patient; discomfort to the medical attendants; difficulty performing cardiopulmonary resuscitation; difficulty monitoring vital signs, and unpleasant and unhygienic conditions should vomiting or diarrhoea occur.

OTHER SUPPORTIVE MEASURES

It is imperative during the cooling period to monitor the vital signs, and to record continuously the core temperature, blood pressure and pulse. Hypotension usually improves with cooling and correction of hypovolaemia. The precise amount and type of fluid to be given will depend on the response of each patient and the results of the laboratory investigations. Central venous pressure monitoring is imporant. If there is oliguria after hydration, consider giving 500 mg of 10% mannitol. Positioning the patient in the semilateral position is important, so as to avoid aspiration pneumonia. The control of convulsions and muscle rigidity is essential to prevent further production of heat, lactic acid and myoglobin.

Acidosis whether pure metabolic or compensated should be corrected and monitored regularly. Hypokalaemia must be corrected. In our experience the majority of patients present with normokalaemia or hyperkalaemia, but once the hypovolaemia is corrected, their potassium level goes down. During the Makkah pilgrimage, some patients presented with very low serum potassium levels less than 2.0 meq l^{-1}.

PREVENTION

Prevention of heat illnesses is crucial since they are potentially lethal. Physicians, health administrators, paramedical personnel, industrial and military leaders, organizers of mass participation and other sporting events must appreciate the risk of heat illnesses. The principle of prevention and management of heat illnesses should be presented to all members of the community starting with children at school.

In our experience, success in prevention of heat illnesses could be achieved through: awareness and education; acclimatization; matching the level of activity to ambient temperature and humidity; liberal water replacement; use of proper clothing and appropriate medical history and physical examination.

Despite the success and substantial reductions in heat casualties, heat illness continues to occur all over the world. Thus physicians must always be sensitive to the possibility of heat illnesses and especially heat stroke and to be ready to provide the appropriate management, if significant mortality and morbidity are to be avoided.

REFERENCES

Al Khawashki MI, Mustafa MKY, Khogali M and El Sayed H (1983) Clinical presentation of 172 heat stroke cases seen in Mina and Arafat. In: *Heat Stroke and Temperature Regulation* (eds M Khogali and JRS Hales), pp 99–108. Sydney: Academic Press.

Bouchama A, Paarhar RS, Er-Yazigi A, Sheth K and Al-Sedairy S (1991) Entoxemia and release of tumor necrosis factor and interleukin-1 alpha in acute heat stroke. *Journal of Applied Physiology* **70**: 2640–2644.

Brinnel H, Cabanac M and Hales JRS (1987) Critical upper levels of body temperature, tissue thermosensitivity and selective brain cooling in hyperthermia. In: *Heat Stress: Physical Exertion and Environment* (eds JRS Hales and DAB Richards), pp 209–240. Amsterdam: Elsevier.

Brock-Utne JG and Graffin SL (1989) Endotoxins and antiendotoxins. *Anaesthesia and Intensive Care* **17**: 49–55.

Caldroney RD (1986) Heat-induced illness. *Hospital Practice* **15**: 48M–48T.

Chao TC (1987) Post-mortem findings in heat stroke. In: *Heat Stress: Physical Exertion and Environment* (eds JRS Hales and DAB Richards), pp 297–302. Amsterdam: Elsevier.

Clark WG and Lipton JM (1991) Drug-related heat stroke. In: *Thermoregulation: Pathology, Pharmacology and Therapy* (eds E Schonbaum and P Lomax), pp 125–177. New York: Pergamon Press.

Editorial (1989) Endotoxins in heat stroke. *Lancet* **2**: 1137–1139.

El Kassimi FA, Al-Mashhadani S, Abdullah AK and Akhtar J (1986) Adult respiratory distress syndrome and disseminated coagulation complicating heat stroke. *Chest* **90**: 571–574.

Hales JRS, Khogali M, Fawcett AA and Mustafa MKY (1987) Circulatory changes associated with heat stroke: observation in an experimental animal model. *Clinical and Experimental Pharmacology and Physiology* **14**: 761–777.

Hopkins PM, Ellis FR and Halsall PG (1991) Evidence of related myopathies in exertional heat stroke and malignant hyperthermia. *Lancet* **338**: 1491–1492.

Kains JP, Dewit S, Close P *et al.* (1983) Exertional heat stress diseases. *Acta Clinica Belgica* **38**: 315–323.

Khogali M (1983a) Heat stroke and heat exhaustion. *Travel and Traffic Medicine International* **1**: 166–169.

Khogali M (1983b) Heat stroke: an overview. In: *Heat Stroke and Temperature Regulation* (eds M Khogali and JRS Hales), pp 1–12. Sydney: Academic Press.

Khogali M (1983c) Epidemiology of heat illnesses during the Makkah pilgrimages in Saudi Arabia. *International Journal of Epidemiology* **12**: 267–273.

Khogali M (1983d) Makkah Body Cooling Unit. In: *Heat Stroke and Temperature Regulation* (eds M Khogali and JRS Hales), pp 139–148. Sydney: Academic Press.

Khogali M and Mustafa MKY (1984) Physiology of heat stroke: a review. In: *Thermal Physiology* (ed. JRS Hales), pp 503–510. New York: Raven Press.

Khogali M and Weiner JS (1980) Heat stroke: report on 18 cases. *Lancet* **11**: 276–278.

Kilbourne EM, Choi K, Jones TS and Thacker TS (1982) Risk factors for heat stroke: a case control study. *Journal of the American Medical Association* **247**: 3332–3336.

King E, Negus K and Vance JC (1981) Heat stress in motor vehicles: A problem in infants. *Paediatrics* **68**: 579–582.

Knochel JP (1989) Heat stroke and related heat disorders. *Disease-a-Month* **35**: 301–378.

Lind AR (1983) Pathophysiology of heat exhaustion and heat stroke. In: *Heat Stroke and Temperature Regulation* (eds M Khogali and JRS Hales), pp 179–188. Sydney: Academic Press.

Mustafa MKY, Omer O, Khogali M *et al.* (1985) Blood coagulation and fibrinolysis in heat stroke.

Rubel CR (1984) Hepatic injury associated with heat stroke. *Annals of Clinical Laboratory Sciences* **14**: 130–136.

Sarvadie E, Prevedorus H, Irish A *et al.* (1991) Heat stroke following rugby league football. *Medical Journal of Australia* **155**: 636–639.

Slovis CM, Anderson GF and Casolaro A (1982) Survival in a heat stroke victim with a core temperature in excess of 46.5°C. *Annals of Emergency Medicine* **11**: 269–271.

Soliman SM, AbuTaleb Z, Khogali M and El Sayed H (1983) Pulmonary aspiration and adult respiratory distress syndrome in 40 cases of heat stroke. In: *Heat Stroke and Temperature Regulation* (eds M Khogali and JRS Hales), pp 129–138. Sydney: Academic Press.

Strother SV, Bull JMS and Branham SA (1986) Activation of coagulation during therapeutic whole body hyperthermia. *Thrombosis Research* **43**: 353–360.

Tek D and Olshaker JS (1992) Heat illness. *Emergency Medical Clinics of North America* **10**: 299–310.

Thrall DE, Page RL, Dewhirst MW *et al.* (1986) Temperature measurement in normal and tumour tissues of dogs undergoing whole body hyperthermia. *Cancer Research* **46**: 6229–6235.

Velamoor VR, Norman R, Caroff SN *et al.* (1994). Progression of symptoms in neuroleptic malignant syndrome. *Journal of Nervous and Mental Disease* **182**: 168–173.

Yarbrough B and Hubbard RW (1989) Heat related illnesses. In: *Management of Wilderness and Environmental Emergencies* (eds PS Auerbach and EC Geehr), pp 119–143. St Louis: CV Mosby Co.

Zhi-Cheng M and Yi-tang W (1991) Analysis of 411 cases of severe heat stroke in Nawjing. *Chinese Medical Journal* **104**: 256–258.

25

Tropical Malabsorption and its Neurological Sequelae

Gordon C. Cook

Hospital for Tropical Diseases, St Pancras Way, London NW1 0PE, UK

INTRODUCTION

Small-intestinal malabsorption is common in most tropical and subtropical countries, but most cases are subclinical (Cook, 1980a). Neurological sequelae (Román *et al.*, 1985) seem uncommon; most descriptions have been associated with postinfective malabsorption (PIM) ('tropical sprue') (Cook, 1984a). Theoretically, the most likely mechanism relates to vitamin (especially B_{12}) deficiencies – known to be severe in a well-established case (Cook, 1980a; Román *et al.*, 1985); ileal involvement is common in PIM (see later).

Classification of Malabsorption in Tropical Countries

PIM (with a long history, and fascinating geographical distribution) dominates tropical malabsorption (Table 25.1). The term 'sprue' (see later) has sometimes been used to embrace gluten-induced enteropathy (coeliac disease). Protozoa (especially *Giardia lamblia*) and helminths are also important; coccidia are relevant in the context of AIDS-associated malabsorption in Africa. *Strongyloides stercoralis* causes malabsorption, but severity seems to vary with different strains; infection is especially common in south-east Asia. *Capillaria philippinensis* is important in the northern Philippines and Thailand. HIV-enteropathy, a major problem in tropical Africa, is increasing in Asia. Ileocaecal tuberculosis accounts for malabsorption throughout the tropics due to: (i) bile salt loss (ileal injury interrupts the enterohepatic circulation), and (ii) a direct effect of unabsorbed bile salt(s) on colonic mucosa. Mediterranean lymphoma occurs sporadically, especially in northern Africa, the Mediterranean and Middle East (Cook, 1980a); it is successfully treated with tetracycline when diagnosed early. Kwashiorkor can be followed by a malnutrition–malabsorption–anorexia cycle. Intestinal resection (and short-bowel syndrome) is relatively common. Chronic calcific pancreatitis (CCP) – first described in 1959 in Indonesia (Cook, 1980b) –

TABLE 25.1 Causes of malabsorption in a tropical/subtropical environment

*Small-intestinal**
   Postinfective malabsorption (PIM) ('tropical sprue')
   Small-intestinal parasites:
      Giardia lamblia
      Cryptosporidium parvum
      Isospora belli
      Sarcocystis spp.   protozoa
      [*Plasmodium falciparum*
      visceral leishmaniasis (Kala azar)]

      Strongyloides stercoralis
      Capillaria philippinensis   helminths
   HIV-enteropathy
   Ileocaecal tuberculosis
   Mediterranean lymphoma (α-chain disease)
   Severe malnutrition (Kwashiorkor)
   Intestinal resection (after intussusception, 'pig bel' disease, trauma, etc.)

Extraintestinal:
   Chronic calcific pancreatitis
   Liver disease (e.g. macronodular cirrhosis)

Specific malabsorption:
   Hypolactasia –   primary (genetically determined)
                    secondary to mucosal damage
   Addisonian pernicious anaemia†

* Gluten-induced enteropathy is probably unusual in tropical/subtropical countries; however, it can present for the first time in travellers to those countries.
† Addisonian pernicious anaemia is uncommon in most tropical countries.

is the commonest cause of overt (clinical) malabsorption in tropical Africa, and also exists in southern India; theories regarding its aetiology and pathogenesis are not universally accepted (Cook, 1980a,b; Nwokolo and Oli, 1980). Chronic liver disease (which rarely achieves clinical significance) can be associated with malabsorption. Specific malabsorption is dominated by hypolactasia; frequently primary (genetic), it may also follow severe jejunal/ileal mucosal damage (secondary hypolactasia) (Cook, 1984b). Addisonian pernicious anaemia is unusual – especially in Africa.

   Subclinical malabsorption is exceedingly common amongst indigenous people in tropical countries. Jejunal mucosal changes are mild (leaf-shaped villi – sometimes forming ridges – predominate, while finger-shaped ones are rare); minor functional abnormalities often coexist (Baker, 1976; Cook, 1980a). Subclinical malabsorption is common where standards of living/sanitation are unsatisfactory; it results from recurrent insults to the jejunal mucosa, caused by a multiplicity of infective agents (including viruses, bacteria and parasites). It rarely accounts for neurological sequelae however (Román *et al.*, 1985).

HISTORY

Malabsorption in the Tropics

Ancient Indian literature contains relevant accounts (Baker and Mathan, 1971). The English physician William Hillary (1766) described an acute, apparently epidemic disease in Barbados, of which the major clinical manifestation was malabsorption; he termed the disease *aphthoides chronica*; it was possibly caused by *G. lamblia* or another intestinal parasitic infection. Grant (1854) wrote on 'hill diarrhoea' at Indian hill stations during the heyday of the British Raj; Simla was rife with this form of malabsorption. During the nineteenth century, many reports were made of malabsorption in tropical countries; Pringle (1764) called it 'the white flux', Chevers (1886) 'diarrhoea alba', Goodeve (1866) 'cachechtic diarrhoea', and Thin (1897) 'psilosis'. Most were aware that it could begin acutely; in some, bloody diarrhoea was the earliest manifestation (Twining, 1835; Manson, 1880); however, this later gave way to: 'copious, paste-like brown [stools] in a state of fermentation; occasionally they [were] frothy, with a subalbid or grey sediment, like a mixture of chalk and beer' (Twining, 1835). Furthermore, 'a portion of the ailment often [passed] through the intestinal canal, indigested; and then the evacuations [were] of various colours'. Twining considered that in this condition the 'belly is generally flat, inelastic, and somewhat retracted; though in a few cases tympanites is a troublesome symptom'.

Patrick Manson (father of modern tropical medicine) working in 1880 in Amoy, China, was aware that Dutch physicians in Java (Dutch East Indies) used the word 'spruw' to describe an entity dominated by malabsorption; he adopted the term (Manson, 1880). (The term had previously been used in the Netherlands and Scottish lowlands to describe a disease in children in which there was gross wasting, associated with aphthous ulceration; with hindsight this was possibly gluten-induced enteropathy or 'coeliac disease'.) With hindsight this was not, however, a homogeneous entity. This was also the view of Chevers who wrote of 'the class of maladies known as "*diarrhoea alba*" ' (Chevers, 1886). It is now clear that *S. stercoralis* infections, which remain common in south-east Asia, can also cause significant malabsorption (O'Brien, 1975; Genta *et al.*, 1988). Since 1880, the term 'tropical sprue' has been widely used to describe *malabsorption in the tropics* – a heterogeneous entity with numerous causes (Table 25.1). During the first half of the twentieth century, there were many descriptions of malabsorption of acute onset in a tropical setting; some were doubtless examples of PIM (Rogers, 1913; Low, 1928; Manson-Bahr and Willoughby, 1930). Prolonged diarrhoea, malabsorption and weight loss caused by *G. lamblia* was not widely recognized (Fantham, 1916; Porter, 1916); however, the second of those writers compared the 'bulky' stools in giardiasis to 'khaki, mud, whipped cream, and putty'. It is now clear that *G. lamblia* infection can give rise to a clinical syndrome identical to PIM. Manson's 'lumping exercise' – while drawing attention to the existence of malabsorption in the tropics – resulted in the bringing together of several diseases under a single 'umbrella' (Cook, 1978a).

Haematological and Nutritional Abnormalities

Anaemia (frequently megaloblastic) is frequently a prominent manifestation of severe PIM and other causes of malabsorption in tropical and subtropical countries; earlier writers were unclear as to whether this had a cause or effect relationship. Goodeve felt that 'the tendency of all chronic diarrhoea is to destroy life by anaemia and exhaustion' (Goodeve, 1866). Sir Neil Hamilton Fairley and his colleagues, working in India during the 1920s and 1930s considered that anaemia resulted from 'sprue toxin' (Fairley *et al.*, 1929; Mackie and Fairley, 1929). Low (1928) had previously considered anaemia to be a result of, rather than a cause of, the disease; he concluded: 'the cure of . . . sprue cures the anaemia'; furthermore, '[in untreated sprue] a picture closely resembling pernicious or Addisonian anaemia develops'. Manson-Bahr and Willoughby (1930) recognized two types of anaemia: the first originated from an 'intestinal toxin', and the second was a true 'pernicious anaemia'. Confusion also surrounded the role of malnutrition. Low (1928) considered that 61% of 150 cases (described in London) had 'a [previous] history of some debilitating illness'.

Neurological Complications of Malabsorption in the Tropics

Early reports of malabsorption in tropical countries (especially India), documented oral signs/symptoms which originated in part, at least, from vitamin deficiencies (Pringle, 1764; Hillary, 1766; Twining, 1835; Manson, 1880; Chevers, 1886; Goodeve, 1866; Grant, 1854; Cook, 1978a; Thin, 1897). In Ceylon (now Sri Lanka), Bahr (1915) described oral changes in advanced disease; these were associated with a 'pernicious' type of anaemia; Begg (1912) stressed difficulty in distinguishing sprue from pernicious anaemia. However, like other early workers, neither of them described neurological sequelae, even in chronic disease (Pringle, 1764; Hillary, 1766; Twining, 1835; Manson, 1880; Chevers, 1886; Goodeve, 1866; Begg, 1912; Grant, 1854; Thin, 1897). Postmortem examinations rarely included a detailed assessment of the central nervous system (CNS); Mackie and Fairley concluded: 'as we have never met with clinical evidence of organic disease of the brain or spinal cord or of the peripheral nerves in any case of sprue during life, the omission of these organs from the necropsy would not appear to be a matter of much importance'. Neither Low's (1928) account of

150 cases, nor that of Manson-Bahr and Willoughby (1930) of 200 cases of 'sprue' (in London) mentioned neurological sequelae. Low failed to record tetany, '. . . described as a common symptom of sprue in all text-books', which was recognized by Manson-Bahr and Willoughby (1930); the latter authors wrote that they had 'never observed nervous changes in true sprue', and that 'cases of sprue anaemia with neuritic changes which have from time to time been reported are referable to the category of subacute combined degeneration of the cord'. Historically, therefore, evidence for neurological sequelae in tropical malabsorption is scanty – despite the presence of severe ileal disease and low vitamin B_{12} concentration.

GEOGRAPHICAL AND EPIDEMIOLOGICAL ASPECTS

Travellers' diarrhoea (TD) (Cook, 1993) seems the usual triggering event for PIM. Begg (1912) reported: 'in one interesting outbreak of sprue in a Chinese port, the evidence pointed strongly to a certain water supply being the cause of all the cases that occurred there'. Outbreaks of PIM have been described in south India (Baker and Mathan, 1968); chronic malabsorption also occurs as part of *G. lamblia* and *Cryptosporidium parvum* infection(s). Historically, PIM was *par excellence* a disease of India and South-East Asia; early reports stressed a very low prevalence in Africa. Low (1928) remarked that certain parts of the world are far more prone to the disease than others: 'It is especially common in the East – China, Cochin China, Manila, Java, Sumatra, Singapore, the Federated Malay States, Burma, India, especially in Bombay. It has been met with in Africa, but is rare there. In the West Indies it is of frequent occurrence in Porto Rico, and also has been noted in some of the other islands. I have also had cases from British Guiana, North Queensland and Mexico.' A similar geographical distribution was described by Manson-Bahr and Willoughby (1930). Within the last two decades, reports of PIM have been made at Lagos, Nigeria (Falaiye, 1970); Harare, Zimbabwe (formerly Rhodesia) (Thomas and Clain, 1976); and Durban, Republic of South Africa (Moshal *et al.*, 1973); some were certainly genuine cases. A report from Birmingham, England, described cases following TD acquired during a visit(s) to the Mediterranean littoral (Montgomery and Chesner, 1985). Geographical distribution has recently been summarized (Cook, 1991).

PATHOLOGICAL CHANGES

Enterocyte Damage

Early descriptions of morphology failed to: (i) include jejunal and ileal biopsy specimens (relevant techniques were only introduced in the 1950s), and (ii) exclude autolysis before postmortem examination. However, Twining (1835) concluded: 'the coats of the small and the large intestines have been found remarkably thin and transparent'. Goodeve (1866) concluded: '[there is] great thinning of all the coats of the small intestines, so that they are quite translucent'. Rogers (1913) also considered that 'the mucous membrane of the small bowel is thinned, and on section shows extensive atrophy of the villi and tube glands, together with a small-celled inflammatory infiltrate'. And Begg (1912), wrote of 'the clear evidence that the morbid process began in the ileum, *and extended from there* [my italics]'. Manson-Bahr (1924) and Fairley (1930) both considered that small-intestinal morphological abnormalities were important in aetiopathogenesis; both also concluded that changes were most severe in the ileum. Recent studies including those of O'Brien (1968a) also documented changes that were predominantly ileal. It is now clear that enterocyte damage becomes more severe as disease progresses, and ileal damage is almost certainly more severe than that in the jejunum (O'Brien, 1968a; Cook, 1980a). However, a 'flat' mucosa (common in gluten-induced enteropathy) is extremely rare. As disease progresses, serum folate concentration declines to a very low level by 4 months. A profound reduction in Na-ATPase concentration (and enterocyte number) has been documented in experimental folate deficiency (Tomkins *et al.*, 1976); in conjunction with luminal bacterial colonization (see later), this doubtless adds to the severity of mucosal injury (Cook, 1984a; Glynn, 1986). Brush-border involvement induces secondary hypolactasia (Cook, 1980a, 1984b).

Haematological and Nutritional Abnormalities

Several early authors had no doubt that the anaemia was classically megaloblastic; a steady decline in folate concentration certainly occurred (see later). A progressive fall in serum B_{12} concentration has also been clearly documented (Sheehy *et al.*, 1961; O'Brien, 1968a); this reaches a trough by 6–12 months. Longstanding vitamin B_{12} deficiency produces neurological sequelae in pernicious anaemia (Abdalla *et al.*, 1986); it now seems probable, however, that by the time such complications become manifest in PIM, most patients have either recovered or died.

Neurological Abnormalities

Postmortem examination of the CNS was not carried out by early investigators (see earlier); it is therefore impossible to assess the true incidence of CNS and peripheral nerve(s) pathology in the 'preantibiotic' era.

In recent reports, neurological sequelae have certainly been unusual (see later), and have usually been reversed by vitamin B_{12} therapy. Nerve conduction studies have only rarely been carried out *in vivo*. Neural biopsies and postmortem examination of CNS are poorly documented.

AETIOLOGY AND PATHOGENESIS OF PIM

Bahr (1915) considered three aetiologies: climatic, dietetic and specific – the last being divided into 'verminous, bacillary and fungoid'; and as Manson-Bahr (1953) wrote: 'the true aetiology of tropical sprue remains one of the outstanding conundrums in tropical medicine'. The last two decades have seen significant advances (Cook, 1978a, 1980a, 1984a).

Ethnological Factors

Under the British Raj in India, the disease was considered specific to British personnel; the Indian population was spared. Manson (1880) claimed: 'I have never recognised it in a native'. Goodeve (1866) concluded, however, that it 'attacked both Europeans and natives, and was not confined to people in poor circumstances'. Bahr (1915) considered that 'all writers are in agreement on one point, namely that sprue is preeminently a disease of the European in the tropics and that the native is only occasionally, if ever, affected'. Michel (1924) wrote of it as a 'white man's disease' affecting those who have lived in the tropics over an extensive period. As recently as 1927, the disease was considered 'obviously rare in Indians as compared with Europeans' (Megaw and Gupta, 1927).

During World War II (1939–1945), numerous observations were made in India; opinion emerged that PIM occurred in Indians in a form indistinguishable from that affecting Europeans (Elder, 1947; Walters, 1947). It was common in British soldiers and in those of Asian origin, but cases in Africans serving with the British Army were few (Cook, 1980a). In epidemics in the Philippines in 1968–1969, the attack rate was lower in the local Filipinos than in the American servicemen (Lindenbaum, 1973). A recent study at Puerto Rico has demonstrated a significant predominance of certain HLA subtypes in cases of 'tropical sprue' compared with controls (Menendez-Corrada *et al.*, 1986).

The fact that only a minority of individuals develops PIM after an acute intestinal infection seems certain to indicate an underlying genetic/ethnic predisposition.

Nature of the Initial Intestinal Infection

Small-intestinal infection (by many different organisms) has long been considered relevant (Bahr, 1915); Begg (1912) recorded 'that the disease is caused by an invasion of microorganisms was first suggested by me in 1890'. Undisputed evidence now indicates that most bacterial and viral infections of the small intestine can be associated with malabsorption which is sometimes severe (Lindenbaum, 1965).

To obtain precise data on the initiating infection(s) a large longitudinal study –

involving several hundred individuals – in an area where PIM is common would be necessary.

Cause(s) of Persisting Small-Intestinal Colonization

Persistence of luminal (present also at the enterocyte surface) Enterobacteriaceae has been demonstrated in PIM (Banwell and Gorbach, 1969; Klipstein *et al.*, 1973; Tomkins *et al.*, 1975); some produce enterotoxins which induce water secretion into the intestinal lumen (Tomkins, 1981), while others possess adherence properties and are cytopathic (Drasar *et al.*, 1980). Cause(s) of persisting colonization are multiple: delayed transit, hypochlorhydria, and pre-existing protein-energy malnutrition are probably important (Cook, 1980a, 1984a; Tomkins, 1981). Vitamin B_{12} deficiency probably results predominantly from luminal bacterial activity, rather than defective absorption by damaged ileum (see earlier).

Small-intestinal motility is normally increased in the presence of bacteria in the small-intestinal lumen (Dixon and Paulley, 1963; Kent *et al.*, 1966; Abrams and Bishop, 1967; Cook, 1984a); however, evidence exists for the reverse situation in PIM (Drew *et al.*, 1947; O'Brien, 1968b; Baker and Mathan, 1971; Cook, 1978b, 1984a). Motility is important in preserving sterility of the *milieu interior* (see earlier); decreased motility with relative stasis is likely therefore to account for significant chronic bacterial 'overgrowth'.

Pre- and post-prandial plasma enteroglucagon and motilin concentrations are greatly elevated in adults with PIM; these return to normal after treatment (Besterman *et al.*, 1979; Cook, 1984a). Intraluminal fat infusion is known to produce hyperenteroglucagonaemia, but in PIM this hormone is also greatly elevated in the fasting state (Cook, 1984a). Enteroglucagon is a trophic hormone (producing mucosal hypertrophy) and is liberated in response to intestinal (especially ileal) mucosal damage and/or resection; it also reduces small-intestinal transit rate. Ileum is more severely damaged than jejunum in PIM (see earlier). The physiological role of motilin has not been clearly established; that of neurotensin has not been fully explored in PIM (Glynn, 1986).

Reduced gastric acidity allows proliferation of small-intestinal bacteria (and some parasites) (Cook, 1994); importance of hypochlorhydria in PIM is, however, unclear. Fairley (1930) demonstrated it to be a common accompaniment of 'sprue'; this fact made differentiation from pernicious anaemia difficult. Other reports in the former half of the twentieth century also referred to its frequent occurrence, a finding corroborated in south India (Baker and Mathan, 1968).

Normal colon absorbs 4–7 l of water, and 100–160 mmol carbohydrate (as volatile fatty acid) per 24 h (Cook, 1984a). Significant colonic abnormalities have been documented in PIM (Ramakrishna and Mathan, 1982; Tiruppathi *et al.*, 1983); these are also common in many colonic bacterial and parasitic infections in 'Third World' countries. Colonic injury results in a relative failure of 'colonic salvage' (Read, 1982), a further factor in the vicious cycle culminating in PIM.

Mechanisms Underlying Chronic Disease

Most historical accounts (see earlier) described a chronic disease originating with acute diarrhoea. A minority described an 'insidious' entity (Cook, 1978a); however, the meaning of this term has almost certainly changed during the last two centuries. (Insidious is derived from the Latin *insidiosus* – used in the English language since the mid-sixteenth century. It originally indicated 'treacherous' rather than 'to proceed secretly' (P. Considine, personal communication). Early authors probably used it in the former sense.) With the notable exception of a small series of cases reported in London in 1971 (Mollin and Booth, 1971; Booth, 1984), recently reported cases have begun acutely; this presentation is entirely consistent with an acute infective aetiology (see earlier). An hypothesis (Cook, 1984a) suggests a vicious cycle: mucosal injury → hyperenteroglucago-naemia → small-intestinal stasis → intraluminal bacterial overgrowth → mucosal injury; this is broken by treatment with tetracycline + folic acid (see later). The additive effect of these two agents is more effective than one alone; this is considered supportive evidence for the hypothesis (O'Brien, 1968a).

CLINICAL FEATURES OF PIM

Dominant features are (i) large bulky, pale, offensive (malabsorption) stools, and (ii) progressive weight loss (Cook, 1980a, 1984a). Low (1928) considered that 'no disease with the exception of cancer, produces such a rapid and extensive loss of weight'. In the 1990s, cases are rarely so advanced that chronic sequelae become manifest; thus, megaloblastic anaemia – caused by folate and later vitamin B_{12} deficiency – is unusual. Hypoalbuminaemia (and resultant oedema) is present only in the most chronic cases. Most patients (unless access to medical care is lacking) now receive treatment before these manifestations become overt. Buccal pathology, folate-deficient megaloblastic anaemia, hypo-albuminaemia and oedema (Cook, 1980a, 1984a), are now therefore unusual. Low vitamin B_{12} concentration (which is apparently common in south India (Baker and Mathan, 1968)) is also very unusual in cases now presenting in the UK.

Neurological Sequelae

Table 25.2 summarizes publications in which neurological symptoms and signs have been clearly attributed to PIM (and other causes of tropical malabsorption). Historical reports contain only limited evidence of neurological sequelae (see earlier). However, Michel (1924) wrote 'the mentality in severe cases may become involved and impaired. The patient becomes dissatisfied, irritable and complains constantly. All the nerve energy is decreased and the special senses are impaired. In some cases paraesthesia is noted on the outside of the upper legs. All reflexes are impaired and sluggish.' Tetanic-like attacks were observed

TABLE 25.2 Evidence for neurological/psychiatric sequelae to malabsorption in a tropical environment

Neurological sign(s)	
Peripheral neuropathy	Walters (1947), Lai and Ransome (1970), Iyer *et al.* (1973), Taori and Iyer (1973), Román *et al.* (1985), Ramachandran *et al.* (1986)
Subacute combined degeneration	Baker and Mathan (1971), Mollin and Booth (1971), Taori and Iyer (1973), Dastur *et al.* (1975) Román *et al.* (1985)
Brachial neuritis	Baker and Mathan (1971), Mollin and Booth (1971), Taori and Iyer (1973), Dastur *et al.* (1975), Román *et al.* (1985)
Psychiatric impairment	Michel (1924), Elder (1947), Walters (1947), Iyer *et al.* (1973)
Neurological symptom(s)	
Paraesthesiae	Michel (1924)
Muscle cramps	Stefanini (1948)
Tetany	Michel (1924), Iyer *et al.* (1973)
'Burning feet syndrome'	Lai and Ransome (1970)
Chronic sequelae	
Peripheral neuropathy	Gibberd and Simmonds (1980)
Optic atrophy	Gibberd and Simmonds (1980)

in some cases' (Michel, 1924). During World War II several large series of cases of PIM were recorded. Despite a high prevalence of B avitaminoses (glossitis, stomatitis, angular stomatitis, and cheilitis [soreness and reddening of the lips]), Elder (1947) failed to encounter significant neurological involvement in a series of 400 cases, 22% of whom had macrocytic anaemia; one and three respectively, became disorientated and hallucinated, or 'extremely depressed'. More than 17% of 1069 cases documented by Stefanini (1948) developed paraesthesiae, and 27% suffered muscle cramps; a few had 'exaggerated tendon reflexes, but as a rule neurological examination was negative'. In a series of 42 severe cases in Indian soldiers (most were vegetarians) described by Walters (1947), however, mild peripheral neuropathy was present in 64%. This usually involved the lower limbs and consisted of tingling, burning and numbness; impaired sensation and sluggish tendon reflexes were present in the majority; 'evidence of degeneration of the long tracts of the spinal cord was never found'. Transient acute psychoses developed in two of them. It seems likely that the vegetarian diet played a significant role.

Recent reports also suggest that peripheral neuropathy is perhaps not as rare as previously suggested (Lai and Ransome, 1970; Taori and Iyer, 1973; Román *et al.*, 1985). In west India, 9% of cases of severe PIM had evidence of peripheral neuropathy (Jeejeebhoy *et al.*, 1968). In south India, nerve conduction studies indicated that 8 out of 24 patients with PIM had a peripheral neuropathy (Iyer *et al.*, 1973); in only one (who also had subacute combined degeneration), however, was objective evidence detectable. Muscle weakness was present in 15; 1 had tetany and 3 mental change(s). Similarly, subacute combined degeneration seems very uncommon despite the fact that serum B_{12} concentration is frequently depressed (Taori and Iyer, 1973; Román *et al.*, 1985); this fact is supported by historical reports (sophisticated investigational techniques were unavailable, and clinical examination was at its zenith). Taori and Iyer (1973) reported two examples of subacute combined degeneration out of 25 cases. Baker and Mathan (1971), in south India, recorded only two cases, despite the fact that vitamin B_{12} concentration was often very low; both responded rapidly to B_{12}. Mollin and Booth (1971) described one case (a 62-year-old retired missionary) in a series of 11 chronic cases of PIM in London; in addition, a 73-year-old woman had a brachial neuritis; both responded to vitamin B_{12}. Eight out of 12 patients with tropical neuromyelopathy (some had ataxia and spastic paraparesis) described at Bombay by Jeejeebhoy *et al.* (1967) had vitamin B_{12} deficiency; neurological sequelae improved after treatment.

It seems possible that a vegetarian diet hastens development of severe vitamin B_{12} deficiency with resultant neurological sequelae; Walters' (1947) observations support this. The experience of Dastur *et al.* (1975) is also consistent; five lactovegetarians with B_{12}-deficient neuromyelopathy (in two accompanied by cord involvement and proximal muscle weakness) responded to vitamin B_{12}. It seems possible also that advanced age is important in exacerbating neurological lesions in the presence of depressed vitamin B_{12} concentration (Román *et al.*, 1985). Interrelationships between B_{12} malabsorption, and folate and other B-complex vitamins are complicated; these warrant further study (Dastur *et al.*, 1975; Román *et al.*, 1985). Folic acid deficiency *per se* has been associated with myelopathy and sensory neuropathy (Román *et al.*, 1985). Metabolic links between folate and cobalamin are close; it is surprising therefore that neurological manifestations are so unusual in PIM.

The possibility that long-lasting neuropathic sequelae follow recovery from PIM has also been addressed (Lai and Ransome, 1970; Gibberd and Simmonds, 1980). Riboflavine deficiency (resulting from malabsorption) is responsible for 'burning feet' syndrome (Lai and Ransome, 1970) (physical signs are absent) – a common symptom in Far East prisoners-of-war (FEPOWs) during World War II; this responds rapidly to vitamin replacement. In a large follow-up study involving 4684 FEPOWs some 20–30 years later, 679 had evidence of neurological disease (Gibberd and Simmonds, 1980) – usually peripheral neuropathy or optic atrophy; in 89, neurological disease developed many years after release from captivity. It is impossible to assess the importance of malabsorption (rather than malnutrition) – either during the south-east Asian exposure, or in subsequent years. Multiple factors might account for neurological changes (Román *et al.*, 1985); vitamin E deficiency has, for example, been associated with spino-cerebellar degeneration in the blind-loop syndrome (Brin *et al.*, 1985).

Neurological Sequelae of Tropical Malabsorption – Excluding PIM

Chronic (non-alcoholic) calcific pancreatitis (CCP) is a common cause of overt malabsorption in tropical countries (see earlier); β-cell and exocrine function are both impaired (Abu-Bakare *et al.*, 1986). Osuntokun (1970) studied 74 patients with CCP in Nigeria, and recorded '. . . no difference in the pattern of neuropathy in this syndrome when compared with the neuropathic complications of diabetes of other (non-pancreatic) causes'; he concluded that this probably resulted from 'a metabolic defect . . . conditioned by acquired insulin deficiency'. In a study incorporating electromyographic and biothesiological observations, Ramachandran *et al.* (1986) recorded clinical evidence of peripheral neuropathy in 6 out of 16 patients with CCP at Madras, India; 9 and 7 had abnormal motor conduction velocity, and subclinical biothesiological abnormalities, respectively. The mechanism of these changes is unclear; vitamin B_{12} concentration was not determined. Out of 40 patients with CCP in India, 13 had evidence of diabetic retinopathy (Mohan *et al.*, 1985).

Neuropathy in CCP seems therefore to result predominantly from pancreatic endocrine deficit rather than malabsorption – resultant on exocrine dysfunction.

INVESTIGATIONS

Serum folate concentration declines as PIM progresses; in a severe case, a very low concentration is demonstrable by 4 months (Cook, 1980a, 1984a); this is frequently associated with megaloblastic bone marrow. However, there is also pronounced reduction in Na-ATPase level and enterocyte number(s). Vitamin B_{12} concentration declines relatively slowly; in a previously well-nourished individual, hepatic stores are substantial. In a vegetarian, however, it is likely that the concentration falls more rapidly; this probably accounts for an increase in neurological disease (see earlier).

Malabsorption of fat, xylose (and a lesser extent glucose) – of varying degree – is present early in the disease (Cook, 1980a, 1984a). Hypoalbuminaemia is often present. Amino acid malabsorption, and protein-losing enteropathy may coexist (Cook, 1980a). In a severe PIM case, reduction in concentration of serum trace elements – manganese and zinc – occurs (Cook, 1980a). Electrolyte (and water) absorption is impaired.

MANAGEMENT

Prevention is dependent on avoidance of acute gastrointestinal infections – virtually impossible in a tropical environment; commonsense measures must predominate. Prophylactic antibiotic therapy is not recommended for travel to a tropical country (Cook, 1993); no antibiotic is without side-effects, and on a broader canvas the widespread use of antibiotics promotes emergence of 'resistant enteropathogens'.

The majority of PIM cases probably remit spontaneously; in a severe case, however, a chronic course with significant mortality (10–20%) may result (Low, 1928; Manson-Bahr and Willoughby, 1930; Cook, 1980a).

A high-calorie, low-fat diet is advisable. Avoidance of lactose and dairy produce is indicated in a severe case. Symptomatic relief of diarrhoea – using an antiperistaltic agent, e.g. diphenoxylate, loperamide and/or codeine phosphate – is occasionally necessary.

Specific Treatment: Antibiotics, Folic Acid, and Vitamin B$_{12}$ Replacement

Claims were made during the 1930s that parenteral vitamin B$_{12}$ produced rapid improvement in a patient with 'tropical sprue' (Sheehy *et al.*, 1961) in contrast to an oral preparation. However, vitamin B$_{12}$ given alone produces a very slow recovery. Folic acid (5 mg three times daily) rapidly reduces severity of diarrhoea and faecal volume within 2 weeks; however, although it produces slow improvement in jejunal morphology (it seems likely that enterocyte recovery is hastened), it rarely cures the disease. An antimicrobial was first used by Rogers (1938); he administered sulphamidochrysoidine to a patient in London, and other sulphonamides were used shortly afterwards. Broad-spectrum antibiotics – initially oxytetracycline – were introduced by French (1955). Tetracycline reduces symptoms, improves jejunal morphology, and cures the disease. In practice, oral tetracycline and folic acid are almost always used in treatment (Cook, 1980a, 1984a). Metronidazole has been insufficiently used to warrant a conclusion regarding efficacy. In south India, antibiotic chemotherapy has proved disappointing (Baker and Mathan, 1971); this might reflect non-bacterial intraluminal flora at that geographical location.

CONCLUSIONS

Mild absorptive defects are very common in tropical and subtropical countries; however, there is no satisfactory evidence that any of the widespread neurological sequelae occurring in tropical countries (Román *et al.*, 1985) are a direct result. The classical entity, postinfective malabsorption (PIM) – formerly designated 'tropical sprue' – is associated with impaired jejunal and ileal function (resulting in vitamin B$_{12}$ deficiency). Other vitamin deficiencies, usually with a dietary origin, are also common. However, significant neurological manifestations, for example, peripheral neuropathy and subacute degeneration of the cord are uncommon in both historical and recent descriptions. This probably reflects: (i) mortality from an unrelated cause before such complications have become apparent (formerly), and (ii) early treatment with antibiotics and/or folic acid which produce rapid cure (in the present day). Many other causes of malabsorption also exist in tropical countries; scant evidence indicates that these predispose to significant neurological sequelae – except on rare occasions.

REFERENCES

Abdalla SH, Corrah PT and Mabey DCW (1986) Severe megaloblastic anaemia due to vitamin B_{12} deficiency in The Gambia. *Transactions of the Royal Society of Tropical Medicine and Hygiene* **80**: 557–562.

Abrams GD and Bishop JE (1967) Effect of the normal microbial flora on gastrointestinal mobility. *Proceedings of the Society of Experimental Biology and Medicine* **126**: 301–304.

Abu-Bakare A, Taylor R, Gill GV and Alberti KGMM (1986) Tropical or malnutrition-related diabetes: a real syndrome? *Lancet* **i**: 1135–1138.

Bahr PH (1915) *A Report on Researches on Sprue in Ceylon:1912–1914*. Cambridge: Cambridge University Press, p 155.

Baker SJ (1976) Subclinical intestinal malabsorption in developing countries. *Bulletin of the World Health Organization* **54**: 485–494.

Baker SJ and Mathan VI (1968) Syndrome of tropical sprue in south India. *American Journal of Clinical Nutrition* **21**: 984–993.

Baker SJ and Mathan VI (1971) Tropical sprue in southern India. In: *Tropical Sprue and Megaloblastic Anaemia: Wellcome Trust Collaborative Study 1961–1969*, pp 189–260. Edinburgh: Churchill Livingstone.

Banwell JG and Gorbach SL (1969) Tropical sprue. *Gut* **10**: 328–333.

Begg C (1912) *Sprue: its diagnosis and treatment*. Bristol: John Wright, p 124.

Besterman HS, Cook GC, Sarson DL *et al.* (1979) Gut hormones in tropical malabsorption. *British Medical Journal* **ii**: 1252–1255.

Booth C (1984) Tropical sprue. *Lancet* **i**: 1018.

Brin MF, Fetell MR, Green PHA *et al.* (1985) Blind loop syndrome, vitamin E malabsorption, and spinocerebellar degeneration. *Neurology* **35**: 338–342.

Chevers N (1886) *A Commentary of the Diseases of India*. London: Churchill, pp 561–583.

Cook GC (1978a) Tropical sprue: implications of Manson's concept. *Journal of the Royal College of Physicians* **12**: 329–349.

Cook GC (1978b) Delayed small-intestinal transit in tropical malabsorption. *British Medical Journal* **ii**: 238–240.

Cook GC (1980a) Malabsorption in the tropics. In: *Tropical Gastroenterology*, pp 271–324. Oxford: Oxford University Press.

Cook GC (1980b) The pancreas in the tropics. In: *Tropical Gastroenterology*, pp 193–202. Oxford: Oxford University Press.

Cook GC (1984a) Aetiology and pathogenesis of postinfective tropical malabsorption (tropical sprue). *Lancet* **i**: 721–723.

Cook GC (1984b) Hypolactasia: geographical distribution, diagnosis and practical significance. In: *Critical Reviews in Tropical Medicine*, vol. 2 (ed. RK Chandra), pp 117–139. New York: Plenum Press.

Cook GC (1991) The small intestine and its role in chronic diarrheal disease in the tropics. In: *Diarrhea* (ed. M Gracey), pp 127–162. Boca Raton: CRC Press.

Cook GC (1993) Travellers' diarrhoea: slow but steady progress. *Postgraduate Medical Journal* **69**: 505–508.

Cook GC (1994) Hypochlorhydria and vulnerability to intestinal infection. *European Journal of Gastroenterology and Hepatology* **6**: 693–695.

Dastur DK, Santhadevi N, Quadros EV *et al.* (1975) Interrelationships between the B-vitamins in B_{12}-deficiency neuromyelopathy. A possible malabsorption–malnutrition syndrome. *American Journal of Clinical Nutrition* **28**: 1255–1270.

Dixon JMS and Paulley JW (1963) Bacteriological studies of the small intestine of rats treated with mecamylamine. *Gut* **4**: 169–173.

Drasar BS, Agostini C, Clarke D *et al.* (1980) Adhesion of enteropathogenic bacteria to cells in tissue culture. *Developmental Biological Standards* **46**: 83–89.

Drew R, Dixon K and Samuel E (1947) Residual defects after sprue: a review of 26 cases. *Lancet* **i**: 129–134.

Elder HHA (1947) Clinical features, diagnosis, and treatment of sprue. *Journal of Tropical Medicine and Hygiene* **50**: 212–218.

Fairley NH (1930) Sprue: its applied pathology, biochemistry and treatment. *Transactions of the Royal Society of Tropical Medicine and Hygiene* **24**: 131–186.

Fairley NH, Mackie FP and Billimoria HS (1929) Anaemia in sprue: an analysis of 67 cases. *Indian Journal of Medical Research* **16**: 831–860.

Falaiye JM (1970) Tropical sprue in Nigeria. *Journal of Tropical Medicine and Hygiene* **73**: 119–125.

Fantham HB (1916) Remarks on the nature and distribution of the parasites observed in the stools of 1305 dysenteric patients. *Lancet* **i**: 1165–1166.

French JM (1955) The aetiology and mechanism of steatorrhoea. *Postgraduate Medical Journal* **31**: 299–309.

Genta RM, Gatti S, Linke MJ, Cevini C and Scaglia M (1988) Endemic strongyloidiasis in northern Italy: clinical and immunological aspects. *Quarterly Journal of Medicine* **68**: 679–690.

Gibberd FB and Simmonds JP (1980) Neurological disease in ex-Far-east prisoners of war. *Lancet* **ii**: 135–137.

Glynn J (1986) Tropical sprue – its aetiology and pathogenesis. *Journal of the Royal Society of Medicine* **79**: 599–606.

Goodeve E (1866) Diarrhoea. In: *A System of Medicine*, vol. 1 (ed. JR Reynolds), pp 82–105. London: Macmillan.

Grant A (1854) Remarks on hill diarrhoea and dysentery with brief notices of some of the Himalayan sanataria. *Indian Annals of Medical Science* **1** (2nd edn): 311–348.

Hillary W (1766) *Observations on the Changes of the Air and Concomitant Epidemical Diseases, in the Island of Barbadoes*, 2nd edn, pp 276–297. London: Hawes, Clarke & Collins.

Iyer GV, Taori GM, Kapadia CR, Mathan VI and Baker SJ (1973) Neurologic manifestations in tropical sprue. *Neurology* **23**: 959–966.

Jeejeebhoy KN, Wadia NH and Desai HG (1967) Role of vitamin B_{12} deficiency in tropical 'nutritional' neuromyelopathy. *Journal of Neurology, Neurosurgery and Psychiatry* **30**: 7–12.

Jeejeebhoy KN, Desai HG, Borkar AV, Deshpande V and Pathare SM (1968) Tropical malabsorption syndrome in West India. *American Journal of Clinical Nutrition* **21**: 994–1006.

Kent TH, Formal SB and Le Brec EH (1966) Acute enteritis due to *Salmonella typhimurium* in opium-treated guinea pigs. *Archives of Pathology* **81**: 501–508.

Klipstein FA, Holdeman LV, Corcino JJ and Moore WEC (1973) Enterotoxigenic intestinal bacteria in tropical sprue. *Annals of Internal Medicine* **79**: 632–641.

Lai CS and Ransome GA (1970) Burning feet syndrome. Case due to malabsorption and responding to riboflavine. *British Medical Journal* **ii**: 151–152.

Lindenbaum J (1965) Malabsorption during and after recovery from acute intestinal infection. *British Medical Journal* **ii**: 326–329.

Lindenbaum J (1973) Tropical enteropathy. *Gastroenterology* **64**: 637–652.

Low GC (1928) Sprue: an analytical study of 150 cases. *Quarterly Journal of Medicine* **21**: 523–534.

Mackie FP and Fairley NH (1929) The morbid anatomy of sprue. *Indian Journal of Medical Research* **16**: 799–826.

Manson P (1880) Notes on sprue. *Medical Reports for the Half-Year Ended 31st March 1880*, 19th issue. Statistical Department of the Inspectorate General Shanghai. China: Imperial Customs II: special series no. 2, pp 33–37.

Manson-Bahr P (1924) The morbid anatomy and pathology of sprue, and their bearing upon aetiology. *Lancet* **i**: 1148–1151.

Manson-Bahr P (1953) The causation of tropical sprue. A hypothesis. *Lancet* **ii**: 389–391.

Manson-Bahr P and Willoughby H (1930) Studies on sprue with special reference to treatment: based upon an analysis of 200 cases. *Quarterly Journal of Medicine* **23**: 411–442.

Megaw JWD and Gupta JC (1927) The geographical distribution of some of the diseases of India. *Indian Medical Gazette* **62**: 299–313.

Menendez-Corrada R, Nettleship E and Santiago-Delpin EA (1986) HLA and tropical sprue. *Lancet* **ii**: 1183–1185.

Michel C (1924) Sprue. In: *Practice of Medicine*, vol. 4 (ed. F Tice), pp 173–195. Hagerstown, Maryland: WF Prior.

Mohan R, Rajendran B and Mohan V *et al.* (1985) Retinopathy in tropical pancreatic diabetes. *Archives of Ophthalmology* **103**: 1487–1489.

Mollin DL and Booth CC (1971) Chronic tropical sprue in London. In: *Tropical Sprue and Megaloblastic Anaemia: Wellcome Trust Collaborative Study 1961–1969*, pp 61–127. Edinburgh: Churchill Livingstone.

Montgomery RD and Chesner IM (1985) Post-infective malabsorption in the temperate zone. *Transactions of the Royal Society of Tropical Medicine and Hygiene* **79**: 322–327.

Moshal MG, Hift W, Kallichurum S and Pillay K (1973) Malabsorption and its causes in Natal. *South African Medical Journal* **47**: 1093–1103.

Nwokolo C and Oli J (1980) Pathogenesis of juvenile tropical pancreatitis syndrome. *Lancet* **i**: 456–459.

O'Brien W (1968a) Acute military tropical sprue in south-east Asia. *American Journal of Clinical Nutrition* **21**: 1007–1012.

O'Brien W (1968b) Clinical presentation and pathology of tropical sprue. In: *Tropical Medicine Conference 1967* (ed. JH Walters), pp 86–95. London: Pitman Medical.

O'Brien W (1975) Intestinal malabsorption in acute infection with *Strongyloides stercoralis*. *Transactions of the Royal Society of Tropical Medicine and Hygiene* **69**: 69–77.

Osuntokun BO (1970) The neurology of non-alcoholic pancreatic diabetes mellitus in Nigerians. *Journal of Neurological Sciences* **11**: 17–43.

Porter A (1916) An enumerative study of the cysts of *Giardia (lamblia)* intestinalis in human dysenteric faeces. *Lancet* **i**: 1166–1169.

Pringle J (1764) *Observations on the Diseases of the Army*, 4th edn, pp 224–294. London: Millar, Wilson, Durham & Payne.

Ramachandran A, Mohan V and Kumaravel T (1986) Peripheral neuropathy in tropical pancreatic diabetes. *Acta Diabetologica Latina* **23**: 135–140.

Ramakrishna BS and Mathan VI (1982) Water and electrolyte absorption by the colon in tropical sprue. *Gut* **23**: 843–846.

Read NW (1982) Diarrhoea: the failure of colonic salvage. *Lancet* **ii**: 481–483.

Rogers L (1913) *Dysenteries: Their Differentiation and Treatment.* London: Oxford University Press, pp 303–323.

Rogers L (1938) The use of prontosil in sprue. *British Medical Journal* **ii**: 943–944.

Román GC, Spencer PS and Schoenberg BS (1985) Tropical myeloneuropathies: the hidden endemias. *Neurology* **35**: 1158–1170.

Sheehy TW, Perez-Santiago E and Rubini ME (1961) Tropical sprue and vitamin B_{12}. *New England Journal of Medicine* **265**: 1232–1236.

Stefanini M (1948) Clinical features and pathogenesis of tropical sprue: observations on a series of cases among Italian prisoners of war in India. *Medicine, Baltimore* **27**: 379–427.

Taori GM and Iyer GV (1973) Neurological complications in tropical sprue. In: *Tropical Neurology* (ed. JD Spillane) pp 73–77. London: Oxford University Press.

Thin G (1897) *Psilosis or 'Sprue': its Nature and Treatment with Observations on Various Forms of Diarrhoea Acquired in the Tropics*, 2nd edn, p 270. London: Churchill.

Thomas G and Clain DJ (1976) Endemic tropical sprue in Rhodesia. *Gut* **17**: 877–887.

Tiruppathi C, Balasubramanian KA, Hill PG and Mathan VI (1983) Faecal free fatty acids in tropical sprue and their possible role in the production of diarrhoea by the inhibition of ATPases. *Gut* **24**: 300–305.

Tomkins A (1981) Tropical malabsorption: recent concepts in pathogenesis and nutritional significance. *Clinical Science* **60**: 131–137.

Tomkins AM, Drasar BS and James WPT (1975) Bacterial colonisation of jejunal mucosa in acute tropical sprue. *Lancet* **i**: 59–62.

Tomkins AM, Badcock J and James WPT (1976) Altered morphology and pathways of DNA synthesis in small intestinal epithelium in dietary folate deficiency. *Proceedings of the Nutrition Society* **35**: 144A.

Twining W (1835) *Clinical Illustrations of the More Important Diseases of Bengal with the Result of an Inquiry into their Pathology and Treatment*, 2nd edn, vol. 1, pp 176–226. Calcutta: Baptist Mission Press.

Walters JH (1947) Dietetic deficiency syndromes in Indian soldiers. *Lancet* **i**: 861–865.

Section 5
SELECTED ASPECTS OF NEUROLOGICAL CONDITIONS

26

Epilepsy

Marcos C. Sandmann and Paulo R.M. de Bittencourt

Services of Neurology and EEG, Hospital N Sra. das Gracas and Unidade de Neurologia Clinica, Rua Padre Anchieta 155, 80410-030 Curitiba, Brazil

INTRODUCTION

About three-quarters of the population of the world live in the tropics, an environment with many common climatic and biological characteristics (Commission on Tropical Diseases of the International League Against Epilepsy, 1994), and at the same time with different socioeconomic features. Most of the regions usually defined as tropical are underdeveloped, and presently included in the so-called Third World.

Many of the causes of epilepsy found in a tropical environment are typical of Third World conditions. Not only microbial and parasitic diseases are common, but also more prevalent are hypoxia due to poor obstetric care, trauma consequent to traffic, work accidents and violence, as well as malnutrition.

Seizures may be acute symptomatic when they take place during active central nervous system (CNS) injury or infection. Epilepsy occurring as a sequel to CNS disease is called remote symptomatic (Commission on Epidemiology and Prognosis of the International League Against Epilepsy, 1993). In some slower and more chronic infections such as neurocysticercosis and HIV these terms may overlap, while they are distinct in the case of acute infections or trauma.

EPIDEMIOLOGY

The majority of epidemiological studies try to identify individuals with seizures, alteration of consciousness or taking antiepileptic drugs in a given region (Sander and Shorvon, 1987). Febrile seizures have been a major complicating factor in epidemiological studies in the tropics. The International League Against Epilepsy recommended that they are included as a subgroup of acute symptomatic (or provoked) seizures, with a high incidence in a specific age population. Single unprovoked seizures have a different prognosis and should not be included in aetiological studies. Epilepsy is a condition characterized by recurrent unprovoked seizures and two seizures are sufficient to characterize recurrence. The inclusion of all of these categories as 'epilepsy' in epidemiological studies may produce biased results, since each has a different prognosis. Only patients with recurrent (two or more) seizures should be included in epidemiological studies of epilepsy (Sander and Shorvon, 1987; Sander *et al.*, 1990).

Studies that try to define incidence are expensive and complex because they include surveillance of defined populations over relatively long periods. The few such reports in the literature usually compare tropical populations to those of developed regions. Age-adjusted incidence rates in Western populations range from 24 to 53 per 100 000 person years (PY) (Commission on Epidemiology and Prognosis of the International League Against Epilepsy, 1993; Sander and Shorvon, 1987; Sander *et al.*, 1990), but the few studies in the tropics have indicated that the incidence of epilepsy, including single and perhaps some febrile seizures, may be above 100 per 100 000 PY (Hauser and Hersdorfer, 1990). Incidences of 30–47.3 per 100 000 PY in the Mariana Islands (Senanayake and Roman, 1993), 114 per 100 000 PY in Chile (Hauser, in press), 122–190 per 100 000 PY in Ecuador (Placencia *et al.*, 1992, 1994) have been reported.

Prevalence rates are more easily found in the epilepsy literature, and they indicate a point prevalence range of 4–8 per 1000 inhabitants in developed environments, and 10–15 in tropical regions (Commission on Tropical Diseases of the International League Against Epilepsy, 1994). Two extensive reviews from the same authors (Senanayake and Roman, 1992, 1993) analyse studies of prevalence of epilepsy in the tropics and discuss methodological aspects used and possible misinterpretations of data. Studies carried out in the tropics reporting areas of low prevalence (below 3 per 1000), have methodological problems (Senanayake and Roman, 1992). The studies that show prevalence

TABLE 26.1 Prevalence of epilepsy in developing countries

Country	Prevalence per 1000 inhabitants*
Latin America	
Brazil	13.3
Colombia	19.5
Ecuador	12.2–19.5
Panama	22.0
Africa	
Ethiopia	5.2
Kenya	18.2
Liberia	28.0
Asia	
Sri Lanka	9.02

* Abstracted in part from Senanayake and Román (1992).

above the upper limit of the generally accepted rate of 9 per 1000, carried out in Africa and South America, also show lack of uniformity in methodology. If these studies had been made as house-to-house surveys with protocols based on WHO guidelines, they may have demonstrated still higher prevalence figures (Senanayake and Roman, 1992). Table 26.1 shows the more recent and well-designed studies of prevalence carried out in developing countries.

Based on these data it is suggested that epilepsy is two to three times more common in tropical and underdeveloped areas as compared to industrialized regions. This excess is a factor of the social, cultural and biological disadvantages in these areas (Senanayake and Roman, 1992, 1993; Hauser, in press).

AETIOLOGY AND PATHOPHYSIOLOGY OF EPILEPSY IN TROPICAL DISEASES

Parasitoses of the CNS

Where epilepsy occurs as a complication of chronic cerebral schistosomiasis, seizures are usually of partial onset and there are other localizing signs (Bittencourt *et al.*, 1988).

Hydatidosis is nowadays a very rare cause of epilepsy, confined to pockets of populations living close to infected sheep, cows or pigs. Very few cases of CNS involvement have been reported in the last decade, in contrast to older reports from Uruguay, southern Europe and South Africa (Arseni and Marinescu, 1974; Bittencourt *et al.*, 1988). Hydatid cysts are frequently very large and lead to raised intracranial pressure and focal neurological deficits, as well as epilepsy.

It has been suggested that neurocysticercosis is the most likely single factor underlying the increased frequency of epilepsy in the tropics (Commission on Tropical Diseases of the International League Against Epilepsy, 1994). Focal CNS signs, hydrocephalus and meningeal irritation, may present in various combinations (Bittencourt *et al.*, 1986a,b, 1988). In more than 50% of the cases there is an isolated parenchymal cyst, granuloma or calcification, but in some there may be countless lesions. Patients with extraparenchymal disease do not have epilepsy. Active mixed parenchymal and extraparenchymal disease has the worst prognosis, with 50% mortality in a few years (Bittencourt *et al.*, 1990a). Some 90% of patients with active parenchymal disease have seizures, two-thirds are partial with or without secondary generalization, but 30% have seizures which are apparently primary generalized. In three-quarters of cases the lesion is located in the hemisphere contralateral to motor or sensory lateralization, but surprisingly in 25% the lesions were found to be ipsilateral (Sotelo *et al.*, 1989). Seizures are more difficult to control in active parenchymal disease, in which bursts of simple partial status and Todd's paralysis are frequent (Goldsmith and Bittencourt, in press). A recent report (Del Brutto, 1995) defines a group of patients presenting with seizures who are shown on CT imaging to have a single parenchymal brain cysticercosis; early treatment with albendazole greatly improves the prognosis. The most vexing question in this field is that of eradication (Commission on Tropical Diseases of the International League Against Epilepsy, 1994). With some 5% infected in populations, the task is enormous and dependent on social and economic development. The combination of mass treatment of pigs and humans augmented by public health campaigns has been used, for example in Southern Brazil. With continued epidemiological surveillance and social progress the long-term results may be positive.

American trypanosomiasis (Chagas disease) is a public health problem in rural areas of Central and South America. The heart, oesophagus and colon are mainly affected but cerebral involvement secondary to embolization of cardiac blood clots is a rare cause of late-onset epilepsy with a high frequency of partial seizures (Jardim and Takayanagui, 1981; Senanayake and Roman, 1993). African trypanosomiasis (sleeping sickness) is widely distributed throughout sub-Saharan Africa. The chronic stage of the disease is characterized by progressive neurological involvement, including generalized and partial seizures. Congenital cases may also occur and manifest as mental retardation and epilepsy (Senanayake and Roman, 1993).

Malaria leads to seizures acutely in two very different settings. *Plasmodium vivax* is possibly the commonest cause of febrile seizures in the world whereas cerebral malaria, caused by *P. falciparum* leads to acute symptomatic generalized tonic-clonic seizures in the context of a severe encephalopathy (Bittencourt *et al.*, 1988; Brewster *et al.*, 1990; Hamer and Wyler, 1993).

Toxoplasmosis leads to remote symptomatic epilepsy in the congenital form (Neto and Bittencourt, 1994) and 40–60% of these patients have seizures (Bittencourt *et al.*, 1988). In adults, toxoplasmosis is a frequent cause of localized symptomatic seizures in the context of HIV infection (Bittencourt *et al.*, 1988). With the increasing incidence of AIDS in the tropics, toxoplasmosis is becoming a more important cause of epilepsy (Senanayake and Roman, 1993).

Bacterial Diseases of the CNS

There are few published reports of the characteristics of seizures and epilepsy in the context of acute bacterial meningitis. In a study of 185 children (Pomeroy, 1990) followed for a mean of 8.9 years after acute bacterial infection, one-third of seizures arose during acute infection, 67% of which had a partial onset. A study of 41 years experience with 200 cases of cerebral abscess showed that 28% presented acutely with seizures. Of the total sample 40% died in the immediate postoperative stage. Of the 40 cases who survived the acute hospitalization, 9 had epilepsy as their major handicap, and 3 died of epilepsy. The authors identified 67 patients between 3 and 40 years after surgery and concluded that both epilepsy and mental deficiency were commoner in children than in adults suffering from cerebral abscess, epilepsy occurring in 20 and 9%, and mental deficits in 33 and 13% respectively (Nielsen *et al.*, 1983). Subdural empyema, a complication of sinusitis, meningitis or neurosurgical procedures, is a rarer cause of acute seizures, and also of chronic epilepsy (Kaufman *et al.*, 1975).

Tuberculosis of the central nervous system presents with basal meningitis, vasculitis, encephalopathy, tuberculoma, spinal meningitis and rarely intraspinal tuberculoma. Meningitis can lead to epilepsy as a late sequel in 8–14% of patients and is frequently associated with hemiplegia. Epilepsy is also a common manifestation of intracranial tuberculomas that present as slow-growing, space-occupying lesions (Senanayake and Roman, 1993).

The reports of seizures associated with childhood shigellosis probably refer to common febrile seizures or perhaps unrelated epilepsy in this population. In a report of 153 cases (Ashkenazi *et al.*, 1987), all seizures occurred with fever, 75% with temperatures above 39°C, 20% had a positive family history, 23% had a previous history of seizures and 87% were younger than 5 years. Furthermore, 80% of seizures were brief tonic-clonic events. The CSF was normal in the 34 cases where lumbar puncture was undertaken.

Viral Diseases of the CNS

Herpes simplex and other viral encephalitides can lead to acute symptomatic seizures and to remote symptomatic epilepsy. Seizures are usually partial and very frequent in the acute phase, and there may be refractory simple or complex partial seizures as a sequela. Partial motor seizures started approximately 5 days after the initial lethargy and low-grade fever in neonatal herpes encephalitis (Arvin *et al.*, 1982).

Cytomegalovirus is a cause of epilepsy in congenital CMV infection, as part of a severe encephalopathy with mental retardation, microcephaly and deafness (Bale, 1984). Patients with clinical encephalopathy at birth have a significant risk of developing West syndrome, and conversely, some 5% of patients with West syndrome have congenital or immediate postnatal CMV encephalopathy (Riikonen, 1978).

Measles encephalitis leads to acute symptomatic seizures in some 50% of cases (Aarli, 1974). Seizures with a localized onset are of poor prognostic significance for the development of subsequent epilepsy.

HIV may lead to epilepsy by direct invasion of the brain, as in HIV encephalopathy, or as a consequence of opportunistic infections. In direct invasion of the brain, seizures are usually myoclonic or other generalized epilepsies in the context of the AIDS-dementia complex. Associated infections such as toxoplasmosis, cryptococcus meningitis, tuberculosis, lymphoma and herpes encephalitis give rise to partial seizures.

In children with HIV-encephalopathy, seizures have been observed in 10–20% (Labar, 1992), and tend to be generalized with spike and wave in the EEG, sometimes with a cortical myoclonic nature. The more advanced the encephalopathy the more severe and frequent are the seizures.

Trauma and Hypoxia

The age-specific incidence of head injury with brain involvement has a trimodal pattern, with a peak in young children, a second peak in the teenager and young adult, and a third peak in the elderly (Hauser and Hersdorfer, 1990). Males are affected almost twice as frequently as females. In a civilian cohort study, brain trauma associated with loss of consciousness has been associated with a three-fold increase in risk for subsequent epilepsy (Hauser and Hersdorfer, 1990) and the risk for epilepsy increased with increasing severity of injury.

Hypoxaemic-ischaemic encephalopathy is the cause of 13–14% of all epilepsy (Bittencourt and Turner, 1990; Senanayake and Roman, 1993). Underlying causes predisposing to hypoxia are prematurity, maternal cardiovascular diseases, placental and umbilical cord diseases, prolonged labour, airway obstruction at birth and dystocic deliveries. Children in underdeveloped countries are predisposed to perinatal damage by poor maternal peri- and post-natal care. Cerebral palsy and mental retardation, frequently associated with perinatal hypoxia should be considered 'markers' for underlying brain abnormalities which are responsible for both the neurological handicap and the epilepsy. The more severe the mental retardation or cerebral palsy, the higher the proportion with epilepsy (Hauser and Hersdorfer, 1990).

Epilepsy and Drug Therapy

Therapy of neurocysticercosis with albendazole or praziquantel decreases the period of disease activity, leading to early parasite death, when epilepsy becomes more easily controlled (Commission on Tropical Diseases of the International League Against Epilepsy, 1994; Kshirsagar and Shah, 1992). It has been shown that dexamethazone, carbamazepine and phenytoin decrease the serum and cerebrospinal fluid (CSF) levels of praziquantel (Vazquez et al., 1987; Bittencourt et al., 1990b,c, 1992). The best possible alternative is to treat patients with frusemide and mannitol for intracranial hypertension, and sodium valproate or benzodiazepines for epilepsy, in order to allow the cysticidal agent, usually praziquantel, to have therapeutic concentrations in the serum, CSF and brain. The effect of carbamazepine and phenytoin on praziquantel appears to be related to their liver-enzyme induction, shared with phenobarbitone and primidone (Bittencourt et al., 1992). Inactive neurocysticercosis warrants no specific therapy.

The treatment of seizures in cerebral malaria is the same as that for status epilepticus of any cause, with short-acting intravenous benzodiazepines followed by longer acting intravenous phenytoin or nasogastric carbamazepine or valproate drugs. It appears that when patients recover from cerebral malaria they do so completely or almost completely, thus the frequency of epilepsy as a long-term complication of cerebral malaria is very low. Generalized seizures have occurred in non-epileptic subjects taking high doses of chloroquine, occasionally with therapeutic doses, and even during prophylactic treatment. Patients with epilepsy or low seizure threshold may be especially prone (Commission on Tropical Diseases of the International League Against Epilepsy, 1994). Inhibition of glutamate dehydrogenase activity is a possible mechanism. Quinacrine and mefloquine have exacerbated tonic-clonic seizures in patients with epilepsy.

The effect of dexamethazone on the outcome of acute bacterial meningitis was verified through a double-blind placebo-controlled study (Odio *et al.*, 1991) in which patients who received 0.6 mg kg^{-1} dexamethazone had less brain damage as shown by the computed tomography (CT) scan. Two of 51 children on dexamethazone had seizures as compared to 7 of 48 on antibiotics only.

It has been suggested that persons living in rural economically depressed areas of tropical countries may need higher oral doses of antiepileptic drugs to achieve a therapeutic response, due to problems in absorption, as well as other factors, such as plasma protein binding, distribution and elimination. Malnutrition may underlie this abnormal pharmacology (Commission on Tropical Diseases of the International League Against Epilepsy, 1994).

The World Health Organization (WHO, 1990) introduced a policy of training primary health workers of developing countries to identify patients with tonic-clonic seizures and treat them with phenobarbitone. This policy has been criticized because of cognitive side-effects and the development of tolerance. Both problems may be decreased with the use of low dosages (Commission on Tropical Diseases of the International League Against Epilepsy, 1994) but usually the opposite occurs, for example in Brazil, where the standard dose of phenobarbitone is 100 mg daily, and frequently children take 50 mg daily, or adults more than 150 mg (Shorvon *et al.*, 1991). Gradually and depending on the economic status, carbamazepine is rising to a prominent position as an anticonvulsant in tropical countries.

In practice, in most developing countries, a significant number of patients are not treated at all. This phenomenon is called 'the treatment gap' and may vary from 10% in more developed regions to some 75% of the epileptic populations in the least developed regions of the world (Shorvon *et al.*, 1991). This fact alone is used to justify the WHO initiative as specified above. Another significant part of the population is treated with barbiturates independent of their seizure disorder or diagnosis. It is only a minority of the population, with financial resources and access to sophisticated medical care, that will be treated with carbamazepine, valproate and the newer drugs (Bittencourt and Turner, 1990; Kshirsagar and Shah, 1992). Large regions of Latin America and Asia have shown substantial economic progress in the last decade, and large segments of the world population now are able to acquire a more sophisticated medical care. It is very likely that this trend will continue in the coming decade. The WHO initiative and the indiscriminate treatment of epilepsy with barbiturates is likely to remain in areas of least development.

ACKNOWLEDGEMENTS

The authors are grateful for the information and help provided by Professor W.A. Hauser and Dr J.W.A. Sander, respectively of New York and London, as well as for the bibliographical search conducted by the National Epilepsy Library of the Epilepsy Foundation of America.

REFERENCES

Aarli JA (1974) Nervous complications of measles: clinical manifestations and prognosis. *European Neurology* **12**: 79–93.

Arseni C and Marinescu V (1974) Epilepsy in cerebral hydatidosis. *Epilepsia* **15**: 45–54.

Arvin AM, Yeager AS, Bruhn FW *et al.* (1982) Neonatal *Herpes simplex* infection in the absence of mucocutaneous lesions. *Journal of Pediatrics* **100(5)**: 715–721.

Ashkenazi S, Dinari G, Zevulunov A *et al.* (1987) Convulsions in childhood shigellosis: clinical and laboratory features in 153 children. *American Journal of Diseases of Children* **141**: 208–210.

Bale JF (1984) Human cytomegalovirus infection and disorders of the nervous system. *Archives of Neurology* **41**: 310–320.

Bittencourt PR and Turner M (1990) Epilepsy in developing countries: Latin American aspects. In: *International Epileptology*, 1st edn (eds M Dam and L Gram), pp 807–820. New York: Raven Press.

Bittencourt PR, Gorz AM, Oliveira TV and Mazer S (1986a) Neurocisticercosis: conceptos básicos de clinica, diagnóstico y tratamiento. Parte I. *Acta Neurologica (Colombia)* **2**: 11–15.

Bittencourt PR, Gorz AM, Oliveira TV and Mazer S (1986b) Neurocisticercosis: conceptos básicos de clinica, diagnóstico e tratamiento. Parte II. *Acta Neurologica (Colombia)* **2**: 11–14.

Bittencourt PR, Gracia CM and Lorenzana P (1988) Epilepsy and parasitosis of the central nervous system. In: *Recent Advances in Epilepsy*, vol. IV (eds TA Pedley and BS Meldrum), pp 123–160. Edinburgh: Churchill Livingstone.

Bittencourt PR, Costa AJ, Oliveira TV *et al.* (1990a) Clinical, radiological and cerebrospinal fluid presentation of neurocysticercosis. A prospective study. *Arquives de Neuro-psiquiatria* **48**: 286–295.

Bittencourt PR, Gracia CM, Gorz AM *et al.* (1990b) High-dose praziquantel for neurocysticercosis: efficacy and tolerability. *European Neurology* **30**: 229–234.

Bittencourt PR, Gracia CM, Gorz AM, Oliveira TV (1990c) High-dose praziquantel for neurocysticercosis: serum and CSF concentrations. *Acta Neurologica Scandinavica* **82**: 28–33.

Bittencourt PR, Gracia CM, Martins R *et al.* (1992) Phenytoin and carbamazepine decrease oral bioavailability of praziquantel. *Neurology* **42**: 492–496.

Brewster RD, Kwiatrowski D and White DH (1990) Neurological sequelae of cerebral malaria in children. *Lancet* **336**: 1039–1043.

Commission on Epidemiology and Prognosis of the International League Against Epilepsy (1993) Guidelines for epidemiology studies on epilepsy. *Epilepsia* **34(4)**: 592–596.

Commission on Tropical Diseases of the International League Against Epilepsy (1994) Relationship between epilepsy and tropical diseases. *Epilepsia* **35(1)**: 89–93.

Del Brutto OH (1995) Single parenchymal brain cysticercosis in the acute encephalitic phase: definition of a distinct form of neurocystericosis with a benign prognosis. *Journal of Neurology, Neurosurgery and Psychiatry* **58**: 247–249.

Goldsmith P and Bittencourt PR (in press) Epileptogenesis in neurocysticercosis: a review. *Epilepsia*

Hamer DH and Wyler DJ (1993) Cerebral malaria. *Seminars in Neurology* **13**: 180–188.

Hauser WA (in press) *Epidemiology of Epilepsy.* New York: Columbia University.

Hauser WA and Hersdorfer D (1990) *Epilepsy: Frequency, Causes and Consequences.* New York: Demos.

Jardim E and Takayanagui OM (1981) Epilepsy and chronic Chagas disease. *Arquivos de Neuropsiquiatria* **39**: 32–41.

Kaufman DM, Miller MH and Steigbigel NH (1975) Subdural empyema: analysis of 17 recent cases and review of the literature. *Medicine* **54(6)**: 485–498.

Kshirsagar NA and Shah PU (1992) Management of epilepsy in developing countries. In: *Recent Advances in Epilepsy* (eds TA Pedley and BS Meldrum), pp 159–176. New York: Churchill Livingstone.

Labar DR (1992) Seizures and HIV infection. In: *Recent Advances in Epilepsy* (eds TA Pedley and BS Meldrum), pp 119–126. New York: Churchill Livingstone.

Neto MC and de Bittencourt PR (in press) Infections and post-infective causes. In: *Epilepsy in Children* (ed. SJ Wallace) London: Chapman and Hall.

Nielsen H, Harmsen A and Gyldenstead C (1983) Cerebral abscess: a long-term follow-up. *Acta Neurologica Scandinavica* **67**: 330–337.

Odio CM, Faingezicht I, Paris M *et al.* (1991) The beneficial effects of early dexamethazone administration in infants with bacterial meningitis. *New England Journal of Medicine* **324 (22)**: 1525–1531.

Placencia M, Suarez J, Crespo F *et al.* (1992) A large scale study of epilepsy in Ecuador: methodological aspects. *Neuroepidemiology* **11**: 74–84.

Placencia M, Sander JWAS, Roman M *et al.* (1994) The characteristics of epilepsy in a largely untreated population in rural Ecuador. *Journal of Neurology, Neurosurgery and Psychiatry* **57**: 320–325.

Pomeroy LS (1990) Seizures and other neurologic sequelae of bacterial meningitis in children. *New England Journal of Medicine* **323(24)**: 1651–1657.

Riikonen A (1978) Cytomegalovirus infection and infantile spasms. *Developmental Medicine and Child Neurology* **20**: 570–579.

Sander JWAS and Shorvon SD (1987) Incidence and prevalence studies in epilepsy and their methodological problems: a review. *Journal of Neurology, Neurosurgery and Psychiatry* **50**: 829–839.

Sander JWAS, Hart YM, Johnson AL and Shorvon SD (1990) National General Practice Study of Epilepsy: newly diagnosed epileptic seizures in a general population. *Lancet* **336**: 1267–1271.

Senanayake N and Roman GC (1992) Epidemiology of epilepsy in the tropics. *Journal of Tropical and Geographical Neurology* **2**: 10–19.

Senanayake N and Roman GC (1993) Epidemiology of epilepsy in developing countries. *Bulletin of the World Health Organization* **71(2)**: 247–258.

Shorvon SD, Hart YM, Sander JWAS and van Andel F (1991) *The Management of Epilepsy in Developing Countries: An ' ICEBERG' Manual.* London: Royal Society of Medicine Services.

Sotelo J, Garcia E and Rubio F (1989) Granuloma en parénquima cerebral. Un modelo humano para el estudio de epilepsia. *Gaceta Medica de Mexico* **125**: 31-35.

Vazquez ML, Jung H and Sotelo J (1987) Plasma levels of praziquantel decrease when dexamethazone is given simultaneously. *Neurology* **37**: 1561-1562.

WHO (1990) Initiative of support to people with epilepsy. Document WHO/MHN/MND/ 90.3. Geneva: World Health Organization.

27

Epilepsy Services and Social Aspects

K.S. Mani and Geeta Rangan

Neurological Clinic, No. 1 Old Veterinary Hospital Road, Basavanagudi, Bangalore 560 004, India

INTRODUCTION

Illustrative Case Histories

A young adult of 25 in a developed country has experienced two unprovoked generalized tonic-clonic seizures (TCS) in 48 hours and is otherwise normal. He is seen by a physician, if not a neurologist, has several investigations, is started on a modern antiepileptic drug (AED) and has a regular follow-up assessment, possibly including serum AED levels. The following five examples are from the unpublished Rural Epilepsy Control Project (Yelandur Study) in a remote rural area of South India, and reveal a marked contrast.

The first example, a 52-year-old female, had focal motor seizures for 3 months involving the left upper limb and associated with weakness of the fingers. There were no facilities for any investigation. She was started on phenobarbitone (PB) with gradually increasing doses, and then changed to phenytoin. During fortnightly follow-up over the next 3 months, the partial seizures continued and increasing weakness of the left hand was noted. She was offered a 150 km trip with an escort to the city for a free EEG and CT scan. This was refused and she stopped her AEDS since she was promised a cure by a local compounder. She died of status epilepticus 18 months after onset of her illness. This was probably a case of brain tumour.

The second case had about 15 diurnal afebrile tonic-clonic seizures to 5 years of age at intervals of 3–4 months. She has been free of seizures for 6 years without any AED treatment, having therefore undergone spontaneous remission. Third, was a 25-year-old man who had two or three TCS each year for 15 years. With PB 30 mg daily he has had 4 years of remission, is fully active and has no sedative side-effects. The fourth is an 82-year-old female has been having TCS about one per month during sleep for 4 years. She refused long-term AEDs and prefers to have seizures which have not interfered with her activities of daily living and is unconcerned about her illness. Her attitude is 'cure me quickly or leave me alone'. Finally, a 26-year-old man has been having episodes for 8 years of altered consciousness in which he sits down, talks irrelevantly is fully recovered in 2–3 minutes. These are precipitated by a hot-water head bath and occur once a week. He has found that reducing the temperature of the water is helpful and does not opt for long-term AED treatment. This is an example of hot-water epilepsy.

None of these patients was subjected to social ostracization in their rural community. They and many like them continue to work, earn their wages, if young marry, have children and if old or mentally retarded, are looked after by the family to the best of their capacity. Their epilepsy is more or less public knowledge in their village.

Except for the example of hot-water epilepsy, the same spectrum of cases would be seen in other tropical countries, but the situation in the urban middle class would more or less be the same as the imaginary example from a developed country where knowledge about the seizures may be confined to immediate family members. Very often teachers, prospective employer or future spouse are not informed, thus keeping the diagnosis hidden for fear of social ridicule and ostracization. This appears to be an urban phenomenon, seldom encountered amongst the rural poor, at least in our area of study.

Services for any illness, but especially if chronic, must be viewed against a background which may vary from one country to another and even within regions or local areas.

EPILEPSY SERVICES

National Priority

Each country must follow its own fiscal priorities, often concentrating on agriculture, irrigation, industry, energy and communication with health occupying a very low position. There is, however, a tendency to improvement in many countries including India, with greater budgetary allotment for education, rural hygiene and health. In most developing countries a majority of the population is rural though urban migration is becoming more common.

Priority in Health Care

Even within the restricted budgets allocated to health, epilepsy is a Cinderella subject. There are more pressing problems such as family planning, control of malaria, leprosy (a fast disappearing disease), tuberculosis, maternal and child welfare and the goal of universal immunization. These measures are slowly improving the rural scene with perceptible changes but there is an urgent need for improved environmental hygiene and sanitation and protected water supply which is still not available for a vast majority in tropical countries. These changes must be accompanied by at least a minimum education for all (Briggs, 1993). It is not surprising that epilepsy, in which, between seizures, 80% of cases are absolutely normal, receives very little attention from health planners.

Epidemiology of Epilepsy

In recent years much epidemiological work has been undertaken in tropical countries. Probably some of the earlier figures from Latin American countries were overestimates. There appears to be a reduction in prevalence figures in India, from 9.8 per 1000 in the 1960s (Mathai, 1969) to around 5 in the late 1980s and early 1990s (Gourie Devi *et al.*, 1987; Bharucha *et al.*, 1988; Mani *et al.*, unpublished series). While the possibility of underestimation cannot be excluded, it appears unlikely since in rural areas it is very difficult to hide epilepsy from neighbours, unlike in an urban population and in developed countries (Zielinski, 1988). Moreover, recent studies have included random sampling and applied requisite corrections. However, more data are clearly needed.

Infections and Infestations

The success of an epilepsy control programme depends on having some idea of the presumed aetiology of the illness. This varies from one country to another and also within a country. Even in hospital and clinic-based series, birth trauma and brain tumours account for hardly 2% of all epilepsies (Mani and Rangan, 1990). However, infections and infestations account for a larger proportion, especially of partial seizures, as noted particularly after the advent of CT scanning (Misra *et al.*, 1994). Cysticercosis, an effective testimonial to standards of public hygiene in the community, leads the list of parasitosis especially in South America and Mexico partly accounting for the high prevalence rates of epilepsy in these areas and possibly parts of India. Many other infections and infestations commonly cause epilepsy (Commission on Tropical Diseases, 1994). Cerebral malaria can be mistaken for febrile seizures especially in parts of Africa, possibly North-East India and South-East Asia.

Perception of Epilepsy as a Disability

This has been referred to in the illustrative case histories. Minimal disability is created by infrequent and/or long-standing TCS or febrile seizures and village folk appear to take these in their stride. They do not consider these as a handicap and do not want the inconvenience and expense of regular long-term drug therapy, in spite of the risks involved in having seizures. This emphasizes the need for a balanced approach in each individual case as well as public education.

Natural History of Epilepsy

We still do not have enough data on the course of untreated epilepsy. There is some evidence to show that 20% of patients attain spontaneous remission (Sanders, 1993; Placencia *et al.*, 1994) and this remission is more or less permanent. Our own observations in the Yelandur Study on inactive epilepsy, seizure free for at least 2 years without AEDs, supports this concept, but treated cases probably remit earlier (Mani *et al.*, unpublished series). Data on a larger number of inactive cases, a neglected aspect of epidemiological studies on epilepsy, need to be collected in developing countries to determine the predictors for spontaneous remission.

Non-rural Areas

While concentrating on rural areas, the urban and semiurban areas may be neglected. Not all rural people are necessarily poor nor all urbanites necessarily rich but as the pace of development proceeds and the economy improves there is an increase in the middle and upper socioeconomic classes, resident often in the cities. In the case of India there is a very large middle class accounting for a third of its huge population of 850 million.

The planning of epilepsy services must take cognisance of these various factors (Watts, 1989; Mani and Rangan, 1990; Shorvon *et al.*, 1991; Meinardi, 1994). The large rural areas in developing countries need to have their basic health services strengthened. For example, this has been achieved to some extent by the barefoot doctors in China, the Primary Health Centre model in India and the involvement of fresh medical graduates in Ecuador. Doubtless there are centuries old traditional systems of medicine, which have their place in the rural order, and there are methods such as fasting, prayers and visits to places of worship to obtain divine grace. It should be borne in mind that these approaches are not necessarily harmful. Similar views have been expressed by Danesi and Adetunji (1994).

Medical Training

An attempt to introduce the Western system of medicine to rural areas requires reorientation of medical teaching and training programmes towards practical down-to-earth aspects of the health problems. Recourse to sophisticated investigations is not feasible. The training given in the medical curriculum for epilepsy is inadequate and has confused priorities. There has been an over-emphasis on aetiology rather than management, with the result that primary-care physicians have been nurturing the mistaken notion that without EEG, CT or blood-level estimation of AEDs, epilepsy cannot be managed. The point needs to be driven home that in the Third World, epilepsy can be tackled fairly successfully at the peripheral level on clinical grounds alone. The aetiological factors seen in a clinic-based series of 3378 cases of epilepsy, showed that in 85% the aetiology was unknown (Mani and Rangan, 1990). Even amongst the known causes obtained from history, examination and investigations in the pre CT era, an altered management strategy was only indicated in 3% of cases. Thus the treatment of epilepsy in rural or peripheral areas has to be mainly clinical with emphasis on follow-up assessment and referral of non-responsive cases to secondary centres. As epilepsy is but a tiny segment of total health care, people's awareness and knowledge of epileptology can be raised in the form of short review articles, booklets or video films. These need to be aimed also at the paramedical workers, the all-important basic human factor in rural health care. They can be involved, after adequate training, in epidemiological studies for identifying epilepsy suspects, drug distribution at nodal points, follow-up and patient and family education and counselling. This needs to be combined with the primary care of other diseases like leprosy, tuberculosis and mental illnesses to make the programme cost-effective. This peripheral decentralized clinical approach, quite different from the developed world, wherein medical aid is taken to the rural door-step, aims at diagnosis and management of epilepsy in its early stages in large numbers of cases.

Drugs

There is a treatment gap of 80–85% in most developing countries (Shorvon and Farmer, 1988), not only from non-availability of drugs, but also breaks in supply, faith in local healers or switching over to alternative systems of medicine. Education of the primary care physicians and the public, including patients and families, is essential for a successful outcome with available inexpensive AEDs. Studies in the Third World have shown the effectiveness of monotherapy with inexpensive drugs like PB or PHT in rural epilepsy control (Feksi *et al.*, 1991; Placencia *et al.*, 1993). In our rural epilepsy control project (Mani *et al.*, unpublished series), in 172 patients using only PB or PHT, complete remission of over 2 years was achieved in 29% and of 1–2 years in 33%, with more than 50% reduction in seizures in 33%, while the seizure frequency was unchanged in 6% and worse in less than 1%. This does not imply that the more expensive drugs are not required, but they are better retained as second-line drugs for resistant cases in rural areas. This hierarchical approach may not be ideal (Shorvon and Farmer, 1988) but stark realities leave no other option in rural epilepsy control. Contrary to popular belief, in the doses employed (seldom above 60 mg in a child or 120 mg in an adult for PB and 150 mg and 300 mg respectively for

PHT) side-effects were very rare; 7% of patients had gingival hyperplasia and 1% somnolence while none was hyperkinetic. Hyperkinesis and impairment of cognitive function with PB or PHT (Trimble and Cull, 1988) need not interfere with rural individuals in their sociocultural and work milieu. This illustrates the need to individualize and not generalize treatment.

In our rural studies, tonic-clonic seizures, primary or secondary, accounted for 84% of cases, and are a potential source of morbidity and mortality. Partial seizures constituted only 16% while absence and myoclonic seizures were rare (Mani and Rangan, 1990). The utility of hyperventilation, a simple bed-side test, as a provocative stimulus for absence seizures is not sufficiently realized and needs to be emphasized. With such a distribution of seizure types the limited role for carbamazepine and valproate in rural epilepsy control becomes obvious.

Brazil, China and India are examples of developing countries with an active pharmaceutical industry, but most others are dependent on expensive imports from developed countries. Whether drugs manufactured in Brazil, China or India would benefit other Third World countries in terms of cost is worthy of attention but requires pharmacokinetic studies. Wherever drugs are manufactured, formulated or imported, the chain of supply from the source to the periphery may be ill-organized with resultant inefficient and interrupted drug delivery. A great sense of commitment in distributors is required. This interruption in supply has been cited as an argument against the use of PB in primary health care (Shorvon and Farmer, 1988), but there does not appear to be any evidence to suggest that failure to take PB as a monotherapy has a greater risk of precipitating status epilepticus than other AEDs, and there is no evidence that PB is a habit-forming drug, or increases the risk of suicide in the Third World. These supposed drawbacks have to be weighed against the advantage of PB/PHT in rural epilepsy control.

Most of the population in developing countries are too poor to afford long-term drug therapy. There is no worthwhile medical insurance in Third World countries and even the nascent insurance scheme in India does not cover epilepsy, although coronary artery disease and by-pass surgery are included. Hence the patients have to fend for themselves. It has been stated that in developing countries family ties are strong and they will even 'donate cattle or treasured items' to afford medical treatment (Shorvon and Farmer, 1988). This may be true for acute illnesses, but whether it will be so for chronic diseases is a moot point. Not infrequently, the poorer people have nothing to sell. Hence it is the government which has to supply the AEDs for free. Non-governmental voluntary agencies for primary health care, well developed in certain countries like India (which has 4500 in number), Indonesia and Sri Lanka, can supplement, but unfortunately cannot replace the government agencies. The large pool of private practitioners, physicians and paediatricians settling down in smaller towns are also an increasingly potent source for primary health care, especially epilepsy. In India they are generally reluctant to maintain case records, but the increasing consumer movement involving the medical profession in its ambit may force them to accept a record system. More efforts need to be made to coordinate the work of these three groups. Refresher courses and lecture demonstrations in smaller towns on practical epileptology are of inestimable value. Practitioners of alternative systems of medicine can also be involved in rural epilepsy control, perhaps under supervision (Danesi and Adetunji, 1994).

There is a need for secondary and tertiary referral centres for epilepsy. Unfortunately the latter act as a repository for unspecified and unselected cases in the outpatient clinics with the result that quality suffers, in spite of the availability of expertise. Institutes for epilepsy care are needed at the national level in each country wherein all the requisite sophisticated services can be offered to the patients including surgery. Such institutes for total care of epilepsy are a distant dream, but day-care centres may be a reality.

SOCIAL ASPECTS

Epilepsy is considered a curse from the social angle in most cultures, but there are exceptions. Certain tribes in Ladakh, Kashmir (Singh, 1981) and Africa (Danesi, 1990) treat these patients as divine. By contrast, in some areas in sub-Saharan Africa, the saliva is considered infectious and most people would not share food with a patient or even rescue him from an open fire during a seizure because of the fear of contagion (Gerrits, 1983; Danesi, 1990). Elsewhere, well-meaning bystanders invariably push something between the teeth to prevent tongue bite or hold the limbs tight to control TCS with the resultant broken teeth or fractures. There is a strong belief in India that taking an iron key to the hand or an old shoe to the nostril of the patient will terminate a TCS. If a person has an attack on the roadside these measures are often followed by those around. In fact this information can be used as a corroborative evidence for a TCS when there is no eye-witness account, just as one with pseudoseizures may grab the key. There is a strong fear among most cultures that epilepsy is hereditary. Hence arranged marriages for these patients in traditional Indian society is a constant source of worry for the parents, who hide the information from the prospective spouse with resultant legal petitions for divorce which are invariably granted. It needs a lot of courage to accept openly that one has epilepsy and most patients and relatives are subject to human frailty and fail in that respect.

The Indian Law is also very much weighted against a patient with epilepsy (Mani and Hegde, 1989). Recurrent attacks of epilepsy at the time of marriage has been introduced as late as 1976 as a negative clause for solemnization of a marriage (Hindu Marriage Act 1955; Special Marriage Act 1954) allowing divorce on these grounds. This absurd legal apartheid is not present in any other country except India and perhaps Brazil. Petitions have been repeatedly submitted from 1987 to the present by the Indian Epilepsy Association to the federal government and there is every possibility that this legislation will be deleted in the near future.

In a collaborative study on epilepsy in India in 1969–1975 in five centres

(Bangalore, Bombay, Calcutta, Delhi and Madras) material was gathered on social aspects of epilepsy and data were available in 3439 patients (Desai, 1989). Adverse effects of the disease on regularity and progress in studies was noted in 28% and 40% respectively. Work status was affected only in 9% but this must be viewed against the common practice of withholding information from a prospective employer. Danesi (1990) in a similar experience found that in Nigeria 90% of those who could be employed had jobs, but a third of these had reduced income because of the illness and surprisingly very few lost their jobs in spite of the employer's knowledge about their illness. In the Indian study, supernatural causation of epilepsy was accepted only in 12%, but 23% of urban and 32% of rural subjects expressed faith in supernatural cure – often in the form of prayers, fasting and other harmless rituals. The patients were all hospital-referred epileptic subjects with a strong urban bias and from traditional Indian society. Similar low figures were noted by Mathai (1969) in South India depending on the rural–urban divide, level of education and other factors. In the Indian series strained social relationships were admitted to in only 1–8% of cases in the five different centres.

Rwiza *et al.* (1993) conducted a Knowledge, Attitude, Practice (KAP) study involving 3256 heads of households in a rural population. One third had never seen a seizure, 68% did not know the cause, 33% mentioned various causes including heredity and witchcraft, 41% believed it was infectious, 37% that it cannot be cured and 17% that it cannot even be controlled. Also, 45% had faith in traditional healers and only 51% in hospital drugs; 33% would not even touch a person during a seizure. In our rural epilepsy control programme in Yelandur, we also conducted a KAP study, involving 372 adult patients or relatives, unlike the Tanzanian series which involved the general population. Our hitherto unpublished observation revealed that 76% had seen or heard about epilepsy (patients excluded) but 69% did not know that it was a disease of the brain. In this study, 28% had visited places of worship and 19% wore amulets, 17% admitted to having had therapy from the village magician and only 4% from an ayurvedic physician. Also, 72% believed that 'English medicine' would cure their illness, but 66% had experienced 'English medicine', albeit briefly, without benefit. A negative psychosocial impact of epilepsy was noted only in 15%.

This study showed that social ostracization because of epilepsy was a very uncommon event in this rural area. Villagers have faith in Western medicine and do not appear to rely any more on the 'medicine man'. Harmless beliefs need not be discouraged, thereby showing respect to local sociocultural ethos, unlike 'city slickers' forcing scientific knowledge on villagers in an unconsidered fashion. The need is highlighted for simple practical methods of training for rural epilepsy control and education of both the primary care physician and the general public.

It is here that lay organizations such as the national chapters of the International Bureau of Epilepsy have a vital role to play and indeed are doing so in several developing countries. For example, the Indian Epilepsy Association, Bangalore chapter has written information booklets on Epilepsy in English and other Indian languages. It has also devised simple flash cards and posters for public education on epilepsy, especially in rural areas. There has been a regular quarterly newsletter from 1984, and radio and TV programmes and video films. Similar projects are undertaken by other branches of the Indian Epilepsy Association, as well as by Epilepsy Associations from Sri Lanka, Kenya, South Africa, Zimbabwe, Colombia, Chile and Ecuador. Public education on epilepsy is heavily dependent on the sociocultural climate and these organizations have been making progress against heavy odds and often on a low budget. They deserve support.

REFERENCES

Bharucha NE, Bharucha EP, Bharucha AE *et al.* (1988) Prevalence of epilepsy in the Parsi community of Bombay. *Epilepsia* **29**: 111–115.

Briggs N (1993) Illiteracy and maternal health. Educate or die. *Lancet* **341**: 1063–1064.

Commission on Tropical Diseases of the International League Against Epilepsy (1994) Relationship between epilepsy and tropical diseases. *Epilepsia* **35**: 89–93.

Danesi MA (1990) Epilepsy in the third world. African aspects. In: *Comprehensive Epileptology* (eds. M Dam and L Gram), pp 795–805. New York: Raven Press.

Danesi MA and Adetunji JB (1994) Use of alternative medicine by patients with epilepsy: a survey of 265 epileptic patients in a developing country. *Epilepsia* **35**: 344–351.

Desai AD (1989) Psychosocial aspects. In: *Epilepsy in India* (ed. PN Tandon), pp 117–143. New Delhi: ICMR.

Feksi AT, Kaamugisha J, Sanders JWAS *et al.* (1991) Comprehensive primary health care – antiepileptic drug treatment program in rural and semiurban Kenya. *Lancet* **337**: 406–409.

Gerrits C (1983) A West African epilepsy focus (letter). *Lancet* **1**: 358.

Gourie Devi M, Rao VN and Prakashi R (1987) Neuroepidemiological study in semi-urban and rural areas in south India. In: *Motor Neurone Disease* (ed. M Gourie Devi), pp 11–21. New Delhi: Oxford and IBM Publ. Co.

Hindu Marriage Act, 1955. Bare Act (1992) Act No. 25 pp 3 Delhi: Delhi Law House

Mani KS and Hegde NS (1989) Epilepsy and law: position in India. 17th International Congress Symposium *Advances in Epileptology*, vol. 17, pp 428–431. New York: Raven Press.

Mani KS and Rangan G (1990) Epilepsy in the third world. Asian aspects. In: *Comprehensive Epileptology* (eds. M Dam and L Gram), pp 781–793. New York: Raven Press.

Mathai KV (1969) Investigation into methods for rehabilitation of persons disabled by convulsive disorders. *SRS Project No. 19-P-56113.* Washington DC and New Delhi: Fol. HEW and ICMR.

Meinardi H (1994) Epilepsy in developing countries: proceedings of a workshop organized by EPICADEC. *Trop Geograph Med* **46** (Suppl): 56.

Misra S, Verma R, Lekhra OP and Misra NK (1994) CT Observations in partial seizures *Neurology (India)* **42**: 24–27.

Placencia M, Sander JWAS, Shorvon SD *et al.* (1993) Antiepileptic drug treatment in a community health care setting in northern Ecuador: a prospective 12 month assessment. *Epilepsy Research* **14**: 237–244.

Placencia M, Sanders JWAS, Roman M *et al.* (1994) The characteristics of epilepsy in a largely untreated population in rural Ecuador. *Journal of Neurology, Neurosurgery and Psychiatry* **57**: 320–325.

Rwiza HT, Matuja WBP, Kilonzo GP *et al.* (1993) Knowledge, attitude and practice towards epilepsy among rural Tanzanian residents *Epilepsia* **34**: 1017–1023.

Sanders JWAS (1993) Some aspects of prognosis in the epilepsies: A review. *Epilepsia* **34**: 1007–1016.

Singh B (1961) Presidential address. In: *Proceedings of National Seminar on Social Aspects of Epilepsy* (eds VS Saxena and KS Mani), pp 12. Bangalore: Indian Epilepsy Association Bangalore Chapter.

Shorvon SD and Farmer PJ (1988) Epilepsy in developing countries: A review of epidemilogical sociocultural and treatment aspects. *Epilepsia* **29**: (Suppl 1): S36–S54.

Shorvon SD, Hart YM, Sander JWAS and Van Andel F (1991) *The management of epilepsy in Developing Countries: An 'ICEBERG' manual*, pp 66. International Congress and Symposium Series 1705. London: RSM Services.

Special Marriage Act, 1954. Bare Act (1992) Act No. 43 pp 2 Delhi: Delhi Law House.

Trimble MR and Cull C (1988) Children of school age: The influence of antiepileptic drugs on behaviour and intellect. *Epilepsia* **29**: (Suppl. 3): S15–S19.

Watts AE (1989) A model for managing epilepsy in a rural community in Africa. *British Medical Journal* **298**: 805–807.

Zielinski JJ (1988) Epidemiology. In: *A Textbook of Epilepsy* (eds AL Richens, J Laidlaw and J Oxley), pp 21–47. Edinburgh: Churchill Livingstone.

28

Multiple Sclerosis

Charles M. Poser

Department of Neurology, Harvard Medical School and Beth Israel Hospital, Boston, Massachusetts, USA

INTRODUCTION

There are tropical diseases and there are diseases of the nervous system which occur in tropical areas. The former are easily defined and consist primarily of helminthic parasitic and fungal diseases. It should be noted that many of those diseases 'which though now are almost confined to torrid zones, in former times were found in temperate zones as well' (Spillane, 1973). In fact, because of increasing mobility of people and rapid transport, some of these diseases are beginning to be observed in temperate zones again. The latter are diseases that occur all over the world but may be modified by the tropical environment. Multiple sclerosis (MS) belongs to that group.

It is therefore necessary to try to define tropical areas. Some specialists in tropical medicine (Dumas, personal communication, 1993) consider black or sub-Saharan Africa as the only 'true' tropical region in the world, but many of the conditions that prevail in those countries also exist elsewhere. It is not sufficient simply to define the tropics as areas of sustained high temperature and humidity. With rare exceptions, these countries share additional characteristics such as poor sanitation, deficient nutrition, overpopulation and urban overcrowding, a largely agricultural depressed economy, lack of adequate health services, and have a large proportion of the population with a very low standard of living existing at or below the poverty level. Thus, although these conditions do describe primarily black Africa, south of the Sahara and north of the Republic of South Africa, similar conditions exist in Thailand, Laos, Cambodia and Vietnam as well as in the Philippines and Indonesia. In the Western hemisphere, southern Mexico, Central America and the countries of the Caribbean basin as well as Ecuador, Colombia, Venezuela and the Guyanas in South America also fulfil these conditions. Delineating these areas for the purpose of this study may seem to be arbitrary but is made because the study of diseases in tropical countries is primarily that of non-Caucasians.

All published studies have indicated that MS is relatively rare in tropical areas, but because there are important differences in cultural, economic and ethnic factors, as well as environmental conditions such as sanitation, nutrition, health care and pollution in these various countries, the study of risk factors for MS may be of particular value.

AETIOLOGY AND PATHOGENESIS

Multiple sclerosis has been known for over 150 years. Despite an immense amount of research, its aetiology remains unknown, its pathogenesis is only partially understood and many of its aspects are controversial. The disease appears to be acquired before puberty (Dean and Kurtzke, 1971) but does not become clinically manifest in most instances until the third and fourth decades. There are some data to suggest that it may have its clinical onset earlier in tropical countries, but this may be related to the generally earlier date of menarche in non-Caucasians. In general, it affects women more commonly than men. Although the disease is progressive, as demonstrated by paraclinical tests (Poser, 1985a; Thompson *et al.*, 1992), in about two-thirds of patients it is characterized by symptomatic remissions and exacerbations. MS is primarily a disease of the white matter that causes the formation of areas of demyelination called plaques in the central nervous system (CNS) which then become glial scars, hence the name of the disease.

A number of hypotheses have been proposed to explain the characteristics of the disease. One theory is that it is due to a virus, most likely one of the so-called slow viruses. Over the past 30 years, reports have appeared purporting to demonstrate the existence of such an organism, the most recent one being HTLV-I, and it was suggested that tropical spastic paraparesis represents the tropical form of MS. Numerous studies (Table 28.1A, B) have refuted this, demonstrating that the frequency with which traces of HTLV-I infection are found in MS patients is the same as that observed in healthy blood donors in endemic areas. Another popular hypothesis is that MS is an autoimmune disease. This has arisen because usually numerous abnormalities of the immune system can be demonstrated in MS patients. Their significance, however, remains questionable since they may represent epiphenomena of the disease rather than pathogenetic factors. Ebers (1993) aptly described the situation when he said that in regard to the role of the immune system in MS, 'a substantial "chicken and egg problem" remains'. It is, however, probable that a combination of viral illnesses and immunological alterations may be the long-sought-after pathogenetic mechanism of the disease (Poser, 1992).

Poser (1992) has delineated a hypothesis of the pathogenesis of MS that attempts to incorporate most of what is known about the various steps of the process.

1. A genetically determined susceptibility to the disease which may be assumed to have originated in Scandinavia and to have been disseminated by the

TABLE 28.1 Multiple sclerosis: HTLV-I positivity
A. Provenance: serum, peripheral blood mononuclear cells
Summary of 91 studies (number of studies) (1 December 1994)

Country		Cases of MS	+	%	Country		Cases of MS	+	%
Australia	(1)	10	0	0	Iran	(1)	2	0	0
Brazil	(4)	51	3	5.9	Italy	(14)	644	5	0.8
Canada	(3)	397	0	0	Japan	(12)	741	81	10.9
Denmark	(1)	101	1	0	Kuwait	(1)	106	0	0
Faroes	(1)	10	0	0	Malaysia	(1)	11	0	0
Finland	(2)	41	6	14.6	Martinique	(1)	8	0	0
France	(4)	163	0	0	Norway	(1)	413	18	4.4
Germany	(4)	175	0	0	Panama	(1)	16	2	12.5
G. Britain	(10)	345‡	0	0	Sweden	(9)	209†	12	6.5
Hungary	(2)	36	0	0	Thailand	(1)	11	0	0
India	(4)	51	1	2.0	USA	(12)	699	20*	2.9
Totals							4148	149	3.6

Methods of detection: Antibodies against HTLV-I or against 'gag' or 'env' proteins in serum and/or PBMC; proviral sequences PCR amplification; *in situ* hybridization; immunoblot studies.
* 10 cases Koprowski, 6 cases Greenberg; † 6 cases not included: Reddy (+) but Fugger (-); also includes 7 cases Koprowski. ‡ 13 cases Afro-Carib-Ind children of immigrants (Elian) and 12 Afro-Carib immigrants (Rudge) to the UK.

B. Source of material: brain and CSF
Summary of 41 studies (1 December 1994)

Country	CSF	+	Brain	+	Cases of MS	+
Australia			3	0	3	0
Brazil	41	1			41	1
Canada	12	0			12	0
Denmark			16	0	16	0
France	58	0			58	0
Germany	27	0	5	0	32	0
G. Britain	66‡	0			66	0
Hungary	15	0			15	0
India	11	0			11	0
Iran	2	0			2	0
Italy	426	7	14	0	440	7
Japan	33	0			33	0
Martinique	7	0			7	0
Panama	9	0			9	0
Sweden	230	7			230	7*
USA	88	1†	30	0	118	1
Totals	1025	16	68	0	1093	16
		1.6%				1.5%

* Cases of Sandberg-Wollheim, same as Reddy's; † case of Koprowski; ‡ 11 Afro-Caribbean immigrants to the UK (Rudge).

Vikings and their descendants (Poser, 1994d). This suceptibility is modified by still unknown environmental factors. The existence of both enhancing and protective factors has been postulated, some of which may be genetic in nature, others environmental, or combinations of both (Poser, 1994c). The most important factor appears to be a genetic one in order to explain the rarity of the disease in non-Caucasians.

2. An environmental factor, almost certainly a viral infection that triggers an immune-mediated response that is characteristically very vigorous and produces a symptomless systemic condition called the MS trait (MST) (Poser, 1994c). Analogous situations exist, as exemplified by sickle cell disease, acute intermittent porphyria and glucose-6-phosphate dehydrogenase deficiency. The MST, a disease waiting to happen, probably affects several siblings in a family. The disease may never progress beyond this stage, and thus the nervous system may never become involved and the individual may never have symptoms.

3. A second viral infection, not necessarily the same as the one that caused the development of the MST, produces an immune reaction that leads to an alteration of the blood–brain barrier (BBB) by a mechanism which is not yet fully understood. The loss of impermeability of the BBB is an obligatory step in the pathogenesis of MS (Poser, 1986). It is probable that this immune response results from the fact that the second viral molecule shares common antigenic epitopes with the first one, the phenomenon of molecular mimicry (Jahnke *et al.*, 1985). Other non-immune mediated events such as trauma or electrical injury may have the same effect in causing this obligatory alteration of BBB impermeability, allowing immune-activated cells and non-cellular constituents of the blood to reach the nervous parenchyma (Poser, 1994b). It is at this stage that MS first affects the CNS, although such involvement will not necessarily produce symptoms. Thus the disease, even after causing damage to the CNS, may remain permanently asymptomatic. In fact, it has been estimated on the basis of autopsy studies (Poser, 1992) that the number of asymptomatic patients may be as large as that of those who have symptoms. These data have been derived from studies carried out in areas of high MS prevalence. It is not known if the same situation exists in tropical countries where no systematic autopsy studies have been carried out.

4. As a result of the alteration of the BBB, oedema and inflammation of the myelin sheath occur that may, but not necessarily will, lead to the formation of a plaque of demyelination that may or may not produce symptoms. The mechanism for the sequence of plaque formation is unknown although there is evidence to suggest an important role for cytokines produced by activated lymphocytes. Plaque formation never occurs in the peripheral nervous system.

5. Because the changes in the BBB do not always return to normal, it is likely that the products of myelin disintegration, such as myelin basic protein, penetrate into the systemic circulation, leading to immune-mediated activation of lymphocytes, thus producing a self-perpetuating pathogenetic circle

which may be one explanation for the progressive nature of this disease (Poser, 1994a).

DIAGNOSIS

Despite the introduction of paraclinical tests such as evoked responses and imaging studies (computer-assisted tomography (CT) and magnetic resonance imaging (MRI)), the diagnosis remains firmly clinical, based on the twin criteria of dissemination in time and in space. The almost universal adoption of the new diagnostic criteria of Poser *et al.* (1983) (Table 28.2) has led to increasing standardization of MS diagnosis in epidemiological and therapeutic studies. Nevertheless, a great deal of confusion still exists because of the inappropriate but increasingly common dependence upon MRI and the failure to differentiate MS from a number of other conditions which often mimic its clinical and laboratory characteristics. The latter include acute, recurrent and multiphasic disseminated encephalomyelitis, chronic fatigue/myalgic encephalomyelitis, neurobrucellosis and neuroborreliosis, and HIV and HTLV-I infections of the CNS.

Another important problem which has affected epidemiological studies in Far Eastern countries has been the use of the Japanese classification of MS (Kuroiwa *et al.*, 1983) that allows the inclusion of Devic's syndrome and a host of other demyelinating conditions. The problem of Devic's syndrome is particularly important, since it appears to be common in tropical countries. Several authors

TABLE 28.2 Diagnostic criteria for multiple sclerosis *

Category	ATT	CLN	PCL		CSF
Clinically definite					
1.	2	2			
2.	2	1	&	1	
Laboratory supported definite					
1.	2	1	or	1	+
2.	1	2			+
3.	1	1	&	1	+
Clincally probable					
1.	2	1			
2.	1	2			
3.	1	1	&	1	
Laboratory supported probable					
1.	2				+

ATT, attack; CLN, clinical evidence; PCL, paraclinical evidence; CSF, OB or IgG.
* Poser C *et al.* (1983).

(Miller and Evans, 1967; Poser, 1985b; Breukelman *et al.*, 1988) have pointed out that it more often represents a form of acute disseminated encephalomyelitis (ADEM). Poser (1994a) has proposed criteria for the definition of Devic's syndrome as MS: a period of at least 6 months must elapse between the optic and the myelitic components, or evidence of a new, separate lesion must appear indicating involvement of the brain itself. For that purpose, CT or MRI may be used. There is no basis for the claim that the disease is different in Orientals in that the optic nerve is much more commonly involved: visual evoked potential studies have demonstrated the extremely common, albeit subclinical, involvement of the optic nerve in Caucasian patients (Drislane, 1995).

GENETIC VERSUS ENVIRONMENTAL FACTORS

For many years a direct relationship between latitude and the frequency of MS has been proposed as evidence of the primary importance of the environment (Kurtzke, 1987). The many exceptions to this rule as shown in Table 28.3 require closer examination of the genetic factor. Indeed, it is now apparent that the latter is as important and probably considerably more so than the influence of nurture (Poser 1994c, d). In the non-Caucasian populations of tropical areas MS is rare and has never been described in ethnically pure north and south Amerindians, Eskimos and Inuits, Lapps, Australian aborigines, Maoris of New Zealand or Pacific Islanders. It is also relatively uncommon among Orientals. Even in North

TABLE 28.3 The world distribution of multiple sclerosis: prevalence and latitude

Location	Lat.	Prev. *	Location	Lat.	Prev. *
Iceland	65N	99.4	Malta	36N	8
Shetland Islands	61N	129	Capetown, RSA	36S	
Winnipeg, Canada	50N	35	Afrikaner		10.9
Seattle, WA, USA	47N	69	'Coloured'/Orientals		3
Switzerland	47N	52	Charleston, SC, USA	33N	14
Parma, Italy	44N	11.6	Newcastle, Australia	33S	32.5
Arles, France	44N	9	Israel (natives)	32N	
Krk, Croatia	44N	44	Sephardi		9.5
Olmsted Co., MN, USA	44N	122	Ashkenazi		35.6
Copparo, Sardinia	44N	31.1	New Orleans, LA, USA	30N	6
Asahikawa, Japan	44N	2.5	Kuwait (Arabs)	30N	
Hobart, Tasmania	43S	68	Kuwaitis		9.5
Htes Pyren., France	43N	39.6	Palestinians		24
Boston, MA, USA	42N	41	Canary Islands	28N	18.3
Sassari, Sardinia	41N	69	Okinawa, Japan	26N	1.9
Alcoy, Spain	39N	17	Hong Kong	23N	0.8
Seoul, Korea	38N	2	Bombay (Parsis)	19N	26

* per 100 000 inhabitants.

America, the south-to-north increase in prevalence rate (PR) for blacks is more likely to be the result of genetic admixture (based on blood group studies) than of whatever environmental factors are represented by latitude (Poser, 1992). Although the evidence for genetic susceptibility is very strong, the exact mechanism of such transmission remains unknown; the HLA system may play an ancillary role in that process. Although it is most likely that genetic susceptibility influences the acquisition of the disease, there is strong evidence to suggest that environmental factors play an important role in determining the clinical onset of the disease. Despite many studies of risk factors, none has emerged as being of specific importance. Nonetheless, several epidemiological studies, in particular the studies of migration from areas of high frequency to those of low incidence, and from low prevalence to those of high prevalence, have suggested the existence of both enhancing and protective environmental factors. This is particularly apparent in Australia, where a true north-to-south gradient does exist, with the prevalence of MS in southern Australia about half that in Tasmania despite the fact that the two populations are ethnically identical. That protective and enhancing factors may be in some way tied to the genetic susceptibility is suggested by the situation in Hawaii, where the prevalence of MS among Hawaiian-born and -raised Japanese-Americans is three times the mean prevalence in Japan, whereas that of Hawaiian-born and -raised Caucasians is about a third lower than that of Caucasians on the mainland (Poser, 1994c). A major argument in favour of the existence of an environmental protective factor in tropical Africa is the fact, as was pointed out by Collomb (1961), that the disease is much less among Caucasians living in West Africa than would be expected in their countries of origin.

MULTIPLE SCLEROSIS IN TROPICAL COUNTRIES

There is no evidence that the disease is any different clinically or pathologically in tropical areas, i.e. in non-Caucasians.

It is difficult to evaluate epidemiological data from tropical areas and developing countries. There are almost no postmortem examinations because of real and imaginary religious as well as cultural restrictions. There are relatively few trained neurologists. Confirmatory test procedures such as evoked response studies, neuroimaging and reliable spinal fluid examinations are generally unavailable and the unquestionable rarity of MS is made even rarer because of the reluctance of physicians to make the diagnosis in non-Caucasians.

In many countries, there are also important cultural problems which render the diagnosis difficult. The general paucity of medical facilities as well as the frequent reluctance of native populations to utilize the ones that are in existence, often due to a distrust of Western medicine and the influence of practitioners of native healing arts, means that only advanced cases of the disease come to medical attention and that the data are based almost exclusively on hospital admissions, which leads to a gross underestimation of the frequency of the disease. In some areas there are also cultural and economic factors which cause a male–female imbalance in admission rates.

Africa

These problems are particularly well illustrated in sub-Saharan Africa. For many years physicians working in Africa claimed that MS did not exist in black Africans (Poser and Vernant, 1993). Several authors have noted that case ascertainment was more hazardous in Africa for a variety of reasons. Rachman (1973) pointed out that for European physicians differences in language and customs, and the existence of taboos, made obtaining histories and performing the neurological examination very difficult. Gelfand (1975) noted that black Africans often find it difficult to perform many of the finer tests used in the diagnosis of a nervous ailment. Clinicians are apt to become discouraged when confronted with patients who cannot understand what is expected of them. Howard (1948) commented that: 'The African can rarely give an objective account of his symptoms and is usually extremely vague as to their duration; in addition he tends to rationalize his symptoms more than the European and often produces very bizarre explanations, so that the difficulty of taking an accurate clinical history makes the diagnosis tend more to depend on the physical findings on examination than on the history of the disease. This is especially unsatisfactory when dealing with nervous diseases, where the diagnosis in many cases depends so much on accurate history.' This applies especially to MS, where the history is considerably more important than the physical examination. The great diversity of tribes and cultures and almost complete ignorance of some of the customs of the smaller tribes makes any survey peculiarly difficult (Muwazi and Trowell, 1944). The attitude of the African is also a severe obstacle. Cosnett (1981) stated that 'Some patients expect no history to be taken. A doctor who needs to ask questions may be considered to lack proficiency. Other patients out of respect for the doctor and in an effort to please, may answer all questions in the affirmative.'

Cases of MS have been reported from black Africa (Table 28.4), but the validity of diagnosis in many of the cases has been in doubt. Gelfand (1975), commenting on the 11 cases reported by Sharp (1938) in Ghana, believed that they all represented instances of acute disseminated encephalomyelitis (ADEM), pointing out that 8 of them had had fever at the onset of their illness. Haddock (1965) mentioned that the diagnosis had been made 133 times in Tanzania, but he was unwilling to accept any of them as true cases of MS, and said that he had never seen a proven case of MS in an African. Haimanot (personal communication, 1988) was unwilling to accept the diagnosis of MS in Lester's (1979) two cases in Ethiopian blacks. He also mentioned that in addition to the case he reported in 1985, he had seen two other well-documented cases.

In Nigeria, Howard (1948) wrote that between 1935 and 1938, out of a total of 3331 cases of nervous diseases treated at the African Hospital of Ibadan in

TABLE 28.4 Multiple sclerosis in black Africans

Country	Cases	Reference		Country	Cases	Reference	
Cameroon	3	Collomb	1961	Nigeria	18†	Howard	1948
Cameroon	1	Mbonda *et al.*	1990	Nigeria	2	Osuntokun	1971
Ethiopia	2*	Lester	1979	Senegal	9	Vigneront	1976
Ethiopia	1	Haimanot	1985	Sierra Leone	1	Lisk	1991
Ethiopia	2	Haimanot§	1988	South Africa	1	Bhigjee	1987
Ghana	11*	Sharp	1938	South Africa	6	Dean *et al.*	1994
Ivory Coast	3	Giordano§	1994	Tanzania	118*	Haddock	1965
Kenya	2†	Goldstein	1946	Uganda	1	Billinghurst	1973
Kenya	2†	Foster and Harries	1970	Uganda	10	Kanyerezi *et al.*	1980
Kenya	9‡	Adam	1989	Zaire	rare	Collomb	1961
Liberia	1	Collomb	1961	Zimbabwe	rare	Lowe *et al.*	1980
Mozambique	6	Collomb	1961	Zimbabwe	7	Dean *et al.*	1994

*, Diagnosis probably incorrect; †, diagnosis uncertain; ‡, includes Mwunzi's three cases; §, personal communication.

Nigeria, there had been 18 cases of disseminated sclerosis. No clinical details were given. The major problem in diagnosis in that country, as elsewhere in Africa, is the differentiation from ADEM. Osuntokun (1971) lists only two cases of MS but 12 of postinfectious encephalomyelitis, 95 of neuromyelitis optica, 11 of retrobulbar neuritis and 23 of acute transverse myelitis. The diagnosis in his first case is probably correct, but his second patient had had only a single episode and must be considered to represent a case of ADEM. The lack of confirmatory laboratory procedures and of postmortem examinations makes it impossible to know how many of the cases diagnosed as neuromyelitis optica, retrobulbar neuritis and acute transverse myelitis may have been cases of MS.

In Kenya, it is probable that one of Goldstein's (1946) two cases is ADEM rather than MS, but Foster and Harries' (1970) two cases are unquestionably MS. Adam (1989) described what he called an epidemic of MS in black Kenyans, reporting six new cases, which fulfilled the criteria of Poser *et al.* (1983), and citing an unpublished report of three other cases by Mwunzi. Other definite cases of MS have been reported recently (Table 28.4). In many instances there is not sufficient clinical detail to determine the exact diagnosis. That is the problem with the ten patients from Uganda (Kanyerezi *et al.*, 1980). Most of the reported cases were seen before it had become possible to diagnose HTLV-I infection, an important consideration in all tropical countries.

In Zimbabwe, Lowe *et al.* (1980) said that the disease was rare in blacks, but Dean *et al.* (1994) discovered clinically definite cases. They also mentioned that seven black African immigrants to London had developed MS. The case of Mbonda *et al.* (1990) in Cameroon, and Lisk's case (1991) in Sierra Leone, are both clinically definite. The reports from Senegal (Vigneront, 1976) (Table

TABLE 28.5 Multiple sclerosis in Senegal (Vigneront, 1976)

Case no.	Age/Sex	Diagnosis	Autopsy	Revised diagnosis*
1	13 M	Schilder		MS
2	15 M	Schilder		MS
3	18 M	Devic		ADEM
4	13 F	Devic	+	MS
5	18 M	Devic		ADEM
6	23 F	MS	+	MS
7	26 M	MS	+	MS
8	54 F	MS	+	MS
9	12 M	MS		MS
10	35 F	MS		MS
11	39 F	MS		ADEM
12	35 F	MS		MS
13	23 F	MS		Vasculitis

* Diagnosis revised based on review of clinical history and according to Poser *et al.* (1983) criteria.
MS, multiple sclerosis; ADEM, acute disseminated encephalomyelitis.

28.5) are unique in that they establish the incontrovertible existence of MS in the black African. In addition to the four autopsied cases, the clinical data in five more are quite convincing. The two cases designated as Schilder's disease are included among the definite MS.

The recent report of an epidemic of six cases in black Kenyans by Adam (1989) is encouraging since it suggests that milder, early cases may be recognized more frequently by better-informed neurologists. Despite its rarity, it is likely that more cases of MS exist but have not been reported. Giordano (personal communication, 1994) mentioned three such well-documented cases which were studied in France in Ivory Coast blacks. Because of the scant number of cases, it is impossible to establish any reliable prevalence data. The fact that the disease does occur in Europeans and Indians living at the same latitude, although undoubtedly in different living conditions, caused Collomb (1961) to state, 'The rarity of MS is not simply due to climate, since MS is much more common among Europeans living in Senegal'. In Senegal, according to Collomb (1961), MS is a hundred times more common in Europeans than in blacks, this figure being based upon the rate of admissions of Europeans versus blacks to the University Hospital in Dakar. He also mentioned that six Europeans with MS had been observed in Mozambique. Osuntokun (1971) noted eight Europeans and one Indian with MS in Nigeria, whereas Lowe *et al.* (1980) in Zimbabwe reported 50 cases of Europeans, all but two of whom had been born outside Africa. Hall (1961) also made the diagnosis in an Indian living in Ethiopia. Billinghurst (1973) observed five Europeans and two Asians with MS in Uganda, and Hutton (1956) reported that he had seen the disease in several Indians born and raised in the same country. The case reported by Boucquey *et al.* (1989) of a Zairean woman of mixed race cannot be counted.

The origin of the disease in black Africans is difficult to trace. Lambo (1956) commented that in the Benin Delta region of Nigeria are individuals with a lighter complexion and narrow noses which may be due to admixture with Caucasians. He pointed out that Portuguese and Arabs had been in contact with the Kingdom of Benin as early as 1472, dealing in ivory and slaves. Haimanot (personal communication, 1988) also observed that his three MS patients are of lighter complexion than the average Ethiopian and suggested some possible European admixture. Thus, as is true in other parts of the world, slavery and European colonization may have introduced the genetic material causing MS susceptibility (Poser, 1994d).

Although South Africa cannot be considered a tropical country, it has a very large black population in whom the disease has always been said to be non-existent or extremely rare. In 1958, Reef *et al.* stated that they had never seriously considered the diagnosis of MS in the exclusively black population served by the Baragwanath Hospital in Soweto, yet in Durban, one of Cosnett's cases (1981) was of probable MS. Eight years previously, Cosnett (1973) had written that in 11 years he had never seen MS in a Bantu (a black South African). Another interesting case reported by Hift and Moodley (1973) is that of a Bantu patient who was diagnosed as having neuromyelitis optica yet who had had two episodes clearly separated by a month and would suggest the diagnosis of MS. More recently, in addition to the case originally reported by Bhigjee (1987), the first case of MS in a South African black, Dean *et al.* (1994) found six new cases. They also mentioned that in the previous 20 years (1973–1993) the neurology unit of the Baragwanath Hospital had considered the diagnosis of MS in five patients, but in all of them there had been evidence of an infection of the nervous system which could well have been the cause of the symptoms. They also referred to two black women in whom MS was given as the cause of death but whose histories could not be checked. There have been a number of definite MS cases reported in South African 'coloured', but their significance is obscured by their mixed genetic background.

The extremely small number of MS cases reported by highly trained observers working in a very good medical care system suggests that the disease is even rarer among blacks in South Africa than in other African countries. Since the Bantu consist of tribal groups (predominantly Zulu and Xosa) who do not live elsewhere in Africa, it is possible that they possess an even lower susceptibility to this disease or have a stronger protective factor. It is not possible to say if there has been an increase in the frequency of MS in black South Africans, or, as is more likely, the disease is being more readily recognized.

Tropical Asia

The tropical areas to be considered include India, Malaysia and Thailand. These countries and their populations are obviously quite different from those of sub-Saharan Africa. In general, although overpopulation certainly is a major problem, the levels of medical care, sanitation, nutrition and general economic conditions are somewhat better in many parts of these countries, although in others, in particular in parts of India, conditions do approach those seen among African blacks. The data for these countries are listed in Table 28.6.

Data from India represent various parts of the country but with the exception of the studies from Bombay, only a few identified the ethnic origin of patients. In Bombay, MS is more prevalent among the Parsis, people of Persian origin who practise the Zoroastrian religion and whose ancestors migrated to the Bombay area starting in the seventh century (Wadia and Bhatia, 1990). Wadia (1973) pointed out that in Bombay many patients are seen who have fair complexions, even light eyes, uncommon in India except among certain sects of Brahmins and other persons of Indo-European origin. In this regard it is interesting that Singhal (1982) mentioned that in the Bombay area the disease seems to affect individuals in the higher socioeconomic group (many of whom are Parsis), whereas in South India (Gourie-Devi and Nagaraja, 1982) the disease appears to affect more persons in the lower socioeconomic strata. Many cases listed as MS include those classified as possible as well as instances of Devic's syndrome. The problem of differentiating the disease from HTLV-I associated paraparesis (HAP) is a very crucial one in India. Mani (1973) who mentions seven cases of MS (including three of Schilder's disease) also recalls 45 cases of HAP in the same period of time.

In Jain and Maheshwari's (1985) review of 30 years' experience with MS in India, they suggest that the disease may be more common in the north, which was settled mostly by Indo-Europeans, than in the south where Tamil and Dravidian populations predominate. They explain the unusual male predominance by the fact that men are more likely to be hospitalized. As well as several other Indian authors, they comment upon the high incidence of optic nerve involvement both at the onset and during the course of the illness. This may, however, be the result of including neuromyelitis optica as cases of MS. The disease has been confirmed by autopsy in several instances.

The MS cases from Malaysia (Selby, 1983; Isler and Balaratnam, 1979; Tan, 1988) (Table 28.6) are of interest because of the striking predominance of ethnic Chinese patients. One of Isler and Balaratnam's three Malay cases is probably ADEM. The disease obviously exists in Thais and autopsy has confirmed this diagnosis in three instances (Vejjajiva, 1982). Whenever the information was available, only definite and probable cases have been listed.

No cases of MS have been reported from the Indochinese peninsula. Kurtzke and Bui's (1980) report of MS developing in three half Vietnamese, half French children who had emigrated to France cannot be counted because of the mixed genetic background.

Tropical Pacific Areas

In the Fiji Islands, Sutherland *et al.* (1972) collected five cases, three in Fijians (PR 2 per 100 000), one in a European and another one in a part-European. No cases were found in Indians, who constitute approximately half the population of

TABLE 28.6 Tropical Asia

Country/region	Number of cases	Ethnic group	Prevalence	% Neurology admissions	Reference	
India: Vellore	17*		0.61†	0.22	Mathew et al.	(1971)
India: south-east	7				Mani	(1973)
India: south-east	12				Nair and Sahasrannam	(1978)
India: north-east	38*			1.1	Chopra et al.	(1980)
India: south	92*			0.6	Gourie-Devi et al.	(1982)
India: Bombay	81*	mixed	1.33†	0.4	Singhal	(1982)
India	194				Jain and Maheshwari	(1985)
India	16	Parsis	30.1		Wadia and Bhatia	(1990)
Malaysia	2	Chinese			Selby	(1973)
Malaysia	3*	2 Malays 1 Chinese		0.5	Isler and Balaratnam	(1979)
Malaysia	30	25 Chinese 3 Malays 2 Indians	2†		Tan	(1988)
Thailand		29 Thais			Vejjajiva	(1982)

*, Hospital admissions; †, ALS/MS ratio.

the island, or among Chinese or other Pacific Islanders. The only report from Indonesia dates back over 40 years, by Verhaart (1951). He described 20 cases, of which 19 are probable. There were 10 Indonesians and 9 ethnic Chinese. Five cases were confirmed at autopsy. The Filipino cases come from two different hospitals in Manila. Navarro *et al.* (1982) found 17 hospitalized cases, and 11 similar cases were reported by Renales *et al.* (1982). The only Guamanian case (Chen, 1982) was in a young man born in Okinawa of a Filipino father and Okinawan mother. No MS cases have been reported in the Carolinian and Chamorro populations of the Mariana Islands.

Hawaii does not conform to the tropical country model outlined above, but the reports from there (Alter *et al.*, 1971; Okihiro, 1982) confirm the fact that Caucasians born in an area of low prevalence have a significantly lower prevalence than those who have migrated there. In regard to the Orientals (nearly all of whom are of Japanese ancestry, born and raised in Hawaii) the prevalence is significantly higher than that in Japan, but almost identical with that found by Detels *et al.* (1982) in Californian Japanese-Americans. This is significantly lower than the prevalence in Caucasians in Los Angeles (Table 28.7). The Hawaiian situation illustrates the paradoxical effect of putative environmental factors on groups of different genetic susceptibility: there appears to be an enhancing effect on Japanese, but a protective factor for Caucasians born and raised in the Islands.

TABLE 28.7 Tropical Pacific

Country	Ethnic group	Number of cases	Prevalence per 100 000	Reference	
Indonesia	Indonesian	6		Verhaart	(1951)
Indonesia	Chinese	3		Verhaart	(1951)
Philippines	Filipino	17H		Navarro *et al.*	(1982)
Philippines	Filipino	11H		Renales *et al.*	(1982)
Guam	Mixed*	1		Chen	(1982)
Hawaii	Japanese (1)	12	6.5	Alter *et al.*	(1971)
Hawaii	Caucasian (1)	3	10.5	Alter *et al.*	(1971)
Hawaii	Caucasian (2)	22	34.4	Alter *et al.*	(1971)
Hawaii	Japanese (1)	17†	7.8	Okihiro	(1982)
California	Japanese (3)	7	6.7	Detels *et al.*	(1982)
California	Caucasian (3)	–	29.9	Detels *et al.*	(1982)

NOTES: H, Hospital admission. (1), Born and raised in Hawaii; (2), immigrants from US mainland; (3), born and raised in California. *, Filipino-Okinawan. †, Not including one each Chinese, Filipino and mixed.

Latin America

Latin American data, in particular from tropical areas (parts of Colombia, Ecuador and Venezuela) are not only fragmentary but are difficult to interpret. Much information is provided by Gomez and Alfert (1975) based on a great deal of unpublished data. Unfortunately no information is available to judge the accuracy of diagnosis. The disease unquestionably exists, since in several countries there have been autopsied cases. In both Brazil and Cuba the disease has been diagnosed in black persons as well as in mestizos. There are 63 cases from Colombia (Constain, unpublished manuscript) who were all admitted to a neurological hospital in Bogota, a city with a very temperate climate which can certainly not be classified as tropical. From personal experience, the author can state that a number of cases diagnosed as MS in Bogota have, in fact, turned out to be instances of ADEM. In a single report from Venezuela (Starosta-Rubinstein *et al.*, 1989), 31 MS patients were identified from hospital records. They evaluated 19, who were classified as 17 clinically definite and 2 laboratory-supported probable. In the most recent report from Cuba, 23 cases were reported (Gomez and Alfert, 1975) with 6 postmortem confirmations. Only 13% of these patients were black and 4% were mestizos, the rest being Caucasians.

Howell *et al.* (1968) described a black woman born in British Guyana who developed MS that was confirmed at autopsy. He cites another case in a black woman in Guyana.

The Caribbean Area

In Curaçao, in the Dutch Antilles, Moffie (1966) reported finding 14 cases, 11 in Europeans, and 3 in persons of mixed black and European ancestry, but only one of which would be considered probable, and another which may well be HAP. In Jamaica, Cruikshank and Montgomery (1961) reported having diagnosed seven cases, three in native Jamaicans. In the subsequent 10 years, they identified ten more cases (Cruickshank, 1973), but the ethnic distribution is not noted. The most recent report comes from the Caribbean (Poser and Vernant, 1993) describing 11 cases of clinically definite HTLV-I negative MS cases in Martinican and Guadeloupean blacks. All but three of these patients had spent the putative years of acquisition, i.e. before puberty, in metropolitan France, suggesting an important environmental influence.

CONCLUSION

The rarity of MS in non-Caucasians in the tropics, in particular in African blacks, is a strong argument in favour of the importance of genetic factors in the acquisition of the disease. It is likely that there are also environmental factors in tropical regions that tend to protect both blacks and genetically susceptible Caucasian MS patients from developing the clinical manifestations of the disease.

REFERENCES

Adam A (1989) Multiple sclerosis epidemic in Kenya? *East African Medical Journal* **66**: 503–506.

Alter M, Okihiro M, Rowley W *et al.* (1971) MS among orientals and Caucasians in Hawaii. *Neurology* **21**: 122–130.

Bhigjee A (1987) Multiple sclerosis in a black patient. *South African Medical Journal* **72**: 873–875.

Billinghurst J (1973) Neurological disorders in Uganda. In: *Tropical Neurology* (ed. J. Spillane), pp 191-206. London: Oxford University Press.

Boucquey D, Sindic C and Laterre C (1989) Clinically definite multiple sclerosis in Zairian woman of mixed race. *Neurology* **236**: 187.

Breukelman A, Polman C, de Slegte R *et al.* (1988) Neuromyelitis optica (Devic's syndrome): not always multiple sclerosis. *Clinical Neurology and Neurosurgery* **90**: 357–360.

Chen K (1982) Multiple sclerosis in the Mariana Islands. In: *Multiple Sclerosis East and West* (eds Y Kuroiwa and L Kurland), pp 159–164. Fukuoka: Kyushu University Press.

Chopra J, Radhakrishnan K, Sawhney B *et al.* (1980) Multiple sclerosis in northwest India. *Acta Neurologica Scandinavica* **62**: 312–321.

Collomb H (1961) La sclérose en plaques en Afrique au sud du Sahara. *Proceedings of the 7th International Congress of Neurology* **2**: 669.

Cosnett J (1973) Neurological disease in Natal. In: *Tropical Neurology* (ed. J Spillane), pp 259–272. London: Oxford University Press.

Cosnett J (1981) Multiple sclerosis and neuromyelitis optica. *South African Medical Journal* **60**: 249–251.

Cruickshank E (1973) Neurological disorders in Jamaica. In: *Tropical Neurology* (ed. J Spillane), pp 426–434. London: Oxford University Press.

Cruickshank E and Montgomery R (1961) Multiple sclerosis in Jamaica. *West Indian Medical Journal* **10**: 211.

Dean G and Kurtzke J (1971) On the risk of multiple sclerosis according to age at immigration to South Africa. *British Medical Journal* **3**: 725–729.

Dean G, Bhigjee A, Bill P *et al.* (1994) Multiple sclerosis in black South Africans and Zimbabweans. *Journal of Neurology, Neurosurgery and Psychiatry* **57**: 1064–1069.

Detels R, Visscher B, Malmgren R *et al.* (1982) Frequency and pattern of multiple sclerosis among Japanese-Americans. In: *Multiple Sclerosis East and West* (eds Y Kuroiwa and L Kurland), pp 171–176. Fukuoka: Kyushu University Press.

Drislane F (1994) Use of evoked potentials in the diagnosis and follow-up of multiple sclerosis. *Clinical Neuroscience* **2**: 196–201.

Ebers G (1993) Multiple sclerosis: new insights from old tools. *Mayo Clinic Proceedings* **68**: 711–712.

Foster R and Harries J (1970) Multiple sclerosis in the African. *British Medical Journal* **3**: 628.

Gelfand M (1975) *The Sick African*, p 577. Cape Town: Juta Press.

Goldstein B (1946) Two cases of disseminated sclerosis in African natives. *East African Medical Journal* **33**: 209–223.

Gomez J and Alfert R (1975) Algunas consideraciones sobre esclerosis multiple en Lationamerica. *Rev. Cub. Med.* **14**: 487–499.

Gourie-Devi M and Nagaraja D (1982) Multiple sclerosis in South India. In: *Multiple Sclerosis East and West* (eds Y Kuroiwa and L Kurland), pp 135–148. Fukuoka: Kyushu University Press.

Haddock D (1965) Neurological disorders in Tanzania. *Journal of Tropical Medicine and Hygiene* **68**: 161–166.

Haimanot R (1985) Multiple sclerosis – a case report in an Ethiopian. *Ethiopian Medical Journal* **23**: 27–29.

Hall P (1961) Neurologic studies in Ethiopia. *World Neurology* **2**: 731–739.

Hift W and Moodley T (1973) A possible case of neuromyelitis optica in a Bantu patient. *South African Medical Journal* **47**: 987–988.

Howard A (1948) Notes on nervous and mental disease encountered in Nigeria. *Transactions of the Royal Society of Tropical Medicine and Hygiene* **41**: 823–828.

Howell D, Jellinek E and Gavrilescu K (1968) Demyelinating disease in a woman from tropical South America with features of multiple sclerosis and neuromyelitis optica. *Journal of the Neurological Sciences* **7**: 115–135.

Hutton P (1956) Neurological disease in Uganda. *East African Medical Journal* **33**: 209–223.

Isler H and Balaratnam C (1979) The 'absence' of multiple sclerosis in Malaysia. In: *Neurological Sciences in Developing Countries* (ed. H Isler), pp 456–463. Kuala Lumpur: University of Malaya Press.

Jahnke U, Fischer E and Alvord E (1985) Sequence homology between certain viral proteins and proteins related to encephalomyelitis and neuritis. *Science* **229**: 282–284.

Jain S and Maheshwari M (1985) Multiple sclerosis: Indian experience in the last thirty years. *Neuroepidemiology* **4**: 96–107.

Kanyerezi B, Kiire C and Obace A (1980) Multiple sclerosis in Mulago Hospital, Uganda. *East African Medical Journal* **57**: 262–266.

Kuroiwa Y, Shibasaki H and Ikeda M (1983) Prevalence of multiple sclerosis and its north–south gradient in Japan. *Neuroepidemiology* **2**: 62–69.

Kurtzke J (1987) Multiple sclerosis in twins. *New England Journal of Medicine* **317**: 51.

Kurtzke J and Bui Q (1980) Multiple sclerosis in a migrant population. 2. Half-Orientals immigrating in childhood. *Annals of Neurology* **8**: 256–260.

Lambo T (1956) Neuropsychiatric observations in the Western region of Nigeria. *British Medical Journal* **2**: 1388–1394.

Lester F (1979) Neurological diseases in Addis Ababa, Ethiopia. *African Journal of the Neurological Sciences* **8**: 7–11.

Lisk D (1991) Multiple sclerosis in a West African. *African Journal of the Neurological Sciences* **10**: 10–12.

Lowe R, Moore H and Briggs B (1980) The histocompatibility (HLA) antigen distribution in multiple sclerosis patients in Zimbabwe. *Central African Medical Journal* **26**: 234–236.

Mani K (1973) Neurological disease in South India. In: *Tropical Neurology* (ed. J Spillane), pp 78–85. London: Oxford University Press.

Mathew N, Mathai K, Abraham J *et al.* (1971) Incidence and pattern of demyelinating disease in India. *Journal of the Neurological Sciences* **13**: 27–38.

Mbonda E, Larnaout A, Maertens A *et al.* (1990) Multiple sclerosis in a black Cameroonian woman. *Acta Neurologica Belgica* **90**: 218–222.

Miller H and Evans M (1967) Prognosis in acute disseminated encephalomyelitis with a note on neuromyelitis optica. *Quarterly Journal of Medicine* **2**: 347–379.

Moffie D (1966) De geografische verbreiding van multipele sclerose. *Nederlandsche Tijdschrift voor Geneeskunde* **110**: 1454–1457.

Muwazi F and Trowell H (1944) Neurological disease among African natives in Uganda. *East African Medical Journal* **21**: 2.

Nair K and Sahasranam K (1978) Multiple sclerosis in Malabar. *Journal of the Association of Physicians of India* **26**: 899–903.

Navarro J, Sobrevega E, Gamez G *et al.* (1982) The clinical manifestations of 51 cases of multiple sclerosis in the Philippines. In: *Multiple Sclerosis East and West* (eds Y Kuroiwa and L Kurland), pp 97–104. Fukuoka: Kyushu University Press.

Okihiro M (1982) Multiple sclerosis in the Oriental population of Hawaii. In: *Multiple Sclerosis East and West* (eds Y Kuroiwa and L Kurland), pp 165–170. Fukuoka: Kyushu University Press.

Osuntokun B (1971) The pattern of neurological disease in tropical Africa: experience at Ibadan, Nigeria. *Journal of the Neurological Sciences* **12**: 417–442.

Poser C (1985a) The course of multiple sclerosis. *Archives of Neurology* **42**: 1035.

Poser C (1985b) Taxonomy and diagnostic parameters. *Annals of the New York Academy of Sciences* **436**: 233–245.

Poser C (1986) The pathogenesis of multiple sclerosis: a critical reappraisal. *Acta Neuropathologica* **71**: 1–10.

Poser C (1992) Multiple sclerosis: observations and reflections – a personal memoir. *Journal of the Neurological Sciences* **107**: 127–140.

Poser C (1994a) The role of the blood-brain barrier in the pathogenesis of multiple sclerosis. In: *A Multi-disciplinary Approach to Myelin Diseases*, II (ed. S Salvati), pp 221–229. New York: Plenum Press.

Poser C (1994b) The role of trauma in multiple sclerosis. *Clinical Neurology and Neurosurgery* **96**: 103–110.

Poser C (1994c) The epidemiology of multiple sclerosis. A general overview. *Annals of Neurology* **36** (supplement 2): 180–193.

Poser C (1994d) The dissemination of multiple sclerosis: a Viking saga? A historical essay. *Annals of Neurology* **36** (supplement 2): 231–243.

Poser C and Vernant J (1993) La sclérose en plaques dans la race noire. *Bulletin de la Société de Pathologie Exotique* **86**: 1–5.

Poser C, Paty D, Scheinberg L *et al.* (1983) New diagnostic criteria for multiple sclerosis. Guidelines for research protocols. *Annals of Neurology* **13**: 227–231.

Rachman I (1973) Neurological disorders in Rhodesia. In: *Tropical Neurology* (ed. J Spillane), pp 237–246. London: Oxford University Press.

Reef H, Lipschitz R and Block J (1958) Neurological disorders at Baragwanath Hospital. *Medical Proceedings* **4**: 292–294.

Renales K, Zaraspe–Yoo E, Perez M *et al.* (1982) Multiple sclerosis among Filipinos. In: *Multiple Sclerosis East and West* (eds Y Kuroiwa and L Kurland), pp 105–116. Fukuoka: Kyushu University Press.

Selby R (1973) Neurological disorders in Malaysia. In: *Tropical Neurology* (ed. J Spillane), pp 299–320. London: Oxford University Press.

Sharp N (1938) A note on some cases of disseminated sclerosis. *Transactions of the Royal Society of Tropical Medicine and Hygiene* **31**: 671–672.

Singhal B (1982) Clinical, profile and HLA studies in Indian multiple sclerosis patients from the Bombay region. In: *Multiple Sclerosis East and West* (eds Y Kuroiwa and L Kurland), pp 123–134. Fukuoka: Kyushu University Press.

Spillane J (1973) *Tropical Neurology*, p 5. London: Oxford University Press.

Starosta-Rubinstein S, Solis O, Fajardo J *et al.* (1989) Multiple sclerosis in tropical America: clinical and MRI features. (abstract) *Neurology* **39** (supplement 1): 180.

Sutherland J, Tyrer J and Eadie M (1972) The prevalence of MS in Australia. *Brain* **85**: 149–164.

Tan C (1988) Multiple sclerosis in Malaysia. *Archives of Neurology* **45**: 624–627.

Thompson A, Miller D, Youl B *et al.* (1992) Serial gadolinium-enhanced MRI in relapsing–remitting multiple sclerosis of varying disease duration. *Neurology* **42**: 60–63.

Vejjajiva A (1982) Some clinical aspects of multiple sclerosis in Thai patients. In: *Multiple Sclerosis East and West* (eds Y Kuroiwa and L Kurland), pp 117–122. Fukuoka: Kyushu University Press.

Verhaart W (1951) Multiple and diffuse sclerosis and related demyelinating diseases in Indonesia. *Folia Psychiatrica Neurologica et Neurochirurgica Neerlandica* **54**: 281–294.

Vigneront F (1976) La sclérose en plaques au Sénégal. Thèse doctorale Université de Nancy.

Wadia N (1973) An introduction to neurology in India. In: *Tropical Neurology* (ed. J Spillane), pp 25–36. London: Oxford University Press.

Wadia N and Bhatia K (1990) Multiple sclerosis is prevalent in the Zoroastrians (Parsis) of India. *Annals of Neurology* **28**: 177–179.

29

Neuro-Behçet's Disease

Mohammed-Zuheir Al-Kawi

Department of Medicine, King Faisal Specialist Hospital and Research Centre, PO Box 3354, Riyadh 11211, Saudi Arabia

INTRODUCTION

Behçet's disease is a chronic systemic illness with a predominating pathological picture of vasculitis. There is evidence for immunological and genetic factors but its aetiology remains unknown. Originally described by a Turkish dermatologist Hulusi Behçet in 1937, to involve oral ulcers, genital ulcers and uveitis, it is now known to affect joints, blood vessels, genitals and the gastrointestinal tract. Involvement of the central nervous system makes a significant contribution to morbidity and mortality.

EPIDEMIOLOGY

Earlier reports on the disease originated in countries of the Mediterranean and Japan. This geographic distribution suggested that genetic suceptibility to the illness was transmitted along the ancient Silk Trade Route. More recent reports from Portugal, Brazil, Ecuador and European countries indicate a more global distribution than previously recognized. Establishing an accurate prevalence of Behçet's disease was hampered by the evolutive nature of its diagnostic criteria, and the absence of a pathognomonic test. Since diagnosis is dependent on recognizing the multisystemic clinical signs, unfamiliarity of physicians in some parts of the world with this disease may lead to underdiagnosis.

Neurological involvement varies in different populations, ranging from 49% (reported from Egypt) to 3.2% (reported from Iran). Most studies show a male predominance (2:1). The median age of onset is in the third decade with a range from early childhood to age 50 in most series.

AETIOLOGY AND PATHOGENESIS

HLA-B5 is over-represented in patients with Behçet's disease and familial cases have been reported. This with the clinical manifestations of an inflammatory nature and the several abnormalities reported in the immune system suggests an immunogenetic pathophysiology. Exogenous triggers such as viral, bacterial, allergic or environmental factors may act on a specific immunogenetic background and trigger a cascade of events which result in the clinical manifestations.

CLINICAL MANIFESTATIONS

The neurological manifestations cannot be considered in isolation of the systemic symptoms and signs which are necessary for the diagnosis. A variety of presentations should lead to the inclusion of Behçet's disease in the differential diagnosis (Serdaroglu *et al.*, 1989).

The involvement of the central nervous system in Behçet's disease can be classified under four categories which are not mutually exclusive: meningitis or meningoencephalitis; vascular; parenchymal; peripheral.

Meningitis or Meningoencephalitis

Aseptic meningitis or meningoencephalitis ranges from asymptomatic or mild to severe. In general, symptoms are non-specific with headache, low-grade fever, psychiatric features and hyper-reflexia. Nuchal rigidity is usually mild or absent but it may rarely be severe. Cerebrospinal fluid analysis reveals mild to moderate pleocytosis with a normal sugar and a slight increase in protein; rarely an acute meningeal reaction may mimic bacterial meningitis with a high cell count and polymorphonuclear predominance. Remission may occur spontaneously or following treatment while persistence of inflammation may lead to focal parenchymal lesions or generalized atrophy in the cerebrum or cerebellum with symptoms of dementia or ataxia.

Vascular

Major vascular thrombosis commonly affects the venous side with dural sinus thrombosis resulting in intracranial hypertension, headache, visual obscuration or visual loss. Papilloedema and retinal haemorrhages may occur. Focal symptoms and signs such as hemiparesis or seizures are usually secondary to venous infarction. Arterial branch occlusion is less common.

Parenchymal

Focal parenchymal involvement due to small-vessel vasculitis tends to affect the diencephalon, brainstem, especially the basal part, and the spinal cord. Consequently, symptoms include paraparesis, quadriparesis, dysarthria, dysphagia, ataxia, cranial nerve palsies, palatal myoclonus, dystonia, tremor, confusion, dementia and pseudobulbar palsy. Subacute progression with stepwise deterioration may mimic multiple sclerosis, but there is a predilection for motor symptoms in contradistinction to the predominance of sensory symptoms and internuclear ophthalmoplegia in demyelinating disease.

Peripheral

The peripheral nervous system may rarely be involved with mononeuritis multiplex, polyradiculitis and neurogenic muscular atrophy. Myositis is also seen.

SYSTEMIC SYMPTOMS

Recurrent oral aphthous ulceration is a major criterion required for the diagnosis. Aphthous ulcers in Behçet's disease have no unique features and are usually whitish spots of different sizes, well demarcated with an erythematous surrounding. A reliable history of genital ulcers is important, especially if past ulcers have healed without a scar. An active ulcer is a painful, punched-out lesion of the scrotum or the labia preceded by induration and itching in some cases. Uveitis may lead to synechiae, cataract and glaucoma with consequent loss of vision (Figure 29.1). Posterior uveitis, retinal vasculitis and episcleritis are also common. Severe involvement may lead to blindness and ocular phthisis. Subclinical involvement of retinal vasculature may be detected by fluorescein angiography which demonstrates leakage from retinal vessels. Involvement of the skin with erythema nodosum, small infarcts and pseudofolliculitis is not infrequent. Other manifestations include arthritis, thrombophlebitis, pulmonary embolism, pulmonary artery aneurysm, intracardiac thrombi with thromboembolic phenomena.

DIAGNOSIS

A high index of suspicion and the recognition of the multiorgan involvement are important in making the diagnosis. The current set of international criteria for the diagnosis of Behçet's disease failed to include nervous system involvement, consequently some cases of early involvement of the nervous system may be excluded until the systemic manifestations appear. Pathergy test results are variable and likely to depend on the technique. The test involves induction of

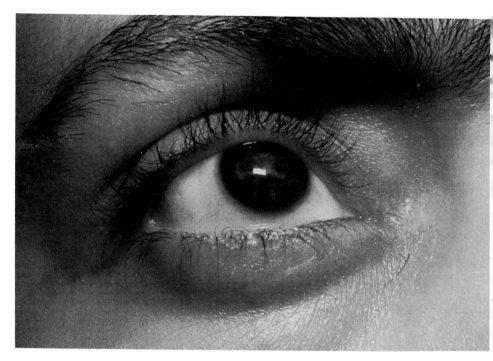

Figure 29.1   Sequelae of anterior uveitis, synechiae, cataract and glaucoma.

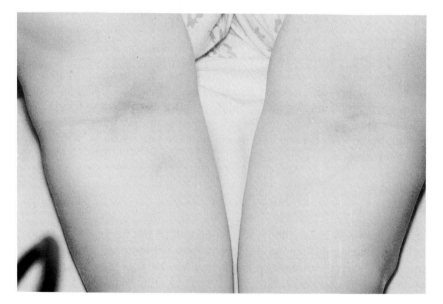

Figure 29.2   Papules at the site of attempted intravenous needle insertion; pathergy phenomen.

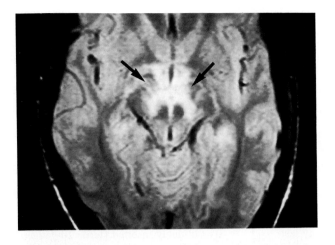

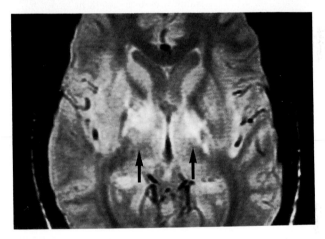

Figure 29.3 Magnetic resonance image showing high signal intensity regions on T2-weighted images affecting the basal midbrain diencephalic regions symmetrically in neuro-Behçet's disease.

a lesion (papule, pustule or ulcer) by traumatizing the skin with a needle. The rate of positivity may correlate with the number of attempts to penetrate the skin and therefore it occasionally occurs at the site of vein puncture (Figure 29.2). MRI in CNS parenchymal involvement shows areas of high signal intensity on T2-weighted images in the thalamic regions, brainstem and/or subcortical white matter; predilection of the basal part of the brainstem and involvement of grey and white matter deep in the hemispheres is characteristic (Al Kawi *et al.*, 1991) (Figure 29.3). Partial or complete resolution of MRI abnormalities can be seen following treatment. MRI is the modality of choice for detecting venous thrombosis. Brainstem auditory evoked potentials are usually normal while magnetic evoked motor potentials are affected. See Table 29.1.

TABLE 29.1 Criteria for diagnosis of Behçet's disease (adopted from the International Study Group for Behçet's Disease (1992)

Recurrent oral ulceration	Minor aphthous, major aphthous, or herpetiform ulceration at least three recurrences in 12 months
Plus two of:	
Recurrent genital ulceration	Aphthous ulceration or scarring
Eye lesions	Anterior uveitis, posterior uveitis, cells in vitreous or retinal vasculitis
Skin lesions	Erythema nodosum-like lesions, pseudofolliculitis, papulopustular lesions; or acneiform nodules (in postadolescent patients not on corticosteroid treatment)
Positive pathergy test	By obliquely inserted sterile 20-gauge needle or smaller, read at 24–48 h

Findings applicable only in absence of other clinical explanation.

TREATMENT

Different forms of immunosuppressive treatment have been tried in Behçet disease. Corticosteroids are the most commonly used during acute exacerbations. Oral prednisolone 1–2 mg kg^{-1} day^{-1} may improve symptoms through its effect on perifocal oedema or its anti-inflammatory action. A short 3–5 days course of intravenous high-dose methyl prednisolone 10–15 mg kg^{-1} once daily can improve symptoms rapidly. Treatment with 1 mg kg^{-1} day^{-1} of prednisolone should be continued from a few to several weeks depending on the severity of symptoms, and the dose then steadily reduced to a maintenance level. To minimize the metabolic effects of the corticosteroids, an alternate day regimen should be used for maintenance whenever possible. Corticosteroids may fail to improve visual symptoms and other immunosuppressive treatment is necessary.

Azathioprine at a dose of 2.5 mg kg^{-1} day^{-1} has been shown to be effective in long-term control of symptoms (Yazici *et al.*, 1990). It has a lower incidence of side-effects than other cytotoxic agents. Chlorambucil 0.1 mg kg^{-1} day^{-1} has been shown to reduce the cerebrospinal fluid pleocytosis in meningoencephalitis and is also effective for ocular symptoms. Cyclophosphamide has also been reported to be effective in ocular symptoms. Cyclosporin-A inhibits the T-helper lymphocytes subset and leads to ocular improvement at a dose of 10 mg kg^{-1} daily. Studies are underway to evaluate the effects of FK-506 and α-interferon.

The treatment of Behçet's disease is difficult and requires considerable skill and judgement over a period of follow-up extending to many years.

REFERENCES

Al Kawi MZ, Bohlega S and Banna M (1991) MRI findings in neuro-Behçet's disease. *Neurology* **41**: 405–408.

International Study Group for Behçet's Disease (1992). Evaluation of diagnostic ('classification') criteria in Behçet's disease – towards internationally agreed criteria. *British Journal of Rheumatology* **31**: 299–308.

Serdaroglu S, Yazici H, Coskun O *et al.* (1989) Neurologic involvement in Behçet's syndrome. *Archives of Neurology* **46**: 265–269.

Shakir RA, Sulaiman K, Khan RA and Rudwan M (1990) Neurological presentation of neuro-Behçet syndrome: Clinical categories. *European Neurology* **30 (5)**: 249–253.

Yazici H, Pazarli H, Barnes CG *et al.* (1990) A controlled trial of azathioprine in Behçet's syndrome. *New England Journal of Medicine* **322(5)**: 281–285.

30

A Perspective on Neurological Rehabilitation

Suranjan Bhattacharji[1] and Michael Saunders[2]

[1]Rehabilitation Department, Christian Medical College and Hospital, Vellore, India;
[2]Northallerton Health Services NHS Trust, UK

INTRODUCTION

Rehabilitation means different things to different people. At one extreme, Oliver (1990) has produced a critique of the medical model describing the activity of a rehabilitation team as the exercise of power by one group over another.

This chapter recognizes the severe limitations of a medical or health care model of rehabilitation but takes the view that there are demonstrable gains from goal-directed activities, one of the best examples being in spinal injuries (Oakes *et al.*, 1990). Difficulties in evaluating rehabilitation outcomes have led to the suggestion that research based on individual case studies may be required to demonstrate positive gain (Morley, 1989). The many ethical issues involved in rehabilitation have been discussed by Saunders (1993); those of justice and access to facilities can be particularly relevant in a tropical environment where resources are limited in many instances.

This chapter concentrates on some of the basic issues and principles involved in rehabilitation and refers in particular to the importance of community-based activities which have major implications for neurological disability throughout the world.

EPIDEMIOLOGY

The estimates of the prevalence of disability are varied and depend on the definition of disability and the characteristics of the population studies. Helander (1993) quotes an average figure of 5.2% as the estimated global prevalence of moderate and severe disability. This implies that there are probably 100 million disabled persons in the more developed and 200 million in the less developed regions of the world. Addressing the need of this huge number of persons within the realities of resource constraints and paucity of trained rehabilitation personnel is a mammoth task. Keeping the solutions flexible enough to address the special needs of disabled women and children, particularly those from a rural background, is even more challenging.

PRINCIPLES OF REHABILITATION

What is rehabilitation? Rehabilitation can be defined as 'all steps taken to mitigate the effects of disability'. Disability is the loss of function due to an anatomical or physiological impairment.

Attempts to reduce any science to its core principles are fraught with danger because in the process of reduction, essential elements may be left out. However, in order that new concepts may be grasped and manipulated an attempt at reduction is necessary. Once these principles are understood their application can be varied to suit different clinical situations.

The five main principles of rehabilitation medicine are: (1) early diagnosis and treatment in a competent centre; (2) management by a multidisciplinary team; (3) maximization of residual potentials; (4) peer interaction; and (5) life-long follow-up. These are discussed next.

Early Diagnosis and Treatment in a Competent Centre

The neurological deficit due to spinal cord injury in a person who has sustained a spinal column fracture is worsened by the second injury of inexpert handling of the unstable spine. Similarly, the neurological deficit in a baby born with a meningomyelocele is often compounded by the injury of the exposed neural tissue due to infection. This means that around the umbra of neurones which have succumbed to a particular insult is a penumbra of surviving but damaged neurones. The course of events after the original insult will determine whether or not these damaged neurones will survive. These second injuries can be prevented by transferring the patient to a competent centre as soon as possible – directly by minimizing further damage to neural tissue and indirectly by preventing other complications like pressure sores, urinary tract infection and respiratory infections which cause local tissue dysfunction and produce further neurological deficit by enhancing the destruction of the damaged neurones in the penumbra region. The effectiveness of a centre is defined not by its size or equipment but by the competence of the staff working in that centre.

To give another example, the brain injury due to birth hypoxia in a newborn child may result in a spastic cerebral palsy. If this is diagnosed early and treated, the child can often be taught how to walk and be restored to a full life. However, if the child is ignored, he grows up to become an immobile adolescent with joint deformities and secondary intellectual and emotional impairment due to a lack of opportunities. The aim of early diagnosis and treatment may not always be met even in developed countries. In poorer countries the difficulties may be insurmountable.

Management by a Multidisciplinary Team

The complexity of the problems which beset a person with a major neurological deficit requires the expertise of many professionals including rehabilitation nurses, physiotherapists, occupational therapists, orthotists/prosthetists, speech therapists, recreation therapists, psychologists, social workers, special educators, vocational counsellors, biomedical engineers, physicians and surgeons. The patient and his family are not mere members of the treating team but central to it. The nature and purposes of a rehabilitation team have been described by Furnell *et al.* (1987).

Rehabilitation medicine offers many options for the solution of a specific disability – the option best suited for an individual can be decided accurately if the patients and their families are part of the decision. For example, to obviate the mobility problems of a person with complete paralysis of both lower limbs, the options available are hand-powered or motor-powered mobility devices. Hand-powered devices could be calipers and crutches or manual wheelchairs; examples of motorized mobility devices are battery-powered wheelchairs, motorized triwheelers or hand-controlled cars. Each option has advantages and disadvantages and the responsibility of the team is to ensure that the patient is able to choose the most appropriate option or options for his or her needs. Comprehensive care is essential as the effort put into just a few aspects of the problem can result in failure of optimal restoration.

Maximization of Residual Potential

Nearly every person with a disability has latent residual potentials. The disability, however, looms so large in front of the patient that the residual potentials are obscured and often remain hidden. The rehabilitation professional needs to evaluate not only the disease or traumatized part of the person but also the normal or undamaged part. After this evaluation, suitable restorative and compensatory intervention can be planned. For example, if a right-handed person were to have leprosy with paralysis due to an ulnar nerve lesion, the ability to write may be compromised. This disability can be compensated for by teaching her to write with the left hand or restoring her writing ability by strengthening exercises and re-education of the weak muscles of the right hand or by stabilizing the weak joints in the hand in an appropriate splint or by replacing lost function of crucial muscles by transferring tendons surgically. The veritable explosion of options (physical, chemical, biological and psychological) available for restoration of ability has resulted in the burgeoning of rehabilitation medicine as an exciting new specialty.

Peer Interaction

Habilitation or rehabilitation is a process of education or re-education by which the disabled are empowered to take control of their lives and fulfil their potentials despite their disability. This process of education occurs best when the newly disabled learn from a person who has already confronted and overcome a similar disability. Whenever this process of learning from peers has been facilitated – as in spinal injury centres and stroke rehabilitation centres – the results have been encouraging. This is especially so, because the battle against disability needs first to be won in the mind – and seeing and talking to someone who is going through or has gone through a similar process is more effective than hours of individual counselling. This learning process can be done in group therapy sessions, either formal or informal, for patients or their families.

Life-long Follow-up

Persons with disability need life-long follow-up because disabilities like muscular dystrophy can be progressive and therefore require new strategies for intervention as the disease progresses. Another reason for the need for life-long follow-up is the special risks that a disabled person may be exposed to that may require close monitoring for complications. For example, a person with paraplegia has a neurogenic bladder which makes him especially at risk for urinary tract infection and renal damage. A regular, life-long follow-up can help to ensure that urinary complications (particularly silent ones) are identified and dealt with early, before irreversible changes occur. Anatomical and physiological changes with maturation in children and ageing in the elderly may result in the development of new disabilities with the passage of time. These needs can be met by a life-long interaction between the disabled person and professionals with appropriate expertise.

Community-based Rehabilitation

The present services available for rehabilitation are mainly institution based. Particularly for less developed countries, there is an urgent need to shift the emphasis to a community-based rehabilitation strategy.

This is defined as a strategy for enhancing the quality of life of disabled people by improving service delivery, by providing more equitable opportunities and by promoting and projecting their human rights (Helander *et al.*, 1989; Helander, 1993). It calls for flexibility and a willingness to learn from the people.

Principles of Community-based Rehabilitation

The principles of decentralization and demystification form the basis for community-based rehabilitation.

Decentralization, or bottom-up approach as opposed to top-down, proposed by David Werner (1988) involves building up the services from the community level and later linking them into a referral system, once the community needs are known and implementation has been tried for a while. Demystification of existing technology involves teaching the essential principles to people who have been educated differently and the preparation of training manuals and modules for medical, educational and vocational rehabilitation needs, in the local languages. Flexible integrated solutions are emphasized, with the disabled persons and their families sharing in the process of restoration and healing (Sethi, 1983).

STRATEGY OF COMMUNITY-BASED REHABILITATION

The models of community-based rehabilitation that have successfully addressed local needs are as varied as the local needs and situations. The general principles of the strategy as set out by Helander *et al.* (1989) are outlined below.

Evaluation of the Problem

This includes a base-line survey to assess the needs of the disabled and their families as well as to learn what local solutions and resources already exist that can be usefully integrated and enhanced.

Planning the Strategy

Having determined a profile of the local need and resources one can set targets and objectives, recruit and train key personnel.

Mobilization of the Community

This step is the key to developing a sustainable programme. It involves a process of sensitization of the community to the fact that disability is common and there are simple methods of training and educating disabled people, that can be applied where they live and that will lead to more independence and better social integration. After the sensitization has been done, the community has to be animated, organized and motivated to discover the hidden potentials that exist in them to evolve local solution. They also need to choose the community workers (local rehabilitation supervisors) who will be the key figures in the ongoing process. Wherever possible it is wise to choose disabled persons themselves for this job because their sensitivity to real needs makes them particularly suitable.

Implementation of the Programme

As the process evolves, the local rehabilitation supervisor or community-level workers and the intermediary-level supervisor or professional would have been selected. These individuals would need to be trained to identify disabilities and evolve appropriate solutions which can be implemented by the family of the disabled. They would then be sent out into the community to work. This process of empowering the disabled and their families would ensure that the rehabilitation is always centred on actual, felt needs of the person with disability rather than the abilities of the professionals advising or treating them. As the implementation proceeds, a referral system would need to be developed as per the local requirements, so that complex rehabilitation problems, particularly those that require evaluation or investigations and advanced training or surgical intervention could be referred to the existing referral centres. Thus a local network would be developed that could be integrated and supportive.

Evaluation at the Local Community Level

This final step is crucial and needs to be part of an ongoing process that ensures that the service is constantly addressing actual needs of disabled persons and reaching out to as many of them as possible. Mid-course corrections of strategy, tailoring modules to address actual problems, rejuvenating workers whose motivation has diminished are some of the obvious gains that can be reaped from this, especially since community-based rehabilitation is a learning process, not a blue-print or a ready-made solution.

One final note – community-based rehabilitation is an expensive process. It is not a low-cost substitute for good institution-based rehabilitation as many understand it to be. It requires an enormous investment of material and human resources. But the end result of having a more caring and just society makes it worthwhile.

REFERENCES

Furnell J, Platt S and Clarke DS (1987) Multidisciplinary clinical teams: some issues in establishment and function. *Hospital and Health Services Review*, January 15–18.

Helander E (1993) *Prejudice and Dignity: An Introduction to Community Based Rehabilitation*, New York: United Nations Development Programme publications.

Helander E, Mendis P, Nelson G and Goerdt A (1989) *Training in the Community for People with Disabilities*. Geneva: World Health Organization.

Morley S (1989) Single case research. In: *Behavioural and Mental Health Research: A Handbook of Skills and Methods* (eds G Parry and FN Watts). London: Lawrence Erlbaum.

Oakes DD, Wilmot CB, Hall KM and Scherk JP (1990) Benefit of early admission to a comprehensive trauma centre for patients with spinal cord injury. *Archives of Physical Medicine and Rehabilitation* **71**: 637–643.

Oliver M (1990) *The Politics of Disablement*. London: Macmillan.

Saunders M (1993) Ethical implications of disablement. In: *Neurological Rehabilitation* (eds R Greenwood, MP Barnes, TM McMillan and CD Ward). Edinburgh: Churchill Livingstone.

Sethi PK (1983) Reaching out in rehabilitation. In: *Proceedings of the Workshop on Extension of Work at Jaipur and Training Programme*. Rehabilitation Research Centre, Jaipur, India.

Werner D (1988) *Disabled Village Children*. Palo Alto, USA: Hesperian Foundation.

Index

Note: Page references in *italics* refer to figures; those in **bold** refer to tables